PROTEIN BIOCHEMISTRY, SYNTHESIS, STRUCTURE AND CELLULAR FUNCTIONS

TRYPSIN

STRUCTURE, BIOSYNTHESIS AND FUNCTIONS

PROTEIN BIOCHEMISTRY, SYNTHESIS, STRUCTURE AND CELLULAR FUNCTIONS

Additional books in this series can be found on Nova's website
under the Series tab.

Additional E-books in this series can be found on Nova's website
under the E-book tab.

MICROBIOLOGY RESEARCH ADVANCES

Additional books in this series can be found on Nova's website
under the Series tab.

Additional E-books in this series can be found on Nova's website
under the E-book tab.

PROTEIN BIOCHEMISTRY, SYNTHESIS, STRUCTURE AND CELLULAR FUNCTIONS

TRYPSIN

STRUCTURE, BIOSYNTHESIS AND FUNCTIONS

KIRK WEAVER
AND
CLAYTON KELLEY
EDITORS

Nova Science Publishers, Inc.
New York

Library of Congress Cataloging-in-Publication Data

ISBN 978-1-61942-319-0

Published by Nova Science Publishers, Inc. † New York

Contents

Preface

Trypsin is a serine protease in the digestive system of humans and animals. This book presents current research in the structure, biosynthesis and functions of trypsin. Topics include the study of trypsins from submammalian vertebrates with special emphasis on fish; the applications of trypsin in food processing; trypsin acting as an activating enzyme in gut innate immunity and protease-activated receptor 2 in the enteric nervous system.

Chapter I - Trypsin is a serine protease with typical molecular weight of 24 kDa. It is synthesized in the pancreas and secreted as an inactive trypsinogen from the pancreatic acinar cells together with chymotrypsinogen and other zymogens. Trypsinogen is activated by enteropeptidase in the small intestine and by the trypsin itself. Trypsin activates chymotrypsinogen and the other pancreatic zymogens (proelastase and procarboxypeptidase), and each active proteolytic enzyme has its substrate specificity.

Chapter II – This article reviews trypsins from submammalian vertebrates including fish, amphibians and birds. A trypsin-like enzyme has been purified from ostrich skeletal muscle.The serine proteases in snake venoms are thrombins and affect platelet aggregation. The trypsins from amphibian sperms and oviducts play a role in fertilization and early development. Trypsins have been isolated from the pylric caeca and intestine of a number of fish species. Some of these trypsins resemble mammalian trypsin in structure.

Chapter III - Trypsin is a serine protease in the digestive system of human and animals. The main function of this enzyme is to hydrolyze proteins into smaller peptides or even amino acids. Trypsin and other digestive proteases such as chymotrypsin are responsible for the digestion of food protein in the small intestine. This proteolytic function of trypsin has been widely used in protein chemistry, proteomics and nutrition research. This function is influenced by the sources of enzyme, and environmental factors such as pH, temperature, and the presence of trypsin inhibitors in the enzymatic reaction medium. In food processing, trypsin or a trypsin preparation which usually contains other enzymes has been used to improve both the functional and nutritional quality of food proteins. This chapter provides a review of the sources of trypsin preparation for food processing and the applications trypsin in food processing to 1) improve the functional properties such as solubility, emulsification, foaming and gelling properties of food proteins, 2) improve the digestibility of vegetable and seed proteins, 3) produce protein hydrolysates and bioactive peptides that are used in infant formulas and for people with special health problems such as hypertension, and 4) reduce the concentration of allergens in some foods. The applications of trypsin in food science research including food protein sequencing, *in vitro* determination of food protein digestibility, and evaluating the impacts of food processing methods on the activity of trypsin inhibitors are also covered in this chapter.

Chapter IV - The polyfunctional properties of carbohydrate-binding proteins, lectins, allow their application to various biological and medical studies as specific agglutinins in blood typing; in synthesis of affine stationary phases for fractionation and analysis of polysaccharides, glycolipids, or glycoproteins; and in cytochemical and histochemical studies of glycoconjugates of tissues and cell surfaces. The hemagglutination reaction, based on specific lectin binding to carbohydrates on erythrocyte surface, is the most common and appropriate test system for the determination of lectin activity and carbohydrate specificity. Treatment with trypsin interferes the pattern of erythrocyte binding by lectins and, therefore, the analytical characteristics of the test-system used for disclosing their carbohydrate-binding properties. Erythrocytes obtained from different organisms differ in carbohydrate determinants, the trypsin-treatment being capable of enzymatic constructing the optimal receptor sites on their surface.

Then the authors turn their attention to the results that their group has obtained over the last ten years. Trypsin-stimulated agglutination of animal (rabbit, horse, ram, bovine) erythrocytes was observed to be appropriate semi-qualitative analytical method for studying the lectin activity and carbohydrate specificity of the agglutinins of basidial mushrooms at the dikaryotic mycelium step. The difference in taxonomic characteristics and in the medium composition on growing the fungal cultures – representatives of xylotrophic basidiomycetes – influenced the hemagglutinating activity to a much lesser extent, as compared with the aggregate state of nutrient medium and the type of erythrocytes in hemagglutination reaction.

Hemagglutinating activity of *Lentinula edodes* intracellular lectins at different morphogenesis steps was explored depending upon the type of erythrocytes, the growth medium, and the grade of proteins purity. The lectin activity under a solid-phase cultivation was appeared to depend on the type of erythrocytes used in a hemagglutination reaction, including the trypsin-treatment of erythrocytes, to a great extent. The sensitivity of the lectins towards trypsin-treated rabbit erythrocytes was no less than a hundredfold higher than towards any other erythrocyte type studied.

The culture of *L. edodes* F-249 occured to synthesize two extracellular lectins. The authors have isolated those from fungal culture liquid and purified to electrophoretic homogeneity. The lectins differ in physicochemical properties, composition, carbohydrate specificity, and ability for agglutination of erythrocytes of various types. The purified extracellular lectins of *L. edodes* are highly selective at recognition of definite structures on the surface of trypsinized rabbit erythrocytes and do not react with the erythrocytes of other animals and humans.

At the same time, a preferable agglutination of human trypsinized erythrocytes compared to untreated ones was not observed under any experimental conditions when exploring the blood-group specificity of the lectins of basidial xylotrophs from different systematic groups. The extent of manifestation of the hemagglutinating activity in respect to human erythrocytes had the peculiarities general for all the cultures along with somewhat differences caused obviously by the individual characteristics of each basidiomycete. The maximal values of hemagglutination titers for all the fungi were on the agar media. Judging from the results of solid-phase cultivation, the agglutinins of *Armillariella mellea* 1346 should be considered to be *H*(*O*) blood-group specific.

Trypsin-treated erythrocytes appeared to be worse test-system for agglutinating ability of mushroom mycelial hemagglutinin, a dimeric membrane-bound 68 kDa-lectin, which we isolated from the surface of dikaryotic mycelium of xylotrophic basidiomycete *Grifola frondosa*. The lectin exhibited high affinity to native rabbit erythrocytes and to human erythrocytes of the *O* blood group, but not to trypsin-treated ones. Only 13.9 μg/ml of the homogeneous preparation of a polysaccharide, a linear D-rhamnan with the definite structure of the repeated component, blocked hemagglutination completely. The lectins specific toward glycoconjugate, but not to any monosaccharide, presumably oppose a trypsin-assisted revision of the erythrocytes surface. Enzymatically lost complex carbohydrate-containing molecules – more or less perfect sites of endolectins binding with erythrocytes – results in poor agglutination and, may be, inadequate conclusions on lectins properties.

Chapter V - The enteric nervous system (ENS) integrates local neuroendocrine signaling with central autonomic input to regulate the motor and secretory function of the gastrointestinal (GI) tract. Exposure to inflammatory mediators such as trypsin or mast cell tryptase is postulated to affect ENS signaling, contributing to both protective and pathologic changes in GI function.

Protease-activated receptor 2 (PAR-2) is a receptor specifically activated by the serine-proteases trypsin and tryptase. Within the mammalian ENS, PAR-2 expression has been identified in neurons of both the submucosal and myenteric plexus. Myenteric neurons respond to trypsin with prolonged depolarization, suppression of fast excitatory post-synaptic potentials, and phospholipase C (PLC) - dependent cytosolic calcium transients. Trypsin also activates PAR-2 in enteroglial cells, causing activation of PLC and sphingosine kinase.

This signaling cascade results in cytosolic calcium transients, subsequent capacitative calcium entry, and c-fos expression. Activation of PAR-2 by trypsin within the ENS may ultimately alter intestinal ion channel permeability and secretory function. PAR-2 may therefore contribute to the physiological function and pathophysiological response in the ENS.

Chapter VI - Digestive enzymes in the human gut play major roles in digesting food so that nutrients can be absorbed through epithelial sheets in the intestinal lumen. Trypsin, one of the digestive enzymes, is mainly produced in the pancreas and secreted in the duodenum. Recent finding have shown that small intestinal epithelial cells produce trypsin peptide, which plays an important role in the human innate immune system. The digestive organs, contributing to the absorption of nutrients on one side and protecting the host from the numerous bacteria residing in the gut microbiota, also protects against external infectious microbes on the other side. Paneth cells, one of the secretory epithelial cells in the small intestine, express and secrete antimicrobial peptide, human alpha-defensin (HD). HD is an innate immune molecule that directly eliminates bacteria to maintain homeostasis in the gut's ecosystem. A specific pattern of trypsin isozymes is also expressed in Paneth cells, and trypsin co-localizes with HD to cleave propeptides to mature forms identical to those isolated *in vivo*. HD is stored in secretory vesicles as a propeptide, but the mature peptides isolated from the intestinal lumen are proteolytically processed forms. HD is produced and stored as a propeptide in Paneth cell granules, secreted in response to stimulation by cholinergic reagents or bacterial antigens, and finally activated by trypsin in the intestinal lumen in order to produce mature functional HD. Therefore, trypsin is involved in the regulation of innate immunity in the small intestine by acting as a prodefensin convertase in human Paneth cells. The activating process is critical for its antibacterial role and it is also a bridge to acquired immunity. This chapter reviews the novel functional role of trypsin which is produced in the small intestine.

Chapter VII - Using cytraconic anhydride and 1,4-cyclohexadione, lysine and arginine of bifunctional inhibitor α-amylase/trypsin from wheat (Triticum aestivum L.) has been modified. These results found that two independent reactive sites are present in the bifunctional wheat inhibitor. The experimental data obtained that the lactoperoxidase-catalyzed reaction is accompanied by oxidation aromatic and sulfur-containing amino acids of the inhibitor. This can point out one of the mechanisms inactivating proteins in sprouting seeds.

Chapter VIII - Proteins, either therapeutic or diagnostic, will become increasingly important in the bio-medical and pharmaceutical field. The major efforts invested in e.g. proteomics, in the recent past, will provide us with many new and promising protein type of target molecules in the coming years. Irrespective whether these proteins are intended therapeutics or endogenous, medically diagnostic molecules, their absolute quantitative measurement will become more and more of an issue. In that respect, immunoassays are of paramount importance. Nevertheless, as in the field of small molecules, alternatives based on chromatography and, inevitably, mass spectrometric detection, are attracting the attention of many investigators. Although more complicated and allowing less sample throughput, (ESI)-LC/MS provides much higher selectivity and thus analytical confidence with respect to the particular measurement. In terms of quantitative target compound analysis, mass spectrometry of intact proteins has the major disadvantage of producing an envelope of multiply charged ions, thus spreading the amount of protein compound over many different species. These results in a major loss of sensitivity as only one of a few species are measured in the (tandem) LC-MS process. In this chapter we report on an alternative approach to analyzing intact proteins based on the proteomic "bottom-up" principle of generating peptides from the protein by proteolysis. These peptides are the stoichiometric representation of the protein and some of them can be selected for LC-MS measurement using the techniques commonly used for small molecules and with comparable analytical complexity. This chapter will focus on the reproducible generation of a number of so called marker-peptides based on enzymatic (trypsin) and especially chemical protein digestion using cyanogen bromide. Reaction conditions for reproducible protein digestion, internal standardization, liquid chromatographic separation, mass spectrometric detection and quantitative evaluation of the approach are discussed using the endogenous human cystatin C protein, a clinically relevant biochemical marker often used in diagnostic settings, as a proof-of-concept protein.

In: Trypsin: Structure, Biosynthesis and Functions
Editors: Kirk Weaver and Clayton Kelley
ISBN 978-1-61942-319-0

Chapter I

Trypsin and its Implementations for Growth, Maturation, and Dietary Quality Assessment

Krisna Rungruangsak-Torrissen[1]
Institute of Marine Research, Ecosystem Processes Research Group
Matre Research Station, Matredal, Norway

Introduction

Trypsin is a serine protease with typical molecular weight of 24 kDa. It is synthesized in the pancreas and secreted as an inactive trypsinogen from the pancreatic acinar cells together with chymotrypsinogen and other zymogens. Trypsinogen is activated by enteropeptidase in the small intestine and by the trypsin itself. Trypsin activates chymotrypsinogen and the other pancreatic zymogens (proelastase and procarboxypeptidase), and each active proteolytic enzyme has its substrate specificity [reviewed in 1].

Trypsin has different isoforms (trypsin isozymes) and the unique intensive studies on trypsin have been performed by Rungruangsak-Torrissen's research team and the works during 1981–1999, especially on trypsin isozymes, have been mainly reviewed in Rungruangsak Torrissen and Male [1]. The first work on identification of genetic differences in trypsin isozyme patterns (trypsin phenotypes) has been published in individual Atlantic salmon, *Salmo salar* L. and rainbow trout, *Oncorhynchus mykiss* Walbaum [2], and later in Arctic charr, *Salvelinus alpinus* L. [3]. The works on biological significance of the expression of trypsin isozymes have been mainly emphasized in Atlantic salmon during sexual maturation [4] and in association with fish size [5], growth rate [6–8], and feed efficiency at different temperatures [7, 9].

Further studies for deeper understanding on digestion and absorption of dietary protein in Atlantic salmon possessing different trypsin phenotypes were performed without success by using a conventional apparent digestibility study [7]. By using a more sensitive technique

[1] E-mail: *Krisnart@imr.no*.

through facilitation of free amino acids (FAA) in plasma and white muscle, the differences in digestion of dietary protein, and absorption and transport of FAA have been observed between different trypsin phenotypes, and higher digestion rate has been shown to associate with faster elevation of essential FAA [10]. For growing Atlantic salmon, the levels of trypsin specific activity and most FAA in plasma and white muscle have been shown to peak at the same time at 6 h post-feeding after subsequent starvation [10]. In addition, it has been observed that the elevation of plasma FAA is not a good indicator. A high absorption of amino acids in the plasma is not always due to high quality feed, as low quality feed could also cause a high absorption of plasma FAA but the transport of FAA to the muscle is not efficient due to amino acid imbalance [10].

Moreover, *in vitro* digestibility study of dietary protein using pyloric caecal crude enzyme extracts has resulted in differences in the digestive ability of different trypsin phenotypes for the same fish meals [11].

This indicates that the simple and practical *in vitro* protein digestibility technique is more sensitive than the conventional apparent digestibility method for differentiation of genetic differences in diet digestion.

Gene expression is dynamic, and the expression of different trypsin phenotypes is dependent on the first environmental condition (i.e. temperature) during the egg incubation and the first feeding period, regardless of the genetic expressions of the parents [9]. Atlantic salmon possessing different trypsin phenotypes also have differences in maintenance ration, protein synthesis capacity, and plasma insulin levels [12].

Relationships between weight specific consumption rate, plasma insulin level and fish growth have been observed. Fish growth has been shown to associate with increased plasma insulin level one month after the increase in trypsin specific activity. The phenotype with higher growth has lower maintenance ration with greater feed utilization ability at a restricted ration and higher capacity for protein synthesis in the white muscle [12], as well as a higher immune response (total serum IgM level) after vaccination [13].

Molecular cloning and characterization of trypsin variants in Atlantic salmon have been performed, and five clones containing near full-length transcripts (four encoded anionic forms and one encoded cationic variant) have been revealed [14]. So far, trypsin clones and trypsin isozymes have never been matched, probably due to too few differences in sequences and the knowledge of gene expression is still limited. However, the real functional genomics study by knowing proteins and their functions are very important and more practical for understanding the biological significance in living organisms.

The aim of this chapter is to review the works during the last decade that have been continuing performed in order to understand more about the unique function of trypsin in relation to the function of chymotrypsin, especially the protease activity ratio of trypsin to chymotrypsin (T/C ratio). Such functional studies, at present, cannot be replaced by studying their genes.

This chapter will demonstrate how trypsin, as well as chymotrypsin and T/C ratio, could be implemented for practical purposes in explaining diet utilization efficiency, growth, and maturation rate, including dietary quality assessment. With unique combinations of different biochemical techniques, the performance qualities of growth and maturation of aquatic animals could be studied both in aquaculture and natural ecosystems where food consumption rate cannot be under control. It could also be a model for other species such as mammals and land-based animals.

Expressions of Trypsin Isozymes

Association with Consumption and Growth

Differences in expressions of trypsin isozymes (trypsin phenotypes) have been studied, first in Atlantic salmon and rainbow trout [2] and later in Arctic charr [3] with designated names described in Torrissen and Barnung [3] and Torrissen et al. [8], as illustrated in Figure 1. Trypsin isozymes could be differentiated in the narrow pH range of 4–6.5 (Figure 1), and cationic isoform(s) of trypsin could exist at pH > 10 [1]. The presence of different trypsin isozymes with variation in isoelectric point (pI) values has been observed in the digestive system of different fish species [reviewed in 1]. Six trypsin isozymes with 10 trypsin phenotypes in Atlantic salmon, 6 trypsin isozymes with 4 trypsin phenotypes in rainbow trout, and 4 trypsin isozymes with 3 trypsin phenotypes in Arctic charr, have been identified (Figure 1). Trypsin isozymes have also been studied later in invertebrates, and 3 trypsin phenotypes have been classified in whiteleg shrimp, *Litopenaeus vannamei* [15–17] and spiny lobster, *Panulirus argus* [18]. Recently, different expressions of trypsin isozymes affected by different feedings have been studied in Nile tilapia, *Oreochromis niloticus* L. [19] as shown in Figure 2, and in Northeast Arctic cod, *Gadus morhua* L. [20] as shown in Figure 3. In Nile tilapia with artificial feeding, 6 trypsin isozymes with 10 trypsin phenotypes have been observed by 12% native-PAGE (Figure 2), and 11 trypsin isozymes have been observed by 15% native-PAGE (Figure 3). In Northeast Arctic cod with natural feeding, 30 trypsin isozymes have been observed with 11 isozymes common to Nile tilapia and 13 isozymes of possibly exogenous trypsin isozyme fragments from prey items (Figure 3). Comparing to Northeast Arctic cod, less numbers of trypsin isozyme expressions observed in Atlantic salmon, rainbow trout, Arctic charr, and Nile tilapia were due to the fishes feeding on artificial diets, and the trypsin isozyme patterns could represent trypsin phenotypes of the individuals. Whereas, in Northeast Arctic cod, the patterns of trypsin isozyme numbers 1–17 might represent their trypsin phenotypes, as 11 trypsin isozymes were common to those of Nile tilapia (see Figure 3). To be certain about trypsin phenotypes, the fish should be fed on artificial diets, and/or the expressions of trypsin isozyme patterns should be studied in the intestinal tissue extracts (without food content) as in Atlantic salmon, rainbow trout, and Arctic charr (Figure 1).

So far, using trypsin phenotypes of individuals for studying temperature dependence of growth rate and feed efficiency have only been performed in Atlantic salmon by Rungruangsak-Torrissen's research team with emphasis on trypsin isozyme patterns 1, 2 and 2' (see Figure 1), which have been mainly studied in Norwegian Atlantic salmon populations. Trypsin isozyme TRP-2*100 was a common isozyme and the isozyme TRP-2*92 was the major variant in Norwegian Atlantic salmon while the isozyme TRP-1*91 was dominant in Scottish Atlantic salmon. These isozymes have been illustrated to have temperature preference for feed efficiency at > 8 °C, ≤ 8 °C (especially below 6 °C), and a wider temperature range (but not ≤ 6 °C), respectively [9]. This has been confirmed by investigating the spatial temperature distribution of the different trypsin isozyme characteristics of wild Atlantic salmon post-smolts in natural marine ecosystems (off the Hebrides and the Norwegian Sea) where more than 80% of the caught post-smolts possessing trypsin phenotypes 1, 2 and 2' [21]. The temperature distributions of the three trypsin phenotypes are illustrated in Figure 4.

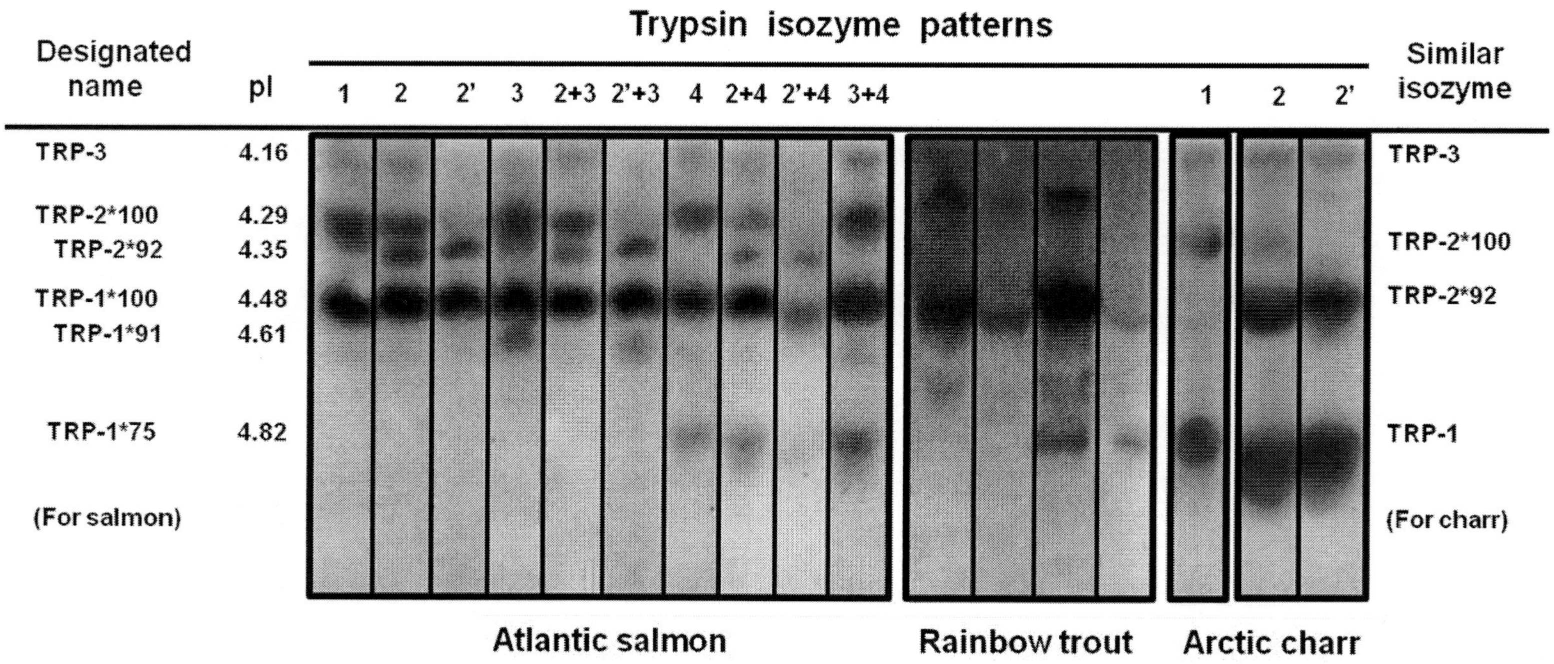

Figure 1. Electrophoretic zymograms of trypsin isozyme patterns (trypsin phenotypes) in the pyloric caecal and intestinal tissue extracts (without food content) of Atlantic salmon, rainbow trout, and two strains of Arctic charr (Skogseid with pattern 1 and Hammerfest with patterns 2 and 2'). Trypsin phenotypes were not defined in rainbow trout. The expressions of trypsin isozymes were revealed by isoelectric focusing on Agarose-IEF gel pH 4–6.5 with benzoyl-L-arginine-p-nitroanilide (BAPNA) as substrate-staining [2]. The designated names and isoelectric points (pI) are illustrated. (Adapted from Rungruangsak Torrissen and Male [1], with permission from CRC PRESS LLC, and based on data from Torrissen [2], Torrissen and Barnung [3] and Rungruangsak-Torrissen et al. [9]).

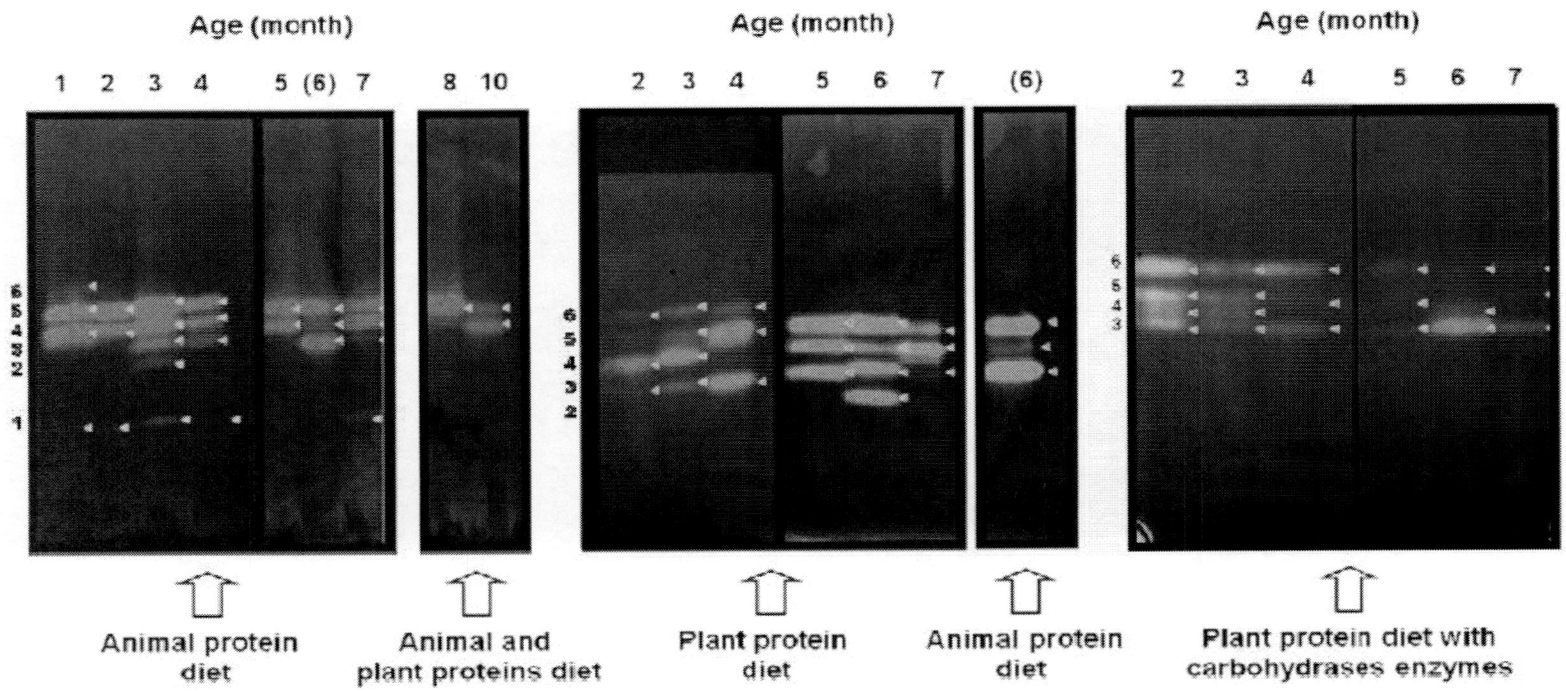

Figure 2. Electrophoretic zymograms (on 12% native-PAGE with *N*-*p*-tosyl-*L*-arginine methyl ester hydrochloride (TAME) as substrate-staining) of trypsin isozymes expressions in the intestinal extracts (with food content) of Nile tilapia feeding on artificial diets with different sources of proteins during the whole experimental periods of 7–10 months. (Adapted from Rungruangsak-Torrissen et al. [19], with the pictures provided by S. Unajak and K. Choowongkomon).

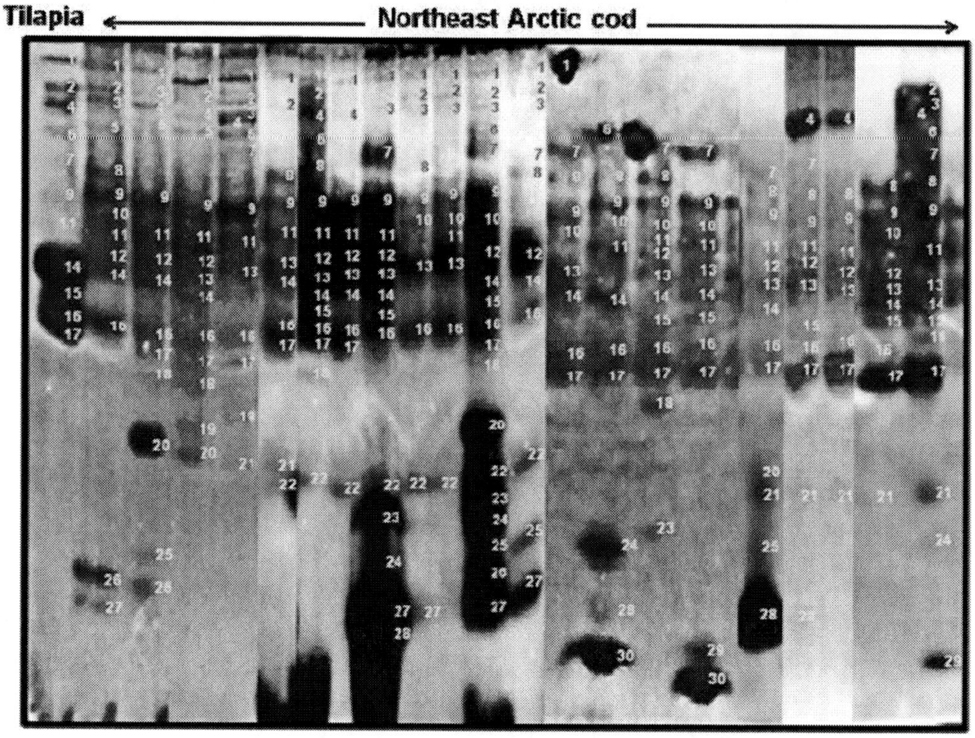

Figure 3. Electrophoretic zymograms (on 15% native-PAGE with N-p-tosyl-L-arginine methyl ester hydrochloride (TAME) as substrate-staining) represented approximately 30 trypsin isozymes observed in the pyloric caecal extracts (with food content) of wild maturing Northeast Arctic cod caught in the Barents Sea in comparison with intestinal extract (with food content) of Nile tilapia cultured with an artificial pellet feed. Trypsin isozymes observed were divided into 3 groups, group 1 (numbers 1–8), group 2 (numbers 9–17), and group 3 (numbers 18–30) of possibly exogenous trypsin isozyme fragments from prey items. The pictures were taken with different camera settings and with the gels on black paper to get dark enzyme activity bands. (Adapted from Rungruangsak-Torrissen et al. [20]).

Off the Hebrides area where the estimated ambient temperature was 10.2 °C with relatively high ichthyoplankton densities (200–2000 at 0–50 m depth), the post-smolts were forced to stay in this area for the feeding opportunity. Because of the high ambient temperature, fish weights observed for the trypsin isozyme patterns 1, 2, and 2' were 63.9 ± 7.1 g, 62.4 ± 3.2 g, and 57.9 ± 4.8 g, respectively (Figure 4).

Contrastingly, in the Norwegian Sea with low ichthyoplankton densities (5–60 at 0–50 m depth) and the thermocline clearly differentiated, fish weights observed for the trypsin isozyme patterns 1, 2, and 2' were 132.6 ± 12.2 g, 136.5 ± 14.9 g, and 234.3 ± 24.9 g, with spatial distribution at estimated ambient temperatures of 9.3 °C, 8.7 °C, and 7.7 °C, respectively (Figure 4). When temperature was high with food abundance, the advantages of the pattern 2' phenotype off the Hebrides area to optimize food utilization and growth were reduced. On the other hand, when foods were limited and the thermocline was clear in the Norwegian Sea, the pattern 2' phenotype distributed in a lower temperature area suitable for optimizing food utilization and growth. Abundance, type, and size of foods may force the fish to stay in the area with high occurrence of food organisms, and this could reduce the advantages of optimizing food utilization and growth in certain phenotypes due to un-suitable ambient temperature.

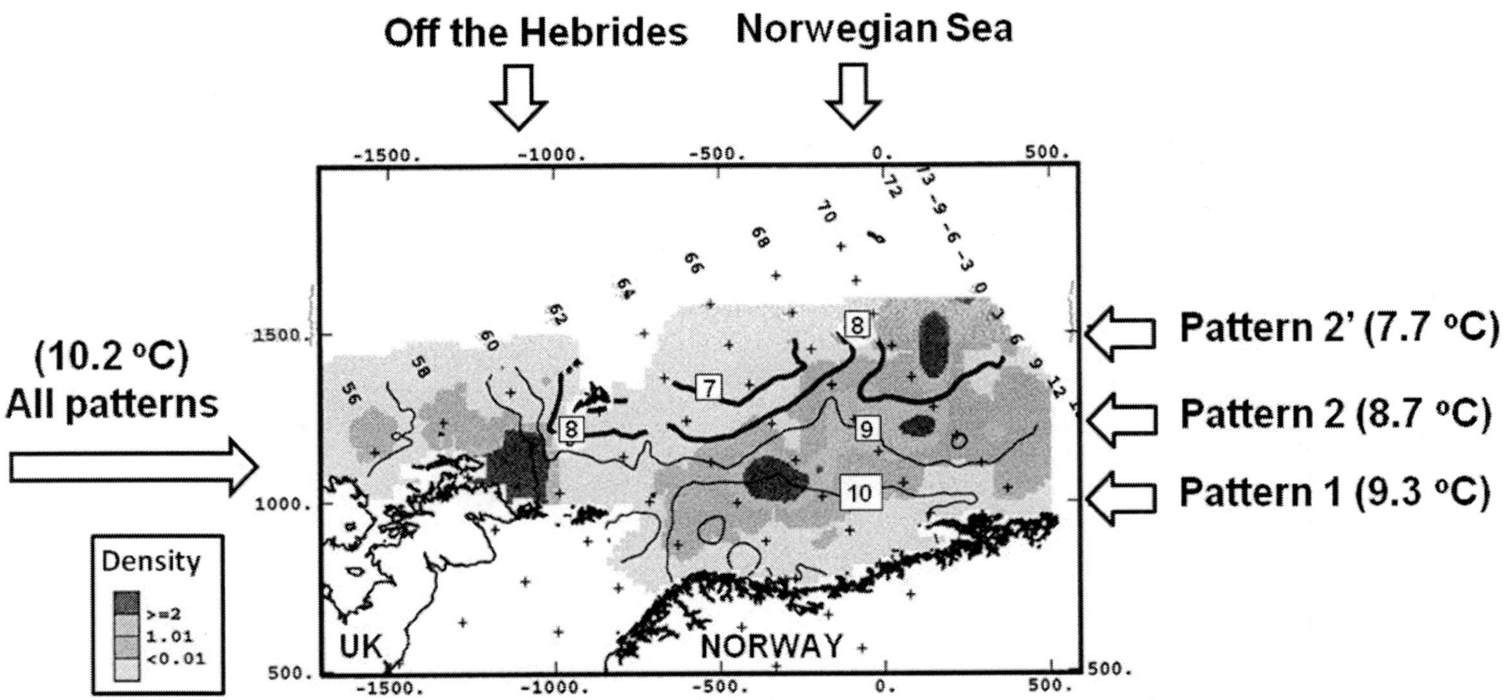

Figure 4. Spatial distribution of Atlantic salmon post-smolts with trypsin isozyme patterns 1, 2, and 2' at different sea temperatures off the Hebrides area and in the Norwegian Sea. Off the Hebrides area, the average weights of the patterns 1, 2 and 2' were 64 g (n = 11), 62 g (n = 22), and 58 g (n = 11), respectively, with estimated ambient temperatures of 10.2 °C. In the Norwegian Sea, the average weights of the patterns 1, 2 and 2' were 133 g (n = 22), 137 g (n = 15), and 234 g (n = 7) with estimated ambient temperatures of 9.3 oC, 8.7 °C, and 7.7 °C, respectively. The isotherms are labeled (°C). Numbers of post-smolts caught per nautical mile are indicated by gray shades. The distance in kilometers is indicated on the frame. Latitudes and longitudes are indicated in the picture. Trypsin phenotypes of pattern 1, pattern 2, and pattern 2' are illustrated in Figure 1. (Data from Rungruangsak-Torrissen and Stensholt [21]).

Association with T/C Ratio, Plasma Insulin, and Free Amino Acids

Further studies were to investigate the effects of trypsin phenotypes on some biological changes that indicate growth performance quality of the fish. Rungruangsak-Torrissen and Sundby [22] have reported the expressions of enzyme specific activities of trypsin and chymotrypsin for digestion of dietary protein, as well as the activity ratio of trypsin to chymotrypsin (T/C ratio) for growth, in relation to the absorption and transport rate of free amino acids (FAA) and secretion of hormone insulin in the plasma, in Atlantic salmon possessing the different trypsin phenotypes reared at different temperatures. The gradient buffer system for the separation of 42 different fluorescent derivatives of amino acids and nitrogen-containing compounds were developed for the studies [22]. Increased plasma insulin secretion was associated with increased total plasma FAA (Figure 5A), especially with essential FAA levels as shown in pattern 1 (Figure 5B). Pyloric caecal T/C ratio levels correlated

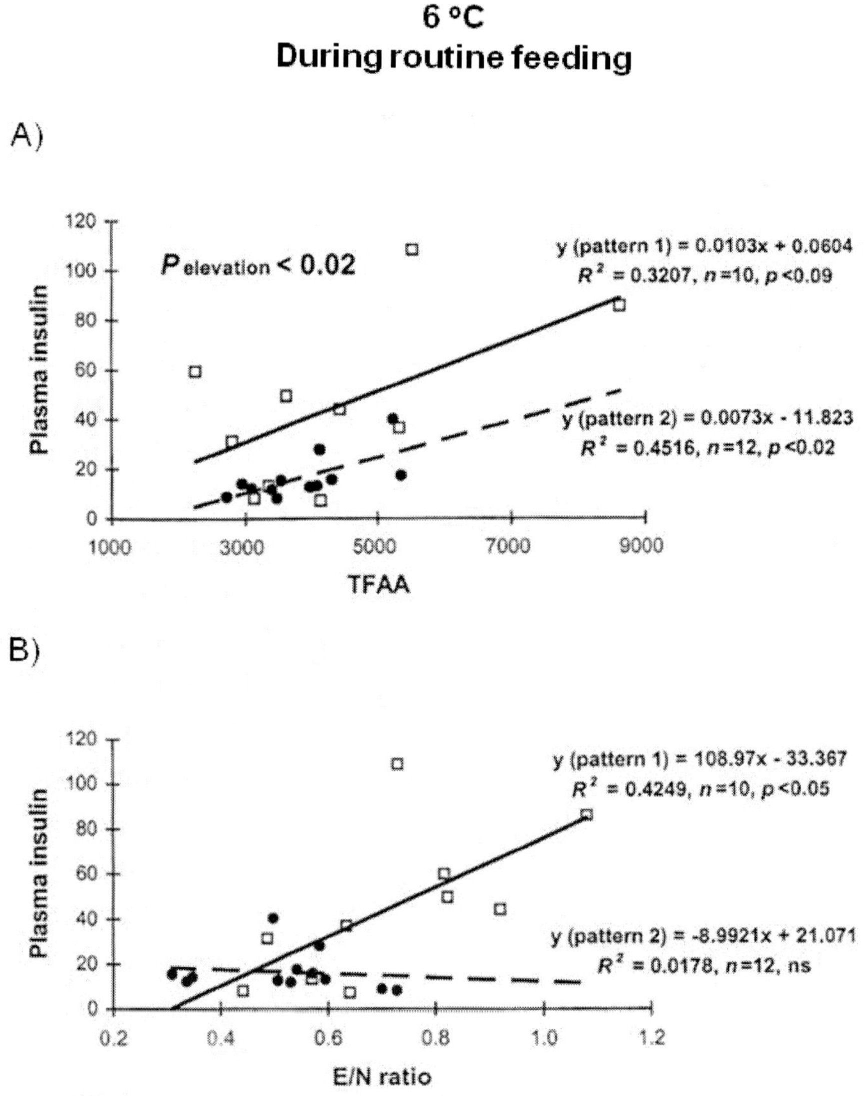

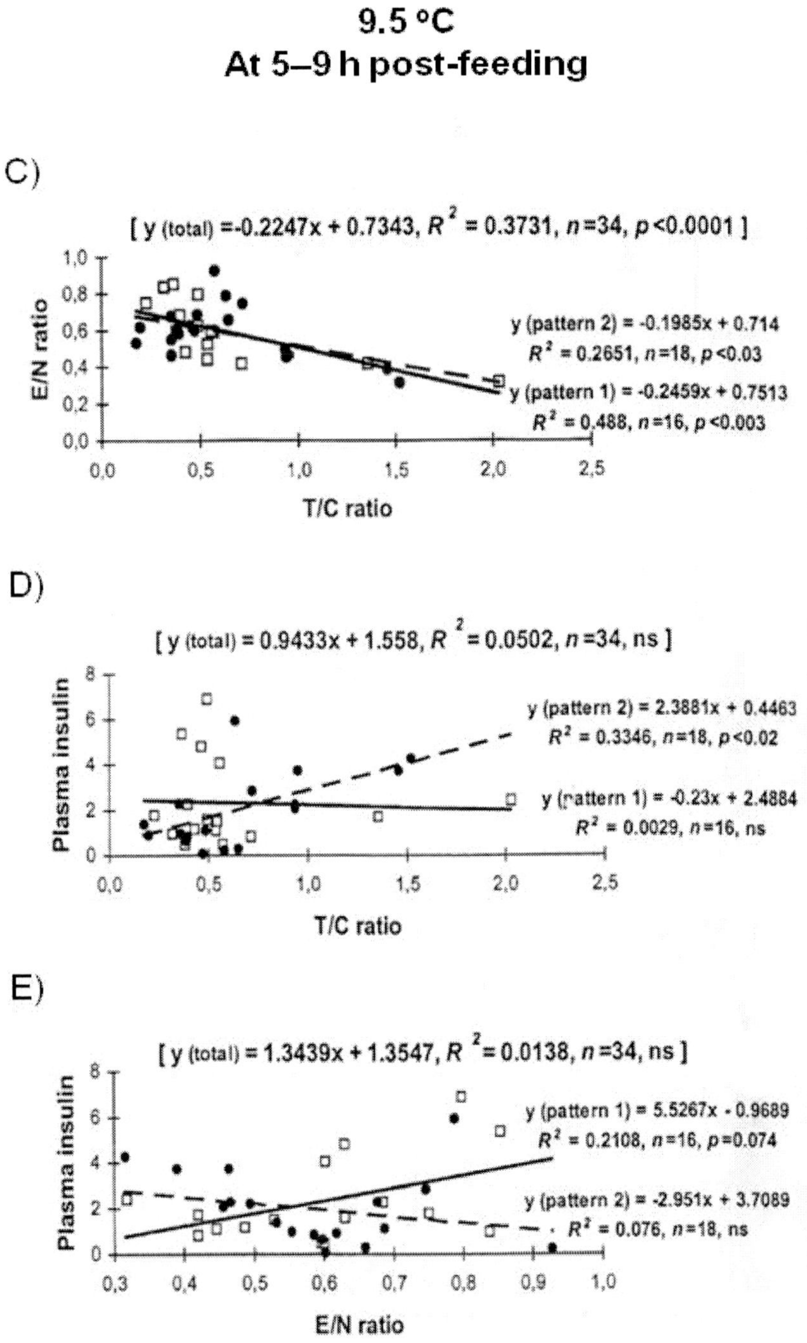

Figure 5. Relationships among plasma total free amino acids (TFAA in nmol ml^{-1}), plasma hormone insulin level (ng ml^{-1}), plasma ratio of essential to non-essential free amino acids (E/N ratio), and the activity ratio of trypsin to chymotrypsin (T/C ratio) in the pyloric caeca, of Atlantic salmon possessing trypsin isozyme pattern 1 (□——□) and pattern 2 (●– –●) reared at 6 °C with the samples collected during routine feeding (A and B) and at 9.5 °C with the samples collected 5–9 h post-feeding after 10 days starvation (C, D and E). The enzyme specific activities of trypsin and chymotrypsin are expressed as µmol *p*-nitroaniline h^{-1} mg $protein^{-1}$ in the pyloric caeca containing food content. Trypsin phenotypes of pattern 1 and pattern 2 are illustrated in Figure 1. ns, not significant.
(From Rungruangsak-Torrissen and Sundby [22], with permission from Springer Corp.).

negatively with the ratio of essential to non-essential FAA (E/N ratio) in the plasma (Figure 5C), and positively with plasma insulin levels as shown in pattern 2 (Figure 5D). Lower elevation of insulin levels (Figure 5A), and no correlation between E/N ratio and insulin levels in plasma (Figures 5B and 5E) observed in pattern 2 at both 6 °C and 9.5 °C, as well as no correlation between T/C ratio and insulin levels in pattern 1 (Figure 5D), suggested faster and/or higher rate of transport of essential FAA for protein synthesis in pattern 2 than pattern 1, as also reported by Torrissen et al. [10, 23]. The results indicate that the higher the T/C ratio value is, the higher is the absorption and transport rate of essential FAA as well as the plasma insulin level for protein synthesis, and the trypsin phenotype of pattern 2 has performed better than pattern 1. The profiles of plasma FAA, plasma insulin, and pyloric caecal T/C ratio during 5–9 h post-feeding after starvation were different between the two phenotypes (Figure 6). A faster secretion of plasma insulin at ≤ 5 h post-feeding with slightly higher pyloric caecal T/C ratio in pattern 2 was observed (Figure 6B2), compared to ≥ 6 h in pattern 1 (Figure 6B1). In addition, high sharp peaks of plasma FAA were observed around 8 h post-feeding in pattern 2 (Figure 6A2) prior to the high insulin peak (Figure 6B2).

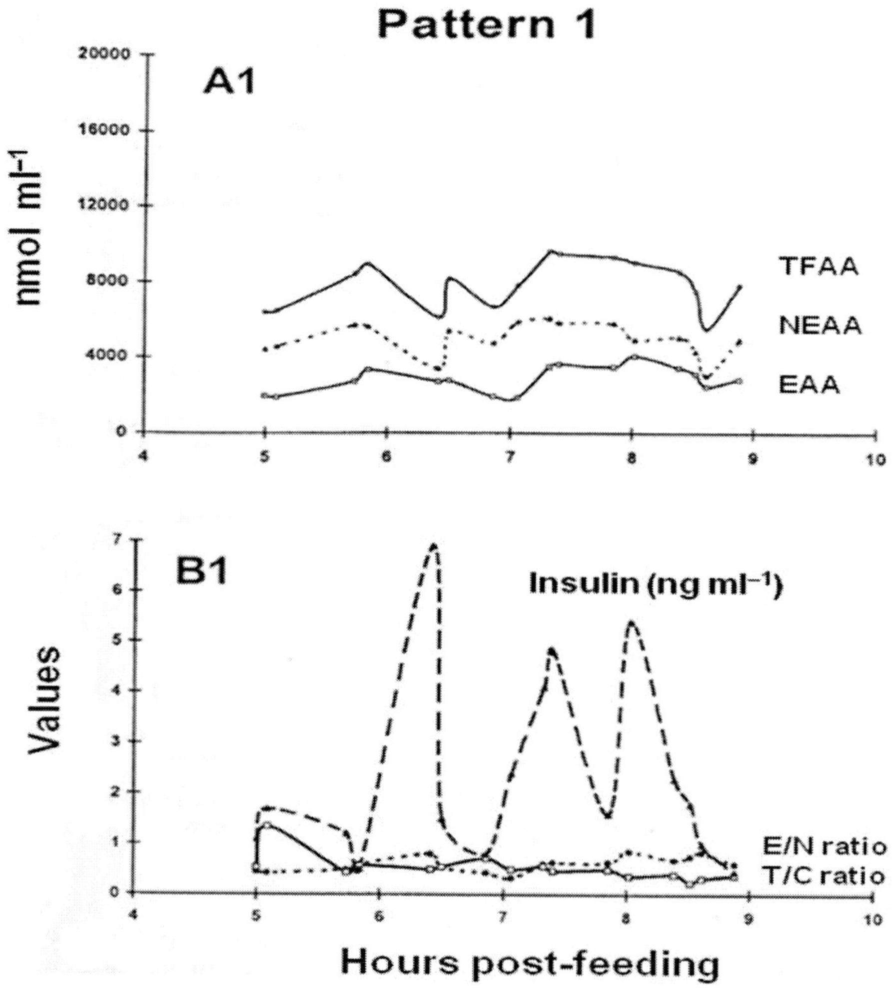

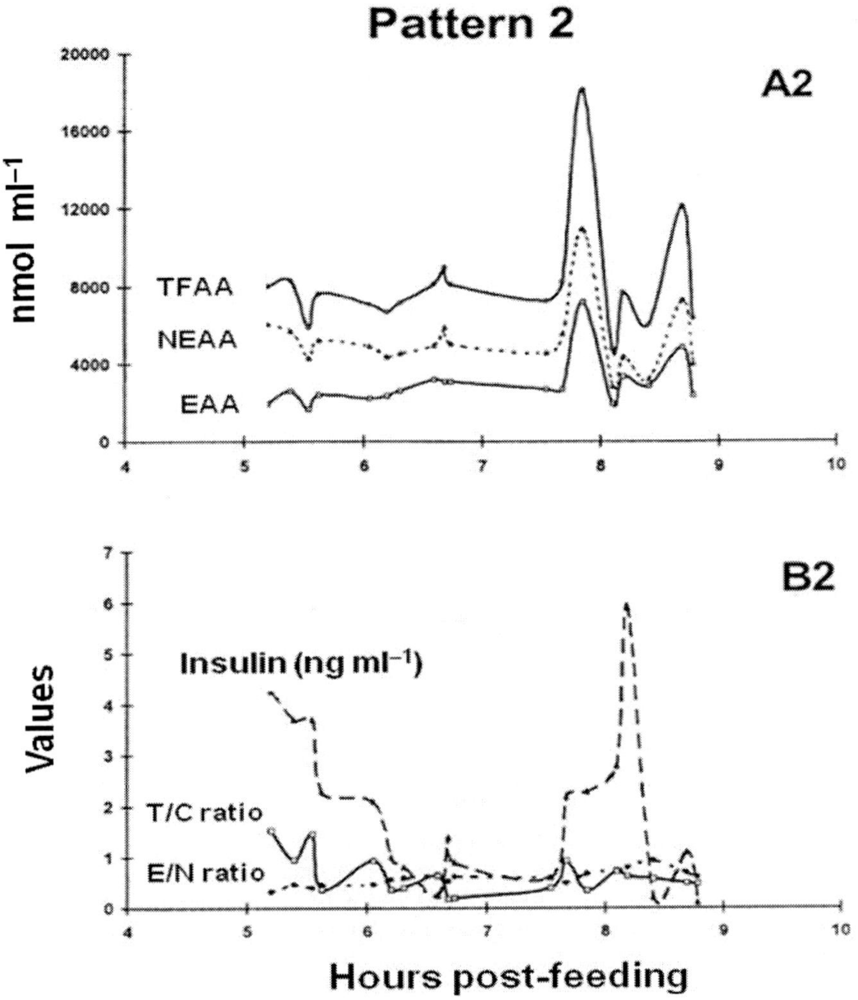

Figure 6. Profiles of total (TFAA), non-essential (NEAA) and essential (EAA) free amino acid concentrations in the plasma, ratio of essential to non-essential free amino acids (E/N ratio) in the plasma, protease activities ratio of trypsin to chymotrypsin (T/C ratio) in the pyloric caeca, and plasma insulin levels, in Atlantic salmon post-smolts possessing trypsin isozyme pattern 1 (A1 and B1) and pattern 2 (A2 and B2) during sampling period from 5 to 9 h post-feeding after 10 days starvation. The enzyme specific activities of trypsin and chymotrypsin are expressed as μmol p-nitroaniline h^{-1} mg protein–1. Trypsin phenotypes of pattern1 and pattern 2 are illustrated in Figure 1. (From Rungruangsak-Torrissen and Sundby [22], with permission from Springer Corp.).

No high sharp peaks of plasma FAA were observed in pattern 1 (Figure 6A1), but the small peaks seemed to be associated with the fluctuation in plasma insulin peaks (Figure 6B1) showing the elevations of plasma FAA were always occurred prior to the elevations of plasma insulinA high amino acid absorption accompany with insulin secretion suggests a higher rate of protein synthesis as observed in the trypsin phenotype of pattern 2, and insulin secretion is stimulated by the elevation of FAA in the plasma.

Studies on trypsin phenotypes have led to deeper understanding of the associations of different biological processes in living organisms.

To establish a practical biological parameter for diet utilization and growth, the relationship between trypsin specific activities and the T/C ratio in the pyloric caeca was studied in Atlantic salmon parr possessing the different trypsin phenotypes of patterns 1, 2 and 2' reared under different temperatures [24]. During routine feeding, the slopes of the regressions between trypsin specific activities and the T/C ratio values were similar among the three phenotypes at 6 °C (Figure 7A), while the slope was higher in the pattern 1 than the patterns 2 and 2' at 10 °C (Figure 7B).

On the other hand, the slope of the post-prandial regressions between trypsin specific activities and the T/C ratio values was higher in the pattern 2' at 6°C, compared to the patterns 1 and 2 (Figure 7C), while the post-prandial regressions were similar among the three phenotypes at 10 °C (Figure 7D).

This was probably due to the amount of feed required for growth at 6°C was less than at 10°C, and a 30 min re-feeding probably reach the requirement at 6°C but not at 10°C. However, the results indicate that the phenotype feeding at suitable temperature will have relatively high diet utilization resulted from high levels of trypsin specific activity and the T/C ratio.

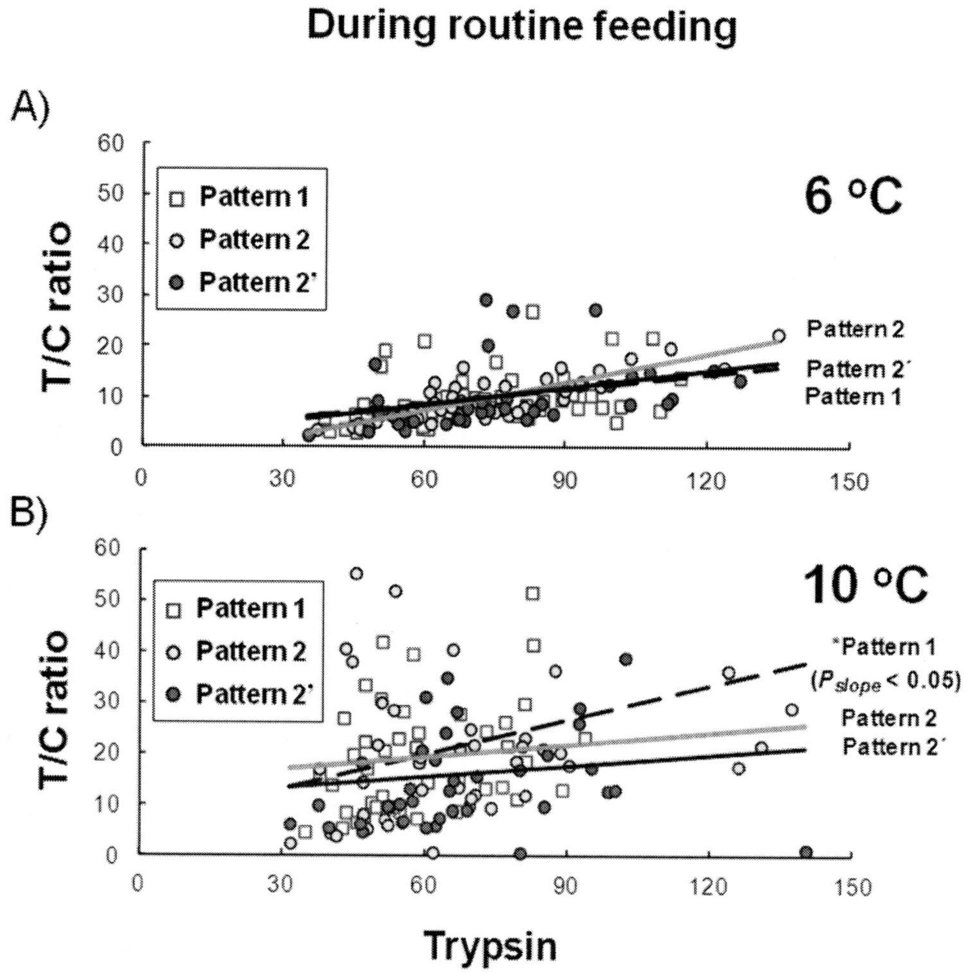

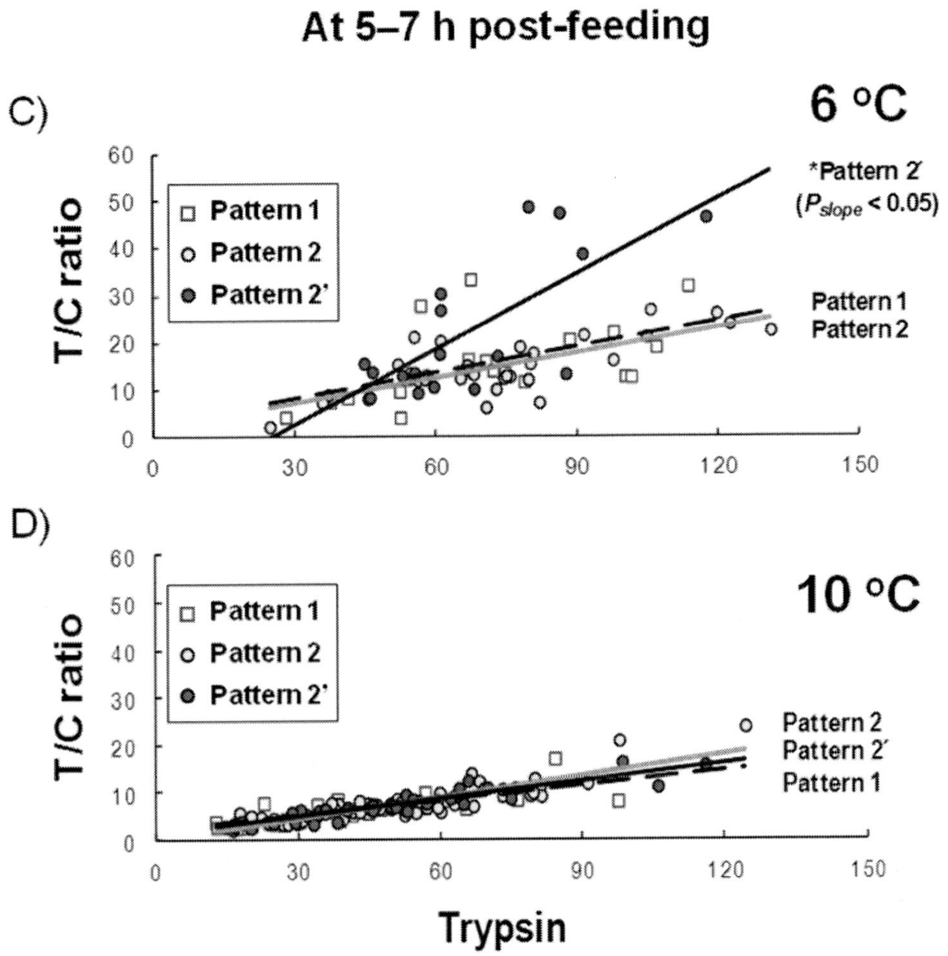

Figure 7. Effects of water temperatures (6 °C and 10 °C) on the relationship between trypsin and the activity ratio of trypsin to chymotrypsin (T/C ratio) in Atlantic salmon parr possessing different trypsin phenotypes of patterns 1, 2, and 2' (see Figure 1). The samples were collected during routine feeding (A and B) and 5–7 h post-feeding after 7 days starvation (C and D). The enzyme specific activities of trypsin and chymotrypsin are expressed as μmol *p*-nitroaniline h^{-1} mg $protein^{-1}$. (From Rungruangsak-Torrissen et al. [24], with permission from Springer Corp.).

Digestion Ability Study

A practical digestibility study has been performed by *in vitro* protein digestion of different fish meal qualities using pyloric caecal crude enzyme extracts from Atlantic salmon possessing the different trypsin phenotypes [11]. The results indicated distinctive characteristics among the three phenotypes in digestion abilities for the same fish meals, whereas the pattern 1 was able to distinguish among different fish meals but the patterns 2 and 2' were unable to distinguish the meals (Figure 8). The pattern 2 was shown to be the most efficient trypsin phenotype in its ability to degrade any type of the studied fish meals and with a relatively higher liberation potential of free amino acids than the other patterns, indicating the advantage of possessing different trypsin isozymes (Figure 8). The technique could differentiate genetic differences in digestive efficiency, which was not possible by using traditional apparent digestibility method. Similar experiment has been performed in spiny lobster possessing different trypsin phenotypes and confirmed the potential differences in protein digestion between individuals with different trypsin isozyme patterns, the advantage of possessing different trypsin isozymes, and the usefulness of *in vitro* digestibility method using crude extracts of digestive organ for sensitivity to small changes in digestion efficiency [25].

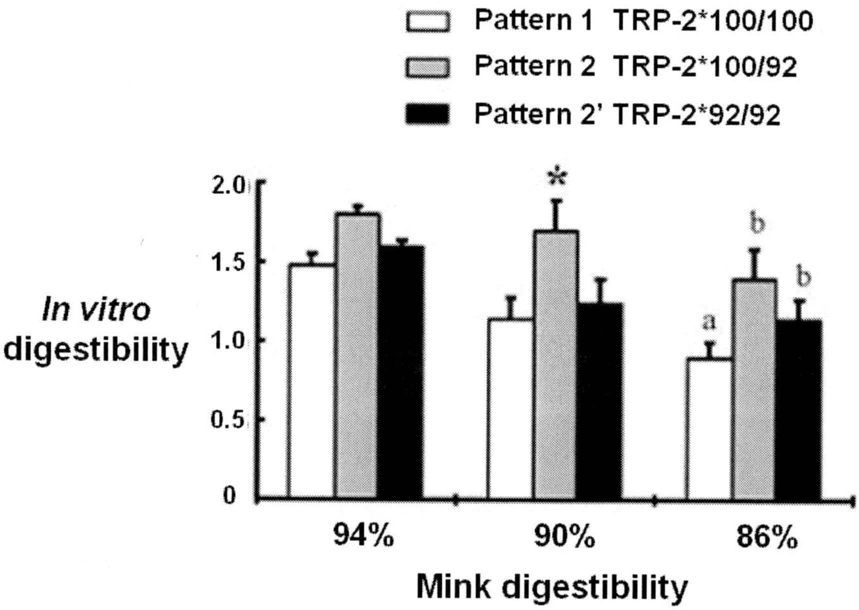

Figure 8. In vitro protein digestion potential (expressed as amino group liberation in 10–4 mol alanine equivalent) of the pyloric caecal crude enzyme extracts from Atlantic salmon possessing trypsin phenotypes of pattern 1, 2 and 2' (see Figure 1), using fish meals as substrates with different quality based on mink digestibility. The bars with the asterisk (*) or with different superscripts are significantly different ($P < 0.05$). (From Rungruangsak Torrissen and Male [1], with permission from CRC PRESS LLC, and based on data from Bassompierre et al. [11]).

Characterization of Trypsin Isozymes

The primary structure of trypsin is available for enormous number of species including fish. Pancreatic cDNA libraries from Atlantic salmon have been constructed and screened, and five clones containing near full-length transcripts have been characterized showing three of them possessing very similar sequences and might be encoded by the same gene locus while the other two were probably encoded by separate gene loci [14].

The charged amino acid distribution showed that four of the Atlantic salmon trypsin clones encoded anionic forms, and the fifth clone represented a cationic trypsin, with around 70% identical primary sequence between anionic and cationic forms [14]. Multiple alignments of amino acid sequences of trypsin from different species, and the relationships between trypsin sequences evolutionally presented as a phylogram are illustrated in Rungruangsak Torrissen and Male [1] and Male et al. [14]. Trypsin has been purified and characterized with the *N*-terminal amino acid sequences identified in different species (Table 1). The purified trypsin isozymes showed the same typical optimum pH around 8 and typical optimal temperature range of 50–60 °C.

Variations in amino acid sequences were observed in different trypsin isozymes and among different species.

Very few trypsin isozymes were purified in each species (Table 1), showing a loss of some isozymes during purification, similar to the observation in Nile tilapia that only one trypsin isozyme was purified while seven trypsin isozymes were observed in crude enzyme extract on native-PAGE with *N*-*p*-tosyl-*L*-arginine methyl ester hydrochloride (TAME) as substrate-staining (S. Unajak and K. Choowongkomon, personal communication). The full paper of Unajak et al. on trypsin isozymes and characterization of purified thermostable trypsin from intestine of Nile tilapia will be published elsewhere.

Table 1. The N-terminal amino acid sequences of purified trypsinisozymes in different species. The different amino acids are shown in bold letters

Species	*N*-terminal amino acid sequence	Reference
Bovine (*Bos taurus*) anionic trypsin	IVGGY**TCA E** NS **VPYQ**VSLN	Reviewed in 1
Bovine (*B. taurus*) cationic trypsin	IVGGY**TCGANTVPYQ**VSLN	Reviewed in 1
Atlantic salmon (*Salmo salar*) anionic trypsins	IVGGYEC**KAY**SQ**THQ**VSLN IVGGYEC**KAY**SQ **PHQ**VSLN	Reviewed in 1
Atlantic salmon (*S. salar*) cationic trypsin	IVGGYEC**R KN**SAS **Y QA**SL**Q**	Reviewed in 1
Spiny dogfish (*Squalus acanthias*)	IVGGYEC**PKHAAPWT**VSLN	Reviewed in 1
Pufferfish (*Fugu rubripes*)	IVGGYEC**RKN**S**VAYQ**VSLN	Reviewed in 1
Winter flounder (*Pleuronectes americanus*)	IVGGYEC**T P H**SQ**AHQ**VSLN	Reviewed in 1
Antarctic fish (*Paranotothemia magellanica*)	IVGG**K**EC**S P Y** SQ**P HQ**VS LN	Reviewed in 1
Plaice (*Pleuronectes platessa*)	I **I** GG**H** EC**AAH**S**RPFMA**SLN	Reviewed in 1
Xenopus (*Xenopus laevis*)	I **I** GG**AT** C**AK S** S**VPY I** V SLN	Reviewed in 1
Sea lamprey (*Petromyzon marinus*)	IVGG**S** E C**AAH**SQ**PWQ**VSLN	Reviewed in 1
Japanese anchovy (*Engraulis japonica*)	IVGGYEC**QAH**SQ**P H T** VSLNS IVGGYEC**Q P Y**SQ**P H Q** VSL**D**S	26
Spotted mackerel (*Scomber australasicus*)	IVGGYEC**T A H**SQ**P H Q**VSLNS	27
Yellow tail (*Seriola quinqueradiata*)	IVGGYEC**T P Y** SQ**P H Q** VSLNS	28
Brown hakeling (*Physiculus japonicus*)	IVGGYEC**PKH**SQ**P H Q**VSLNS	28
Jacopever (*Sebastes schlegelii*)	IVGGYEC**KPY**SQ**P H Q**VSLNS	29
Elkhorn sculpin (*Alcichthys alcicornis*)	IVGGYEC**T P H**SQ**AHQ**VSLNS	29
Walleye Pollock (*Theragra chalcogramma*)	IVGGYEC**TKH**SQ**AHQ**VSLNS	30
Skipjack tuna (*Katsuwonus pelamis*)	IVGGYEC**QAH**SQ**P P Q**VSLN**A** IVGGYEC**QAH**SQ**P P Q**VSLNS	31
Atlantic cod (*Gadus morhua*)	IVGGYEC**TKH**SQ**AHQ**VSLN	Reviewed in 1
Pacific cod (*Gadus macrocephalus*)	IVGGYEC**TRH**SQ**AHQ**VSLNS	32
Saffron cod (*Eleginus gracilis*)	IVGGYEC**PRH**SQ**AHQ**VSLNS	32
Masu salmon (*Oncorhynchus masou*)	IVGGYEC**KAY**SQ**PHQ**VSLNS	33
Pacific saury (*Cololabis saira*)	IVGGYEC**QPH**-	34

Different trypsin isozymes possess differences in their catalytic efficiency (k_{cat} / K_m) and the distribution of charged amino acids appears to be responsible for different substrate-binding preferences, and it has been suggested that the cold-adapted enzyme contained decreased number of salt bridges, lower overall hydrophobicity, and increased surface hydrophilicity, giving an overall more flexible structure compared to the warm-adapted enzyme [reviewed in 1].

So far, the knowledge of the protein structures of different trypsin isozymes in relation to their biological functions has never been revealed. However, the works on trypsin phenotypes in Atlantic salmon on some important biological characteristics, as described above, have led to understanding for further practical studies of food utilization efficiency, growth, and maturation of aquatic animals (Figure 9), as well as for dietary quality assessment, which are described in the following sections.

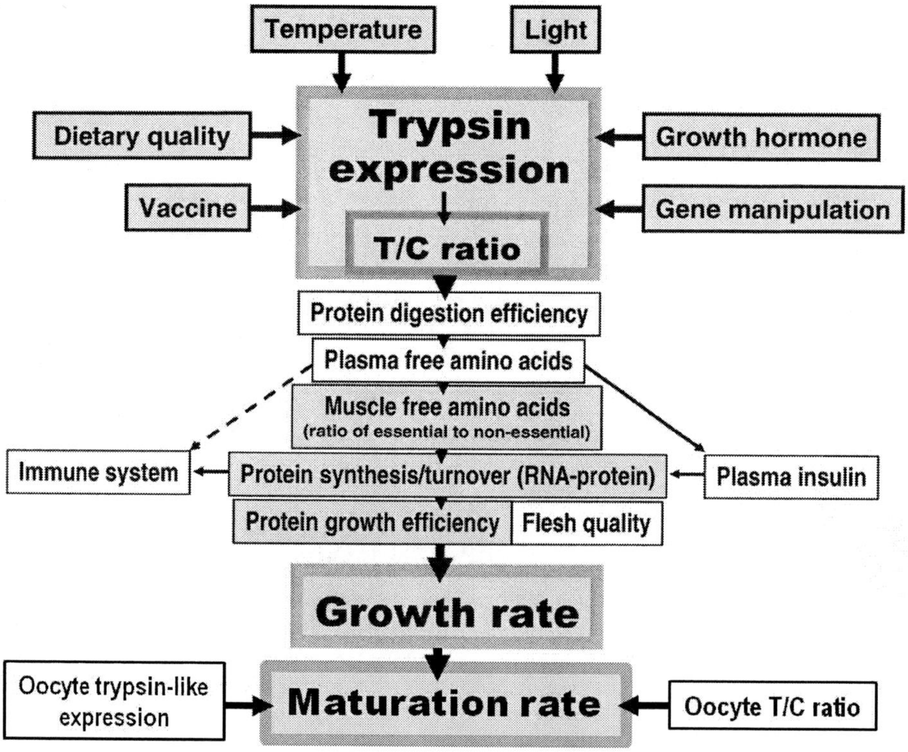

Figure 9. Diagram showing the importance of trypsin for a series of growth mechanisms through its role as the key enzyme in protein digestion process. Trypsin expression and the protease activity ratio of trypsin to chymotrypsin (T/C ratio) in the pyloric caeca (affecting nutrient influx that subsequently influences capacity for protein synthesis and immune system and growth) is influenced by temperature and dietary quality [1, 24, 35] as well as by light regime [36, 37], growth hormone [37, 38], gene manipulation [36, 39], and vaccine type [37]. Transport rate and level of free amino acids to target tissues (affecting plasma insulin secretion and protein synthesis in the white muscle) indicate protein utilization efficiency and flesh quality of the fish. Details of the effects of trypsin expression and the T/C ratio on protein utilization and muscle capacity for protein synthesis and growth were described in Rungruangsak Torrissen and Male [1] and Sunde et al. [35, 36], and on maturation in Rungruangsak-Torrissen [40], Rungruangsak-Torrissen and Fosseidengen [41] and Rungruangsak-Torrissen et al. [20, 42]. (Adapted from Rungruangsak-Torrissen et al. [24], with permission from Springer Corp.).

Food Utilization Efficiency and Growth Studies

Trypsin and Hormone Secretions

Growth of living organisms is dependent on the levels of consumption and how well the diets are utilized. Growth performance quality is, in addition, dependent on the dietary quality that leads to protein deposition in body and muscle, and results in health and maturation processes.

The series of growth mechanism and external effects are illustrated in Figure 9. Rungruangsak-Torrissen et al. [12] have reported that the effect on growth was observed with an increase in trypsin specific activity accompanied by an increase in plasma insulin level, at least one month before an enhanced growth could be found (Figure 10).

Trypsin specific activity peaked faster in fish with a higher growth than those with lower growth (Figure 10) resulting in faster elevations of plasma free amino acids (FAA) that stimulated the secretion of plasma insulin to influence protein synthesis and growth in higher growth fish. This corresponds with the observation by Rungruangsak-Torrissen and Sundby [22] that the secretion of plasma insulin was stimulated by the elevation of plasma FAA resulted from dietary protein digestion by proteases (Figure 6).

Moreover, the profiles of trypsin expression as well as chymotrypsin expression [37] were similar to the profiles of plasma growth hormone levels [43] in the same experiment. These works indicate the associations between the expressions of digestive proteases of trypsin and chymotrypsin specific activities including the activity ratio of trypsin to chymotrypsin (T/C ratio), FAA influx, and hormone secretions (insulin, growth hormone), for protein synthesis and growth.

Thus, trypsin expression and T/C ratio are the primary key factors affecting different levels of nutrient influx for stimulating a series of growth mechanisms including hormone secretions for promoting fish growth, as shown in Figure 9.

Trypsin, Chymotrypsin, and T/C Ratio

Growth is regulated by a series of controls, and food digestion has been shown to be a primary control mechanism (see Figure 9). In animal cultivation, food consumption rate can be controlled and measured, but not in natural ecosystems. Therefore, it is important to find a factor that could explain dietary utilization and growth both in cultivation and natural ecosystems, and the protease activity ratio of trypsin to chymotrypsin (T/C ratio) in the digestive tract (pyloric caeca or intestine) is the unique biological factor. The T/C ratio was first established in association with digestion rate of dietary protein by Rungruangsak-Torrissen and Sundby [22] where the increase in the T/C ratio was due to an increased trypsin specific activity and also with a decreased chymotrypsin specific activity (Figure 11).

Growth rate has been shown to be influenced by variations in two internal factors (trypsin phenotypes, life stages) and three common external factors (starvation, feeding, temperatures), whereas the interaction between trypsin phenotype and start-feeding temperature could affect specific activity of trypsin but not of chymotrypsin [24]. During starvation (limited food), specific activities of trypsin (and also of pepsin) decreased and maintain at low levels while those of chymotrypsin increased and maintain at high levels, and this resulted in low levels of the T/C ratio (Figure 12). After diet deprivation, a decrease in trypsin activity is a common phenomenon in living organisms [24, 44–50], while both decrease [44, 45, 49, 51] and increase [24, 52, 53] in chymotrypsin activity could be observed.

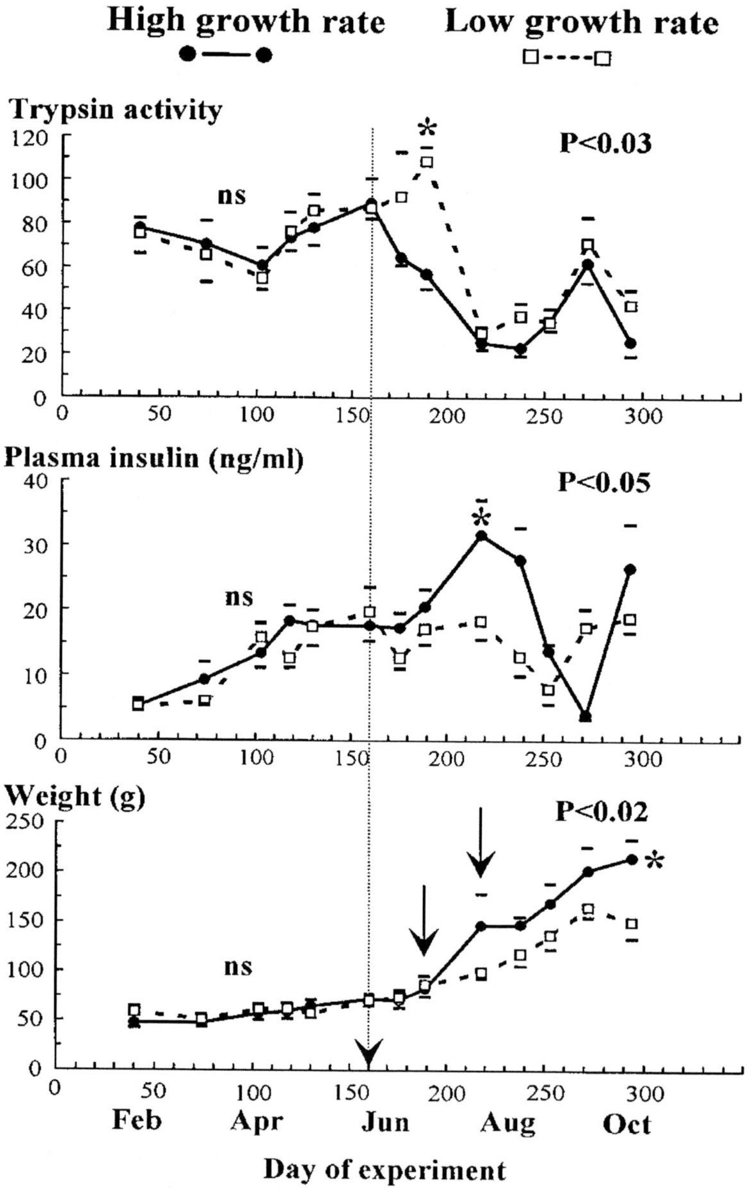

Figure 10. The association between trypsin activity (μmol p-nitroaniline h^{-1} mg protein–1) and plasma insulin levels (ng ml^{-1}) in Atlantic salmon of different growth rates. The arrows indicate the change in growth rate occurred one month later than the changes in trypsin activity accompanied with plasma insulin levels. The sign * indicates significant differences between the two groups at that time ($P < 0.05$ by Student's t-test). Probability values indicate significant differences compared between paired data sets of the whole period during days 160 to 294 (ns, not significant). (From Rungruangsak-Torrissen et al. [12], with permission from Springer Corp.).

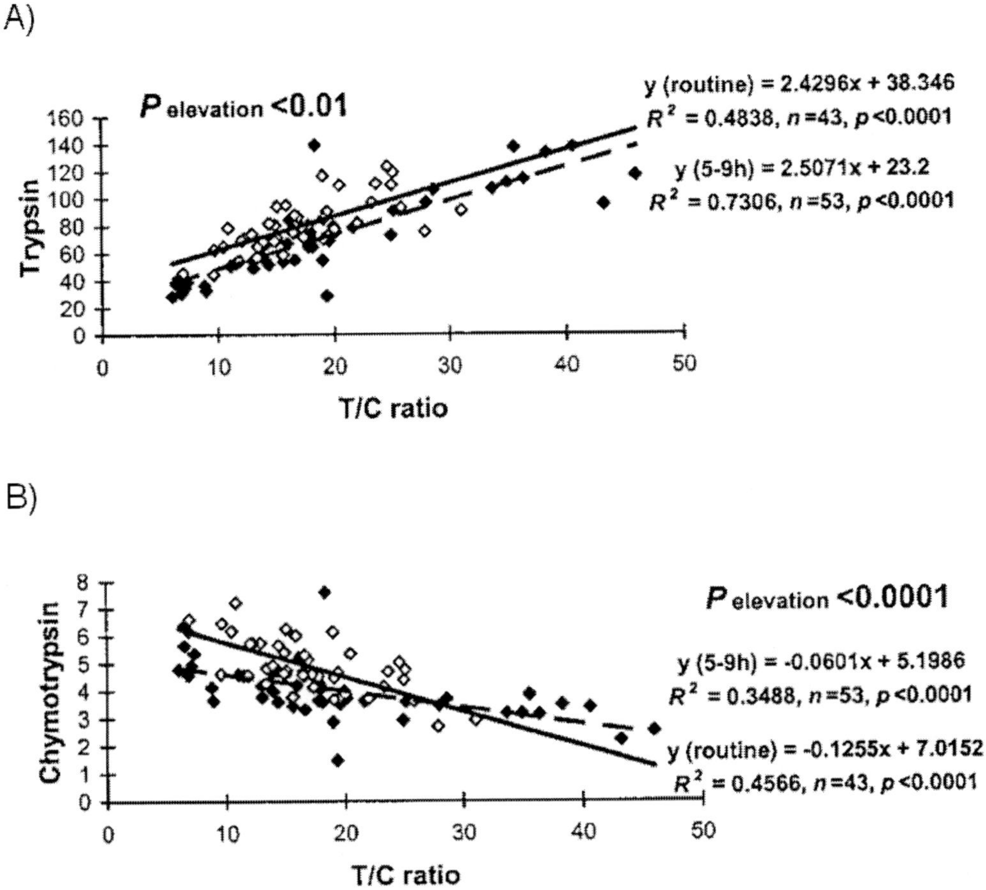

Figure 11. Relationships between the activity ratio of trypsin to chymotrypsin (T/C ratio) (A) with trypsin activity and (B) with chymotrypsin activity, in Atlantic salmon during routine feeding (◊——◊) and at 5–9 h post-feeding after 10 days starvation (♦– –♦). The enzyme activities are expressed as μmol p-nitroaniline h^{-1} mg $protein^{-1}$ in the whole pyloric caeca containing food content. (Adapted from Rungruangsak-Torrissen and Sundby [22], with permission from Springer Corp.).

The increase in chymotrypsin activity after diet deprivation was due to the fishes still had consumption from the natural food supply through water, as they were kept in sea cages [24, 52] and probably also due to the use of circulating water [53]. Therefore, the activity of chymotrypsin could increase when there was a reduction in growth rate [24, 37, 42, 53], which was an unexpected mechanism observed in aquatic animals.

The T/C ratio value would be higher in fish with higher growth potential if they were at a growing phase [24, 36], while during a reduced or steady growth phase, the fish with higher growth would show a lower T/C ratio value due to a relatively higher increased chymotrypsin specific activity [41, 42]. For easy understanding, the phenomena of trypsin and chymotrypsin expressions in fish could be explained in a similar way as car driving that higher acceleration (trypsin specific activity) is needed to increase car speed (fish growth), and higher braking capacity (chymotrypsin specific activity) is necessarily for stopping a car (fish) with higher speed (higher growth) [41].

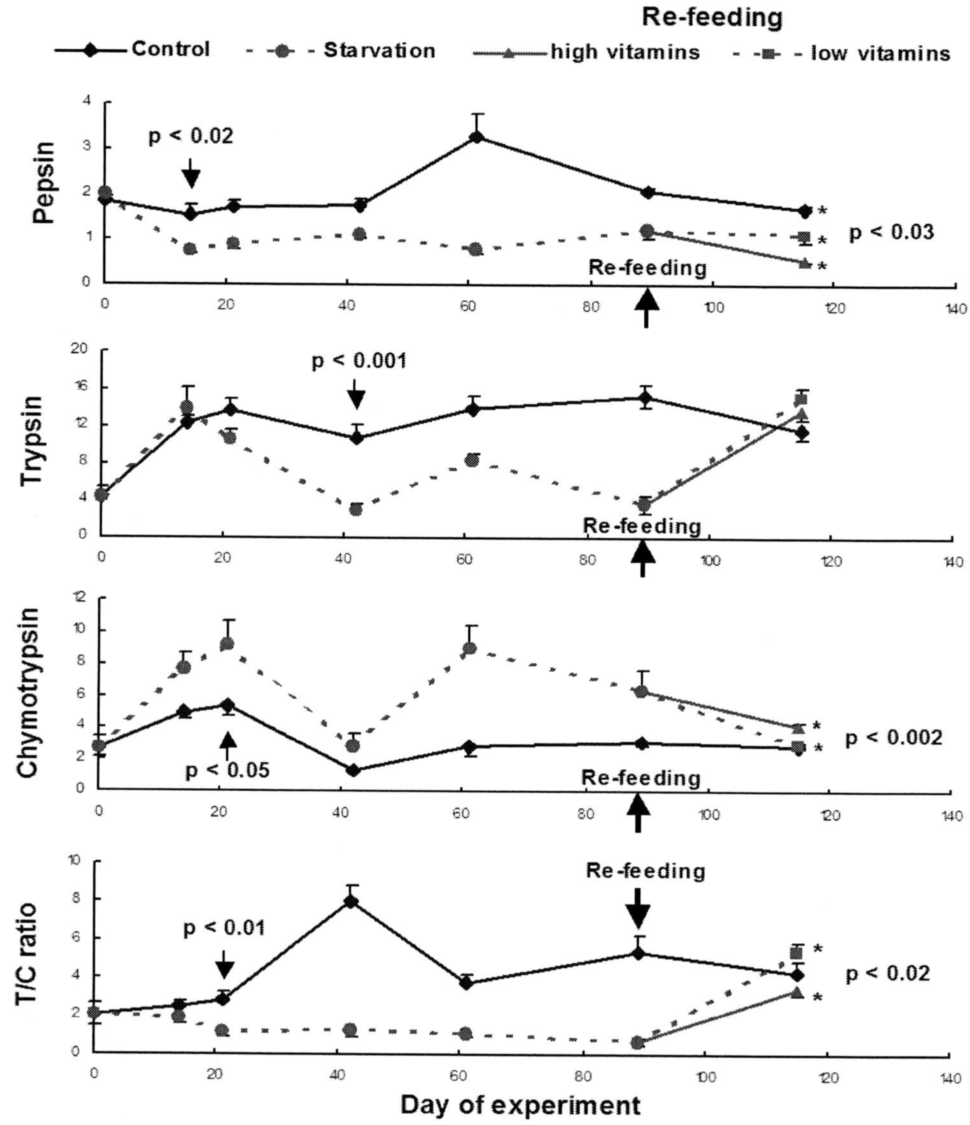

Figure 12. Effect of starvation (limited food) on expressions of pepsin, trypsin, and chymotrypsin in the digestive tract of Atlantic salmon. Arrows with probability values indicate first observations of significantly changing in the enzyme expressions. The values with asterisk (*) are significantly different ($P < 0.05$). The enzyme specific activities are expressed as μmol tyrosine h–1 mg protein^{-1} for pepsin in the stomach, and as μmol p-nitroaniline h^{-1} mg protein–1 for trypsin and chymotrypsin in the pyloric caeca. (From Rungruangsak-Torrissen et al. [24], with permission from Springer Corp.).

A severe influence of starvation period on chymotrypsin activity after re-feeding has been reported, as 3-week-starvation resulted in significantly higher chymotrypsin activity after 12 days post-feeding, compared to 1-week- and 2-week-starvation, without affecting trypsin activity [49]. After *ad lib* re-feeding for five weeks, the 3-week-starvation group showed the lowest chymotrypsin activity with a significantly lower level than the control group, and with similar trypsin activity [49] and final weight to the other groups due to higher feed intake [54]. Unfortunately, Imani et al. [49] did not calculate the T/C ratio values.

Otherwise, a significantly higher T/C ratio would have been seen in the 3-week-starvation group that would indicate its growth rate compensation at the end of the experiment. The other indication showing increasing chymotrypsin specific activity during slower growth is illustrated in Figure 13. During ordinary routine feeding and growth, trypsin activated higher chymotrypsin at 6 °C than at 10 °C (Figure 13A) while the T/C ratio values were higher at 10 °C than at 6 °C (Figure 13B). The relationship between specific activities of trypsin and chymotrypsin could be observed when growth was limited [40], during food deprivation [1, 24], and during maturation [41, 42], while the relationship disappeared at post-feeding after starvation [1] and during growing phase (Figure 13A). According to different studies [20, 24, 37, 40–42], the relationship between trypsin and the T/C ratios (as shown in Figure 13B) could indicate growth status of the fish whether it is growing phase (positive relationship), steady growth phase (no relationship), or reducing growth phase (negative relationship). In order to avoid animal sacrifice, these protease parameters (specific activities of trypsin and chymotrypsin, T/C ratio) have also been studied in the faeces, and they could also indicate fish digestive efficiency, but could not predict fish growth status [40].

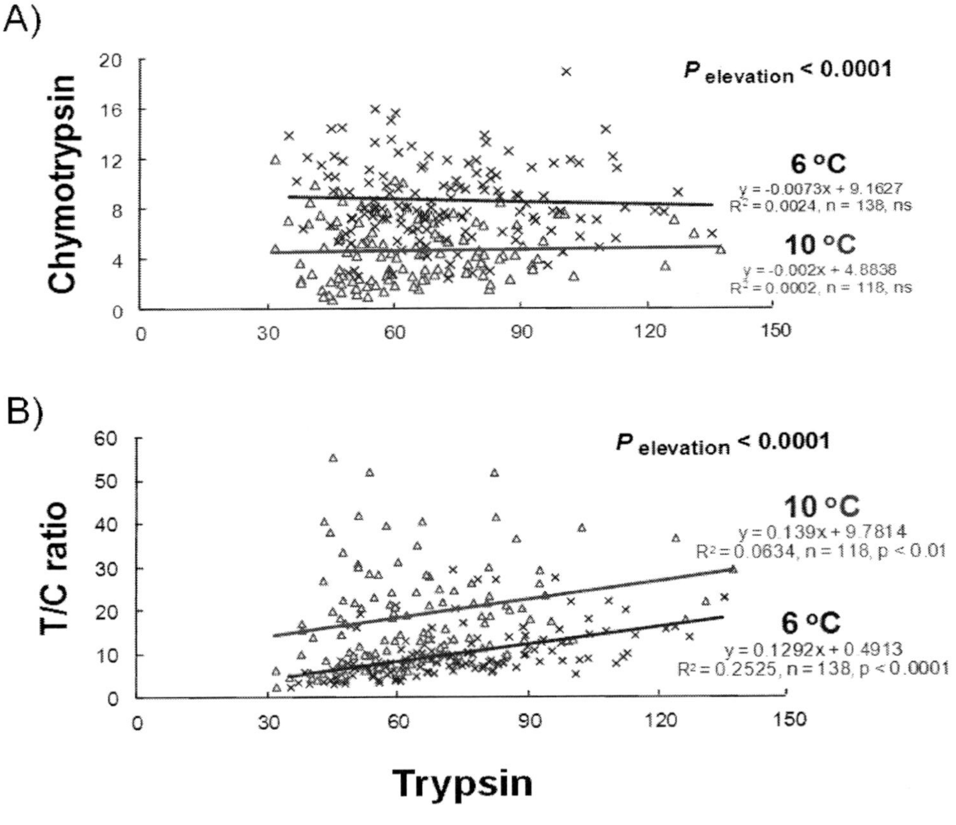

Figure 13. Effect of water temperatures on the relationships of trypsin (A) with chymotrypsin and (B) with the activity ratio of trypsin to chymotrypsin (T/C ratio), in Atlantic salmon parr reared at 6 °C (×) and 10 °C (Δ). The enzyme specific activities of trypsin and chymotrypsin in the pyloric caeca are expressed as μmol p-nitroaniline h^{-1} mg $protein^{-1}$. ns, not significant. (Adapted from Rungruangsak-Torrissen et al. [24], with permission from Springer Corp.).

An interesting T/C ratio study during a molting cycle of adult blue swimming crab, *Portunus pelagicus*, has been recently performed (P. Chamchuen and B. Pratoomchat, personal communication), as shown in Figure 14. Before starting a new molting cycle for growth, the crab had a low growth rate indicated by a low T/C ratio value (stage B). The T/C ratio values increased at different molting stages toward the end of the molting cycle (stages C1–D4). After finishing molting, a higher growth rate with a higher T/C ratio value were observed (stage D4), compared to the last cycle (stage A). High food consumptions were observed at stages C2 and D1, indicated also by high levels of trypsin and chymotrypsin specific activities (Figure 14). The levels of both trypsin and chymotrypsin decreased toward the end of molting cycle (Figure 14) due to less consumption (P. Chamchuen and B. Pratoomchat, personal communication). The increases in the T/C ratio values are independent on the specific activity levels of trypsin and chymotrypsin [24, 36, 37, 39, 42, 55], as also shown in Figure 14. The work confirms the importance of the T/C ratio value as a growth indicator, and the specific activity levels of trypsin and chymotrypsin as indicators of diet consumption (and protein consumption [42]), in living organisms. The full paper of Chamchuen et al. on development of digestive enzymes during growth and molting period of the blue swimming crab will be published elsewhere.

The T/C ratio values could also be obtained as slope T/C ratio by calculating from the regression between specific activities of trypsin (y) and chymotrypsin (x) in each studied group, as illustrated in Figure 15. The direct calculation from the two enzyme activities of individuals provided the T/C ratio values that indicate fish growth rates over a period of 1–2 months, while the slope T/C ratios indicated fish growth rates at sampling [37]. Moreover, the advantage of studying the slope T/C ratio is to differentiate the studied fish groups whether they have been feeding under overlapping environments as indicated by crossed regressions (Figure 15A) or under distinct environments as indicated by parallel regressions (Figure 15B). An observation of parallel regressions with similar slope T/C ratios has also been observed between two populations of Northeast Arctic cod living in distinct environments in the Barents Sea [20].

The studies of T/C ratio and slope T/C ratio are unique and challenged. Although this biological secrecy has been studied and revealed during the last decade by Rungruangsak-Torrissen's research team, most researchers are still not familiar with and do not really utilize these practical biological factors yet. The T/C ratio and slope T/C ratio could provide more precise information on food utilization efficiency and growth while the specific activities of trypsin and chymotrypsin provide the information on diet and protein consumption levels.

Trypsin, T/C Ratio, and Free Amino Acids

Trypsin and chymotrypsin specific activities are related to dietary protein levels [42], and the activity ratio of trypsin to chymotrypsin (T/C ratio) is related to intestinal weight [42] and growth rate independent of the protease specific activities levels of the two enzymes [24, 36, 37, 39, 42, 55]. Despite the changes (increase or decrease) in the activities of trypsin and chymotrypsin, the T/C ratio is always associated with feed efficiency [19, 35, 36, 40, 55] and fish growth rate [19, 24, 36, 37, 39–42] over a period of 1–2 months [37, 42]. The T/C ratio value is affected by different external factors, and its associations with other biological parameters in a series of growth mechanisms are illustrated in Figure 9. Changes in the T/C ratio values could influence the levels of free amino acids (FAA) such as essential FAA, total FAA, and the ratio of essential FAA to non-essential FAA (EAA/NEAA) in the plasma [36], as well as the white muscle levels of free hydroxyproline [36], RNA [19, 20], and protein [19].

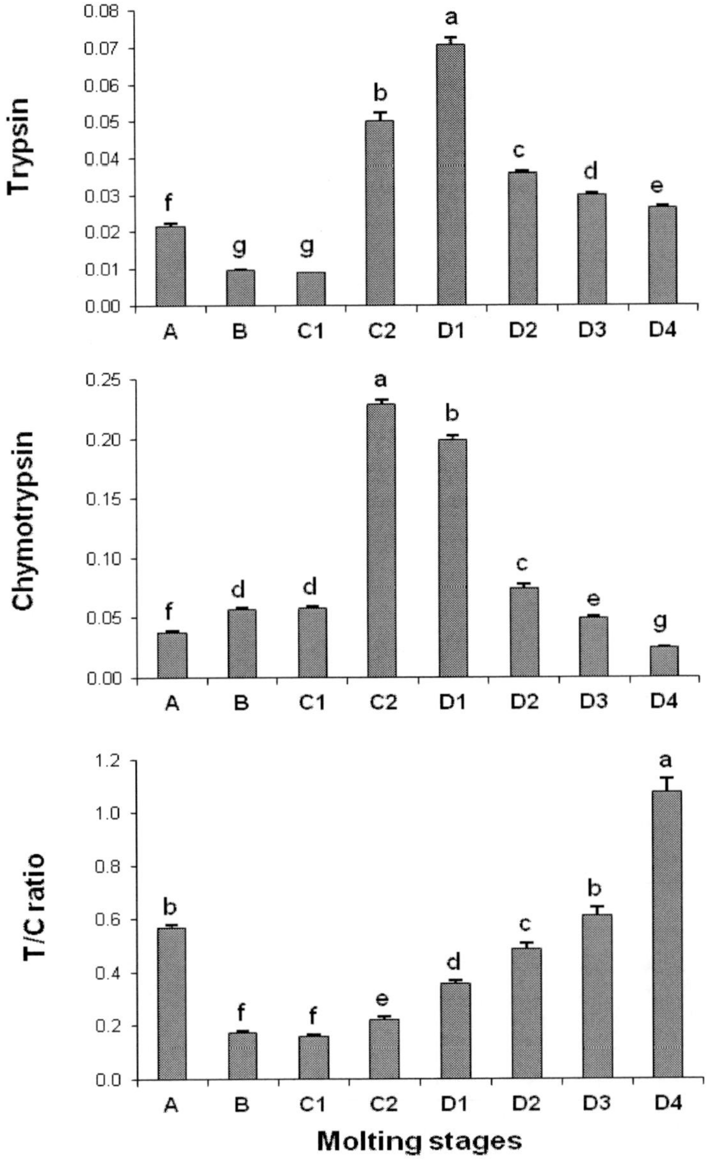

Figure 14. Specific activities of trypsin and chymotrypsin, and the activity ratio of trypsin to chymotrypsin (T/C ratio) of adult blue swimming crab, P. Pelagicus, during a molting cycle; early postmolt (A), postmolt (B), intermolt (C1), late intermolt (C2), early premolt (D1), mid premolt (D2), late premolt (D3), and very late premolt (D4). The enzyme specific activities of trypsin and chymotrypsin are expressed as μmol p-nitroaniline min^{-1} mg $protein^{-1}$. The bars with different superscripts are significantly different ($P < 0.05$). (P. Chamchuen and B. Pratoomchat, personal communication with the figures provided.).

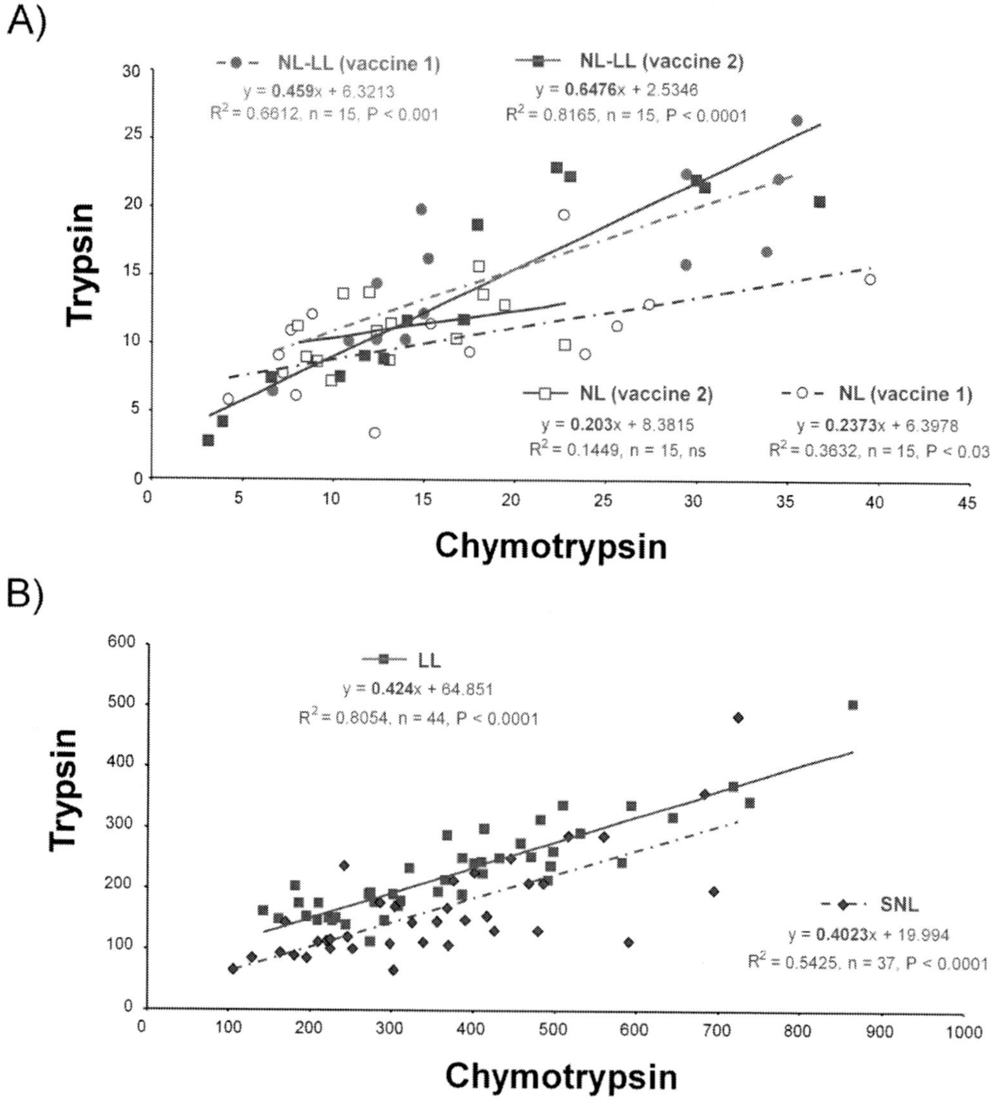

Figure 15. Relationships between trypsin and chymotrypsin specific activities (expressed as μmol p-nitroaniline h^{-1} mg $protein^{-1}$) in the pyloric caeca of Atlantic salmon, (A) overlapping environments: effects of different light regimes [natural light (NL) or natural light with additional continuous light (NL-LL)] and vaccine types, and (B) distinct environments: effects of simulated natural light (SNL) and continuous light regime (LL). The slopes of the regressions indicated the activity ratio of trypsin to chymotrypsin (slope T/C ratio). ns, not significant. (From Rungruangsak-Torrissen et al. [37], with permission from Springer Corp.).

Depending on growth performance in protein synthesis and turnover, the changes in the T/C ratio values could have a negative effect on the white muscle levels of RNA, the ratio of EAA/NEAA [36] and the ratio of RNA to protein [19, 36]. In addition, the T/C ratio values in the digestive tract has been observed to correlate negatively with the T/C ratio (protease activity ratio of trypsin-like to chymotrypsin-like) in the oocytes of maturing females due to slow growth at high maturation rate [20], and could correlate positively [20] or negatively

[19] with the levels of protein to lipid ratio in the oocytes depending on lower or higher stage of maturation, respectively.

Oocyte Maturation Studies

Proteomic Study

During maturation, minimum-feeding behaviour has been observed in order to reduce somatic growth and optimise oocyte maturation process [41, 56]. Both synthesis and degradation of proteins have to be under control during oocyte development [40]. The water uptake during final oocyte maturation seemed to be driven osmotically, not only by uptake of ions but also by hydrolysis of yolk protein to free amino acids [57–59]. During oocyte maturation, hydrolysis of yolk protein to free amino acids (FAA) reserved as food for offspring after hatching has been investigated, and a breakdown of oocyte protein was observed in the presence of protease(s), as trypsin-like specific activity was associated with the levels of total FAA [41] and inversely associated with protein concentrations in the oocytes from females with different feedings [40, 41].

Proteomic study indicated that the expression levels of proteins were higher in the oocytes than in the mature eggs, as protein spots on 2D-gels from the oocyte samples could be observed by Coomassie-staining (Figure 16A) while the protein spots from the mature egg samples could only be observed by the more sensitive Silver staining (Figure 16B). Silver-stained 2D-gels also visualized very low protein expression levels in matured eggs, compared to those in the oocytes (Figure 16B). Twenty-five spots were excised from the Coomassie-stained 2D-gels of oocyte samples for further protein identification (Figure 16A). Fourteen spots were identified with observed molecular masses smaller than the theoretical ones (Table 2). Eleven spots of un-identified proteins were subjected to CAF–MALDI–TOF/TOF MS/MS analysis, and the amino acid sequences of tryptic-digests were identified in nine of them with molecular masses below 25 kDa (Table 3). By searching for short and nearly exact matches using NCBI BLAST, the proteins of the nine spots were predicted (Table 4). They were mainly degraded vitellogenins, phospholipase, a hypothetical protein (probably phosphotransferase), and a conserved hypothetical protein (probably trypsin) (Figure 16 and Table 4).

It is interesting to note that protein spot 6 (Figure 16) was expressed at a very high level in oocytes, and degraded in mature eggs (Figure 16B). It was an unknown protein similar to human keratin and rice hypothetical protein (Table 2). The observed peptides of protein spot 6 had covered both *N*- and *C*-terminal parts. Since this protein had not been identified in Atlantic cod oocytes, the protein spot 6 was probably an "oocyte keratin". The disagreement between the observed and the theoretical masses and pI should be due to the degraded or not full-length proteins of the picked spots.

Variations in expression patterns and expression levels of oocyte main proteins were visualized between different females (Figure 16A), which might be affected by different degradation rate of proteins. Changes of expression patterns of oocyte proteins and protein phosphorylation during acquisition of maturational competence and signal transduction of oocyte maturation in medaka, *Olyzias latipes*, have been observed [60].

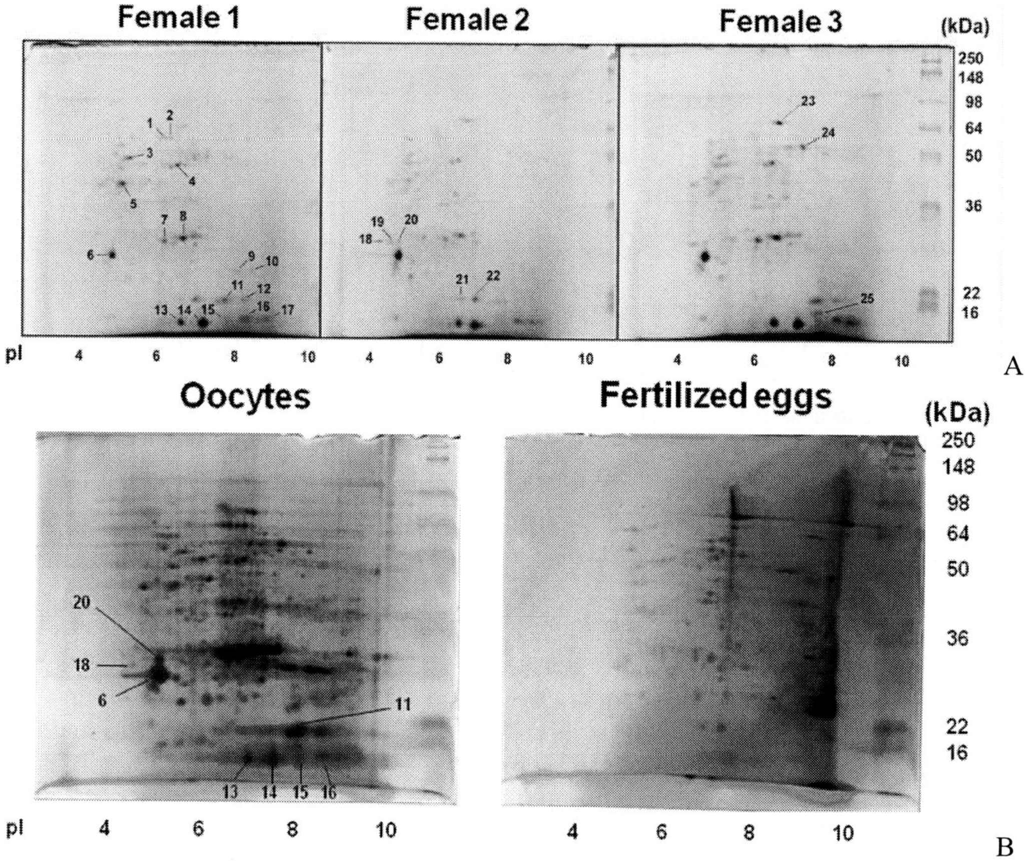

Figure 16. (A) Coomassie-stained 2D-gels of cod oocytes (240 μg protein loaded) from three maturing females, and (B) 2D-gel electrophoresis (240 μg protein loaded) of cod oocytes and fertilized eggs (> 8 cells) detected by Silver staining. The numbers of excised gel-spots for protein identification or *de novo* amino acid sequencing are shown. The identified proteins are listed in Table 2. Amino acid sequences of peptides of un-identified proteins are shown in Table 3, and the predicted proteins are listed in Table 4. (Rungruangsak-Torrissen [unpublished data]).

A comprehensive survey of thousands of genes involved in maturation and development of oocytes in rainbow trout has been reported [61].

It should be noted that the NCBI BLAST identified spot 21 as trypsin from mammals, besides from a conserved hypothetical protein of *Bacillus thuringiensis* serovar konkukain str. 97-27 (Table 4). The CAF-fragment 2389.2 m z^{-1} from spot 21 (Table 3) represented trypsin fragment.

Although most CAF-derivatized proteins did not show this CAF-fragment, it could not be excluded the possibility that the trypsin identified might be taken up from the porcine trypsin used for in-gel tryptic digestion. However, trypsin-like activity has been observed in the oocytes of different fish species [19, 20, 40, 41]. Trypsin has also been observed in non-pancreatic tissues such as rat brain that was inducible by infection with influenza viruses [62], and the presence of a maternal trypsin transcript in reproductive tissues (ovaries, oviducts, and oocytes) in adult female salmon louse, *Lepeophtheirus salmonis* [63] as well as the trypsinogen genes in human β T cell receptor locus [64] has been revealed.

Table 2. List of proteins from cod oocytes (Figure 16) in categories, identified after 2D-gel electrophoresis by MALDI–TOF/TOF MS or MS/MS analysis. (Rungruangsak-Torrissen, unpublished data)

Spot number	Protein identification	Species homology	Accession number	Score	Number of mass values matched	Sequence Coverage (%)	Mass (M_r)	pI	Mass detected (Da)	pI detected
Nuclear										
12	PREDICTED: similar to chromosome 20 open reading frame 4, partial	*Bos taurus*	XP_612731	83	14	47	42293	6.23	17000	8.25
17	COG1595: DNA-directed RNA polymerase specialized sigma subunit	*Haemophilus somnus* 2336	ZP_00131828	87	7	66	16054	6.32	12000	8.85
Cytoskeleton										
3	Simple type II keratin K8b (S2)	*Oncorhynchus mykiss*	CAA6330	97	21	31	58997	5.14	48000	5.24
5	gamma-Actin	*Mus musculus*	CAA31455	80	13	43	41335	5.56	40000	5.03
6	Keratin 1 Hypothetical protein P0004D12.20 (or P0004D12.28)	*Homo sapiens* *Oryza sativa* (japonica cultivar-group)	AAG41947 NP_914826 (or BAB92676)	82 46	15 –	32 8	66198 28328	8.16 8.75	26000	4.78
18	Keratin 10 Type I keratin S8	*Homo sapiens* *Oncorhynchus mykiss*	AAH34697 CAC45059	79 ns	14	26	59020	5.09	29000	4.38
20	Keratin 10; cytokeratin 10	*Homo sapiens*	NP_000412	79	17	25	59020	5.09	29000	4.76
Transport										
1	Serotransferrin		Q92079	211	29	50	69523	6.12	57000	6.15
2	Serotransferrin		Q92079	203	23	39	69523	6.12	57000	6.28
7	Ribose transport ATP-binding protein RbsA	*Vibrio fischeri* ES114	YP_204828	94	18	42	55554	5.20	28000	6.15
19	Serotransferrin		Q92079	115	–	19	69523	6.12	29000	4.54
Egg-specific										
4	Vitellogenin A	*Melanogrammus aeglefinus*	AAK15158	56	–	13	183758	9.08	46000	6.49
8	Vitellogenin B	*Melanogrammus aeglefinus*	AAK15157	103	–	10	179983	9.11	29000	6.63
Other										
24	Unnamed protein product	*Tetraodon nigroviridis*	CAG08839	80	16	44	57068	7.67	53000	7.26

ns, not significant.

Table 3. List of peptides of un-identified proteins from cod oocytes (Figure 16). Amino acid sequences were analysed by chemical associated fragmentation (CAF) method following by MALDI–TOF/TOF MS/MS analysis. (Rungruangsak-Torrissen, unpublished data, with amino acid sequences provided by H. K. Garberg)

Spot number	Protein spot detected		CAF fragment (m/z)	Amino acid sequence identification
	Mass (Da)	pI		
9	24000	8.04	1222.6	NI/LEDI/LI/LAEK
			1569.8	I/LAANI/LDI/LTEGNFR
			1643.8	FI/LGQEI/LAFANI/LDK
			1841.0	I/LQAI/LPVAV(226)AGI/LATVR
10	24000	8.47	1222.6	NI/LEDI/LI/LAEK
			1569.7	I/LAANI/LDI/LTEGNFR
			1643.8	FI/LGQEI/LAFANI/LDK
			1841.0	I/LQAI/LPVAV(226)AGI/LATVR
11	17000	7.74	910.5	FI/LVI/LI/LK
			2269.1	I/LDRI/LI/L(198.5)ANI/LPYQH..??
			2638.3	E/Q(170)AI/LHA(184)HGI/LQEVFI/LDANTI/LK
			2824.4	I/LWGI/LAI/LHA(184)HGI/LQEVYI/LDAN?
13	11000	6.59	944.5	F/M_{OX}F/M_{OX}VI/LI/LK
			1550.8	DNI/LEQNWI/LNVK
			1720.9	(170)DNI/LEQNWI/LNVK
			2285.1	I/LADI/LDI/LDI/LYPENDNFI/LVK
			2545.3	SDW(170)SVYAASHGI/LHEVY(262)R
14	11000	7.16	1550.7	DNI/LEQNWI/LNVK
			1720.8	DNI/LEQNWI/LNVK
			2307.0	ANI/LDI/LDI/LY(226)NDNFI/LVK
			2545.0	SDW(170)SVYAASHGI/LHEVY(262)R
15	11000	7.78	910.5	FI/LVI/LI/LK
			944.5	F/M_{OX}F/M_{OX}VI/LI/LK
			1550.8	DNI/LEQNWI/LNVK
			2269.2	I/LRI/LI/L(198)ADI/LPYQH(213)VK
16	12000	8.25	910.5	FI/LVI/LI/LK
			2269.2	I/LDRI/LI/LPTANI/LPYQH..??
			2638.4	E(171)AI/LHA(184)HGI/LQEVFI/LDANTI/LK
			2824.5	I/LW(170)AI/LHA(184)HGI/LQEVYI/LDAN??K
21	17000	6.59	1209.6	VFQI/LQ(212)GK
			2389.2	I/LWHN/I/LI/LDVI/LEGNEEFI/L.??
			2479.3	VAFI/LI/LAQN/DSGI/LVEVEEWI/LVGK
22	17000	7.16		Un-identified sequences
23	72000	6.75		Un-identified sequences
25	14000	7.61	910.5	FI/LVI/LI/LK
			2263.2	I/LDRI/LI/L(198)ANI/LPYQH…??

The sign / indicates un-differentiable amino acids.
The signs .. and ? indicate unknown numbers of amino acids.
The number in parenthesis represents mass of two unknown amino acids.
ox, Oxidized amino acid.

Table 4. List of proteins from cod oocytes predicted from the amino acid sequences of the peptides of un-identified proteins shown in Table 3. The proteins were searched for short and nearly exact matches using NCBI BLAST. (Rungruangsak-Torrissen, unpublished data)

Spot number	Protein identification	Species homology	Accession number	Number of amino acids	Score	Identities (%)	Positives (%)	Gaps (%)
9 and 10	Hypothetical protein APE2178	*Aeropyrum pernix* K1	NP_148440	289	80	41	46	39
	229aa Long hypothetical protein	*Sulfolobus tokodaii* str. 7	BAB67080	229	78	49	54	18
	Hypothetical protein UM02833.1	*Ustilago maydis* 521	XP_758980	336	76	61	76	4
	Phosphoenolpyruvate-dependent sugar phosphotransferase system EIID, probable fructose specific	*Lactobacillus johnsonii* NCC 533	NP_964593	277	75	68	87	0
11	Vitellogenin B	*Melanogrammus aeglefinus*	AAK15157	1643	111	54	58	38
	Vitellogenin precursor	*Liza aurata*	AAN05023	137	89	51	53	35
13	Vitellogenin A	*Melanogrammus aeglefinus*	AAK15158	1665	170	41	49	48
	Vitellogenin	*Rivulus marmoratus*	AAQ16635	1711	103	39	50	41
14	Vitellogenin A	*Melanogrammus aeglefinus*	AAK15158	1665	149	48	51	45
15	Vitellogenin A	*Melanogrammus aeglefinus*	AAK15158	1665	121	39	42	56
	Vitellogenin	*Verasper moseri*	BAD93695	1628	102	37	40	56
16	Vitellogenin B	*Melanogrammus aeglefinus*	AAK15157	1643	139	58	60	36
	Vitellogenin precursor	*Liza aurata*	AAN05023	137	99	53	53	45
21	Conserved hypothetical protein	*Bacillus thuringiensis* serovar konkukain str. 97-27	AAT59873	206	77	72	72	22
	Trypsin precursor	*Sus scrofa*	P00761	231	73	70	76	23
	Trypsinogen C	*Homo sapiens*	AAC80208	247	67	64	76	23
	Trypsinogen 10	*Mus musculus*	AAB69058	246	67	64	76	23
	Try12	*Macaca mulatta*	AAW69365	247	67	64	76	23
25	Phospholipase D / Transphosphatidylase	*Psychrobacter cryohalolentis* K5	ZP_00653309	479	71	45	57	37

These results indicate an importance of trypsin as the key protease in protein digestion process, not only for food utilization and growth but probably also for health and oocyte development. Although cathepsins have been implicated in the yolk protein processing during oocyte maturation [65–67], trypsin may also involve in the process.

Trypsin-Like Specific Activity and Free Amino Acids

The study of trypsin-like specific activity in oocytes in relation to oocyte development has been preliminary investigated in Atlantic cod, *G. morhua* (Rungruangsak-Torrissen, unpublished data), and the works have been performed later in different fish species such as Nile tilapia [19], Northeast Arctic cod [20], Atlantic salmon [40], and Atlantic mackerel [41]. Variations in oocyte trypsin-like specific activity could affect the levels of essential free amino acids (EAA) and the ratio of essential to non-essential free amino acids (EAA/NEAA ratio) in the oocytes, and this influenced the levels of protein synthesis (RNA concentration) and turnover (RNA/Protein ratio) in the oocytes [41]. Artificially fed Atlantic mackerel, with significantly higher oocyte trypsin-like specific activity, showed significantly higher levels in these free amino acid values but with significantly lower levels in protein synthesis and turnover in the oocytes, compared to the naturally fed mackerel (Table 5).

At the same time, the levels of protein were lower with higher protein turnover rate in the white muscle of artificially fed mackerel (Table 5), suggesting a higher mobilization of white muscle protein to the oocytes of these fish, compared to the naturally fed mackerel. The concentrations of most free amino acids (FAA) in the white muscle and oocytes were higher in the artificially fed mackerel (Table 5). Moreover, some FAA were only observed in the artificially fed mackerel, especially free hydroxyproline, which were not detected in either white muscle or oocytes of the naturally fed mackerel (Table 5). Hydroxyproline is a product from the hydrolysis of collagen, a connective tissue which has a directive role in development and remodeling of tissues [68].

The level of free hydroxyproline in the white muscle has been observed to associate with fish growth [10], and related with trypsin specific activity and the activity ratio of trypsin to chymotrypsin (T/C ratio) in the pyloric caeca, as well as with specific growth rate of Atlantic salmon [36] as shown in Table 6. These results suggest that fish with different feedings have differences in development and quality of the gametes [40, 41]. Further studies should be performed to observe whether the differences could have any effects on hatching success of the offspring.

Trypsin-Like Specific Activity, T/C Ratio, and Protein Turnover Rate

Variations in trypsin-like specific activity and protein turnover rate in the oocytes could indicate variations in rate and quality of oocyte development [20, 40, 41]. During maturing process, protein synthesis (RNA concentration) and turnover (RNA/protein ratio) were higher in the oocytes than in the white muscle [20, 41, 42], as shown in Table 5, and decreases in oocyte trypsin-like specific activity were observed [20]. Oocyte trypsin-like specific activity was related positively with oocyte protein turnover rate, and negatively with oocyte protein level (Figure 17).

Table 5. Concentrations of free amino acids (FAA) and nitrogen-containing compounds (nmol g^{-1}), and capacity for protein synthesis in the white muscle and oocytes, as well as oocyte trypsin-like specific activity (µmol *p*-nitroaniline h^{-1} mg protein^{-1}), from maturing Atlantic mackerel without and with artificial feeding. Significant differences are indicated by bold values ($P \leq 0.05$). (From Rungruangsak-Torrissen and Fosseidengen [41], with permission from John Wiley and Sons, Inc.)

Parameters (*n* = 4–7)	White muscle			Oocytes		
	Without	With	*P*	Without	With	*P*
Essential FAA (EAA)						
Histidine	9330 ± 942	11787 ± 2362	ns	537 ± 27	1504 ± 180	**< 0.004**
Isoleucine	121 ± 5	163 ± 15	**< 0.03**	571 ± 122	2378 ± 676	< 0.082
Leucine	176 ± 32	184 ± 45	ns	99 ± 33	183 ± 13	**< 0.02**
Lysine	133 ± 23	270 ± 76	ns	111 ± 16	84 ± 18	ns
Methionine	120 ± 6	187 ± 19	**< 0.01**	324 ± 53	1576 ± 419	< 0.056
Phenylalanine	1376 ± 192	1643 ± 375	ns	1145 ± 133	4023 ± 563	**< 0.005**
Threonine	167 ± 63	478 ± 49	**< 0.001**	767 ± 91	1555 ± 491	ns
Valine	249 ± 8	284 ± 35	ns	810 ± 154	2790 ± 701	< 0.069
Non-essential FAA						
(NEAA)	2121 ± 104	1686 ± 201	< 0.097	2842 ± 521	5724 ± 172	ns
Alanine	2982 ± 125	2793 ± 452	ns	1638 ± 140	2484 ± 290	< 0.067
β-Alanine + Sarcosine	nd	205 ± 146		nd	nd	
γ-Aminobutyric acid	223 ± 126	4330 ± 642	**< 0.0001**	nd	244 ± 138	
Anserine	106 ± 35	281 ± 51	**< 0.02**	1029 ± 294	3326 ± 435	**< 0.006**
Arginine	nd	130 ± 100		3865 ± 453	1584 ± 450	**< 0.01**
Asparagine	nd	5 ± 3		479 ± 72	1009 ± 281	ns
Aspartic acid	nd	nd		nd	nd	
Carnosine	nd	nd		nd	862 ± 565	
Citrulline	79 ± 60	1859 ± 576	**< 0.02**	908 ± 133	1160 ± 93	ns
Creatinine	99 ± 36	594 ± 189	**< 0.04**	2015 ± 594	852 ± 271	< 0.07
Cystathione	7 ± 2	9 ± 1	ns	24 ± 4	16 ± 3	ns
Cysteine	nd	522 ± 246		443 ± 226	161 ± 30	ns
Cystine	769 ± 91	1030 ± 103	< 0.083	1795 ± 342	2533 ± 474	ns
Glutamic acid	4 ± 2	28 ± 7	ns	78 ± 19	253 ± 73	ns
Glutamine	1273 ± 92	856 ± 130	**< 0.03**	3179 ± 897	2046 ± 423	ns
Glycine	nd	nd		62 ± 13	312 ± 118	< 0.091
Hydroxy-lysine	nd	205 ± 55		nd	24 ± 15	
Hydroxy-proline	nd	nd		nd	39 ± 25	
1-Methyl-histidine	29 ± 14	nd		251 ± 26	167 ± 39	**< 0.04**
3-Methyl-histidine	146 ± 45	303 ± 39	**< 0.02**	1018 ± 158	3644 ± 912	< 0.064
Ornithine	37 ± 16	76 ± 37	ns	3239 ± 1910	1992 ± 480	ns
Phosphoethanolamine	nd	nd		nd	nd	
Phospho-serine	253 ± 72	1212 ± 289	**< 0.02**	959 ± 117	1866 ± 423	ns
Proline	235 ± 55	220 ± 40	ns	1350 ± 324	4171 ± 1349	ns
Serine	3326 ± 306	1750 ± 211	**< 0.0002**	11846 ± 659	17280 ± 820	**< 0.002**
Taurine	102 ± 5	108 ± 12	ns	370 ± 157	1113 ± 298	ns
Tyrosine						
Total FAA (µmol g^{-1})	23.71 ± 1.31	34.81 ± 11.21	ns	42.73 ± 0.48	69.86 ± 9.06	**= 0.05**
EAA (µmol g^{-1})	11.68 ± 2.05	14.78 ± 5.10	ns	4.36 ± 0.29	14.09 ± 2.91	**< 0.04**
NEAA (µmol g^{-1})	12.04 ± 0.76	20.03 ± 6.30	ns	38.37 ± 0.25	55.77 ± 6.21	ns
EAA/NEAA ratio	1.02 ± 0.26	0.71 ± 0.12	ns	0.11 ± 0.01	0.24 ± 0.03	**< 0.02**
RNA (µg g^{-1})	2044 ± 43	1876 ± 71	ns	8309 ± 570	5355 ± 404	**< 0.0001**
Protein (mg g^{-1})	187.8 ± 24.1	99.3 ± 12.8	**< 0.0001**	167.2 ± 13.3	157.5 ± 8.0	ns
RNA/Protein ratio (µg mg^{-1})	11.46 ± 1.56	20.87 ± 2.96	**< 0.0001**	50.64 ± 5.34	34.49 ± 3.02	**< 0.0001**
Trypsin-like specific activity	–	–		6.33 ± 1.59	15.38 ± 2.48	**< 0.0001**

Tryptophan was not reliably detected by the method. nd, not detected. ns, not significant.

Table 6. Correlation coefficient (*r*) between different parameters studied in Atlantic salmon cultured under different light regimes. The values with significant correlation are written in big bold numbers ($P < 0.05$). (From Sunde et al. [36], with permission from Springer Corp.)

Parameters ($n = 78$)	SGR	T	C	T/C	Plasma (P)			White muscle (M)					
					EAA	E/N	TFAA	EAA	E/N	TFAA	Hyp	RNA	P
Specific growth rate (SGR)	1												
Trypsin (T)	**0.34**	1											
Chymotrypsin (C)	0.05	**0.76**	1										
T/C ratio	**0.39**	**0.25**	**–0.38**	1									
P-Essential FAA (EAA)	**0.39**	**0.24**	–0.04	**0.43**	1								
P-EAA/Non-EAA (E/N)	0.17	–0.01	–0.19	**0.25**	**0.65**	1							
P-Total FAA (TFAA)	**0.37**	**0.40**	0.13	**0.37**	**0.82**	0.12	1						
M-Essential FAA (EAA)	–0.09	–0.08	–0.14	0.05	0.13	**0.29**	–0.04	1					
M-EAA/Non-EAA (E/N)	**–0.45**	**–0.27**	–0.10	**–0.26**	–0.07	**0.27**	**–0.28**	**0.74**	1				
M-Total FAA (TFAA)	0.06	–0.01	–0.13	0.15	0.19	**0.27**	0.05	**0.97**	**0.55**	1			
M-Free Hydroxyproline (Hyp)	**0.74**	**0.31**	0.05	**0.35**	**0.24**	–0.03	**0.32**	0.11	**–0.44**	**0.30**	1		
M-RNA (R)	**–0.46**	**–0.25**	0.03	**–0.37**	–0.21	0.02	**–0.25**	0.02	**0.41**	–0.13	**–0.55**	1	
M-Protein (P)	0.23	0.18	0.04	0.16	0.15	0.01	0.18	–0.22	**–0.36**	–0.13	0.17	–0.16	1
M-RNA/Protein (R/P)	**–0.41**	**–0.30**	–0.01	**–0.37**	**–0.28**	–0.07	**–0.31**	0.13	**0.39**	0.02	**–0.36**	**0.63**	**–0.77**

Variations in protein synthesis and turnover as well as the levels of trypsin-like specific activity at different stages during egg development are shown in Figure 18, indicating higher levels of these parameters in the oocytes than in mature eggs. After fertilization, protein turnover rate increased significantly in the fertilized eggs (Figure 18).

Increased trypsin-like specific activity in the oocytes might indicate an abnormal development, as detected in ovarian cancer [69] and in oocytes from fish fed on diet containing too high replacement of fish meal with krill meal as an alternative protein source [40]. Under normal condition, oocytes showed higher trypsin-like specific activity than mature eggs (Figure 18). Thus, an observed higher oocyte trypsin-like specific activity also indicated less development of the oocytes.

In addition, it has been observed that maturing Northeast Arctic cod having higher maturation rate with lower oocyte trypsin-like specific activity as well as oocyte chymotrypsin-like specific activity showed a higher level of the activity ratio of trypsin-like to chymotrypsin-like (T/C ratio) in the oocytes [20].

It is interesting to note that the T/C ratio is very important studied factor, as higher levels of the T/C ratio in the pyloric caeca [20, 24, 35, 37, 40] and in the oocytes [20] indicate higher development in somatic growth and in oocyte maturation rate, respectively, independent of the specific activity levels of the two proteases.

The implementation of using trypsin-like specific activity and the T/C ratio level in the oocytes to indicate oocyte maturation rate is unique and challenged. The parameters have been recently developed by Rungruangsak-Torrissen's research team, and are useful for studying maturation rate of females both in aquaculture and natural ecosystem.

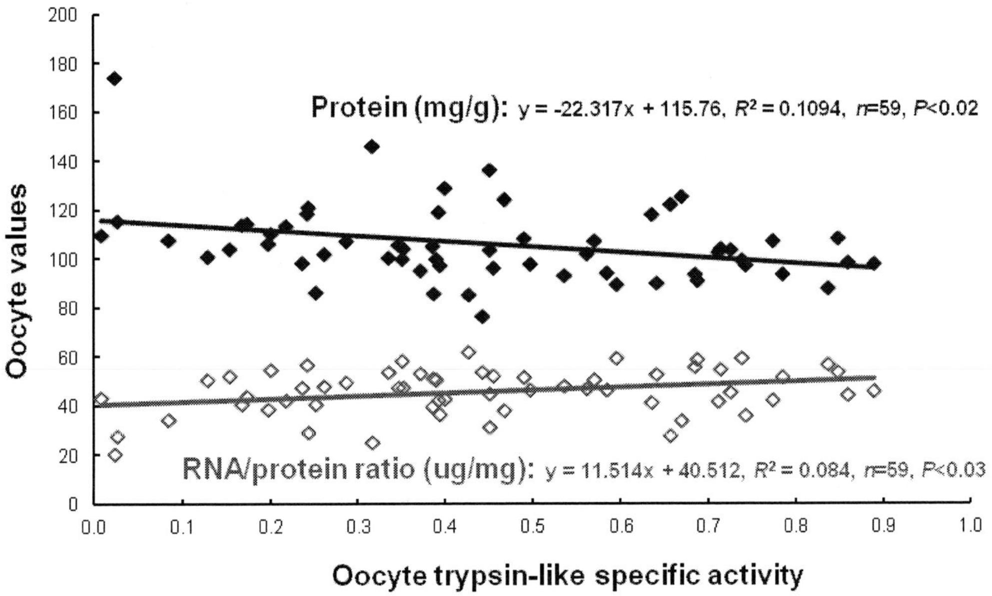

Figure 17. Relationships between trypsin-like specific activity with protein concentration and with protein turnover rate (RNA/protein ratio) in the oocytes from Atlantic salmon. The trypsin-like specific activity was expressed as μmol p-nitroaniline produced h^{-1} mg $protein^{-1}$. ◆—◆ indicates protein concentration, and ◇—◇ indicates RNA/protein ratio in the oocytes. (From Rungruangsak-Torrissen [40], with permission from John Wiley and Sons, Inc.).

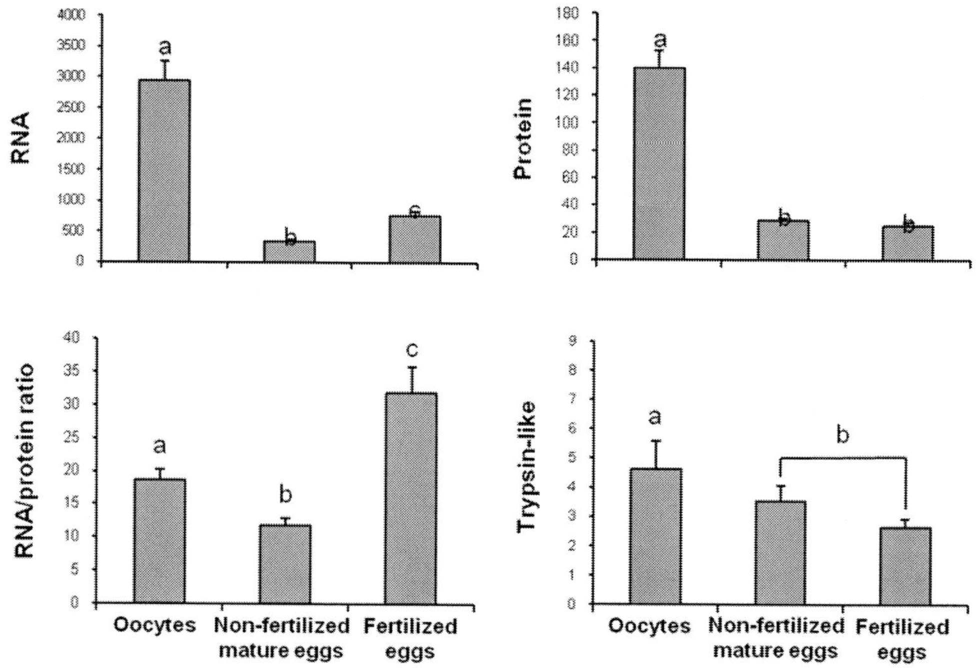

Figure 18. Concentrations of RNA (μg g^{-1}), protein (mg g^{-1}), RNA/protein ratio (μg mg^{-1}), and trypsin-like specific activity (μmol *p*-nitroaniline h^{-1} mg $protein^{-1}$), of oocytes, non-fertilized mature eggs, and fertilized eggs with more than 8 cells, from Northeast Arctic cod. The bars with different superscripts are significantly different ($P < 0.05$). (From Rungruangsak-Torrissen et al. [20]).

Dietary Quality Assessment

In Vitro Digestibility of Dietary Protein

In vitro digestion method has been used to predict the quality of experimental feeds, and the most efficient and practical technique is to use intestinal fluid or caecal enzymes for *in vitro* digestibility study of dietary proteins [11, 70–72]. The technique has also been used for investigation in invertebrates [25, 73, 74]. Among *in vitro* digestibility studies of different main nutrients (protein, carbohydrate, lipid), protein digestibility is apparently the key factor determining food quality followed by carbohydrate digestibility as the second factor [73, 74] while lipid digestibility has never been found to associate with feed efficiency and the quality of the lipid itself [73]. The *in vitro* protein digestibility technique is very sensitive and could differentiate between animals with genetic differences in growth capacity [42] and protein digestion (different trypsin phenotypes) [11, 25]. In rainbow trout, the enzyme extracts from families with high growth capacity have resulted in higher *in vitro* protein digestibility values than the extracts from low and medium growth capacity families [42]. In Atlantic salmon [11] and in spiny lobster [25], the phenotypes possessing more trypsin isozymes are less sensitive to changes in dietary protein quality, while the phenotypes lacking a trypsin isozyme are more sensitive to changes in protein quality and could discriminate between different fish meals. An example is illustrated in Figure 8. By standardizing the crude enzyme extracts with regard to trypsin activity, the *in vitro* protein digestibility values could be comparable among different samples within the same species [25, 40, 42, 55] and also between different species [55]. More informations are described in later section.

In Vitro Protein Digestibility and Protein Quality

The level of *in vitro* protein digestibility is directly dependent on the biochemical structure of dietary protein such as the contents of reactive sulphydryl (SH) group and disulphide (S–S) bond [55] and the concentration of *D*-aspartic acid [75, 76]. The method, for the determinations of SH group and S–S bond of complex proteins such as fish feeds, was first developed [55].

Variations in food processing conditions (temperature, pH, oxygen pressure, moisture) could affect the quality of dietary protein by changing the nature of protein structure and resulting in changing the *in vitro* digestibility of the dietary protein (Figure 19). In addition, aspartic acid racemization from *L*-Asp to *D*-Asp has been observed under different processing conditions [75, 76]. Therefore, the *in vitro* protein digestibility values of food materials were related positively to the reactive SH group content (Figure 19) and the content ratio of SH/S–S (Figure 20A), and negatively to the content of *D*-Asp (Figure 20B). Moreover, the *in vitro* protein digestibility technique has been applied to study the quality of Atlantic salmon filet under different treatments with a non-toxic substance (with anti-oxidant property) to prevent autolysis (Rungruangsak-Torrissen, unpublished data).

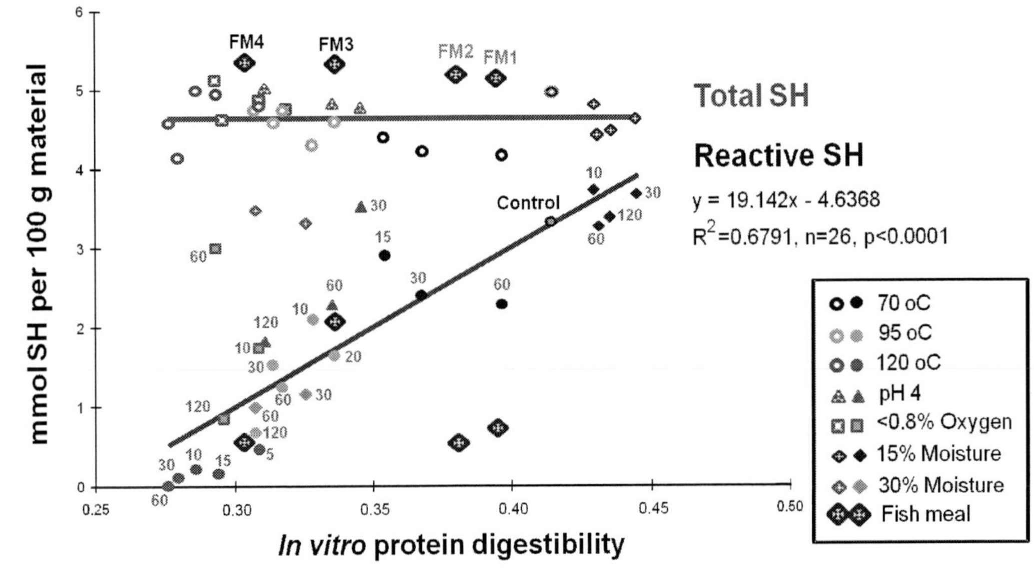

Figure 19. Effect of reactive SH content in 27 fish materials produced under different processing conditions on in vitro protein digestibility (μmol DL-alanine equivalent liberated reactive amino group of peptides produced per 100 μg fish material) by Atlantic salmon pyloric caecal crude enzyme extract. The values of different fish meals (FM1–FM4) are also illustrated, but not included in the regressions. The numbers indicate time of treatment in min. (From Rungruangsak-Torrissen et al. [55], with permission from John Wiley and Sons, Inc.).

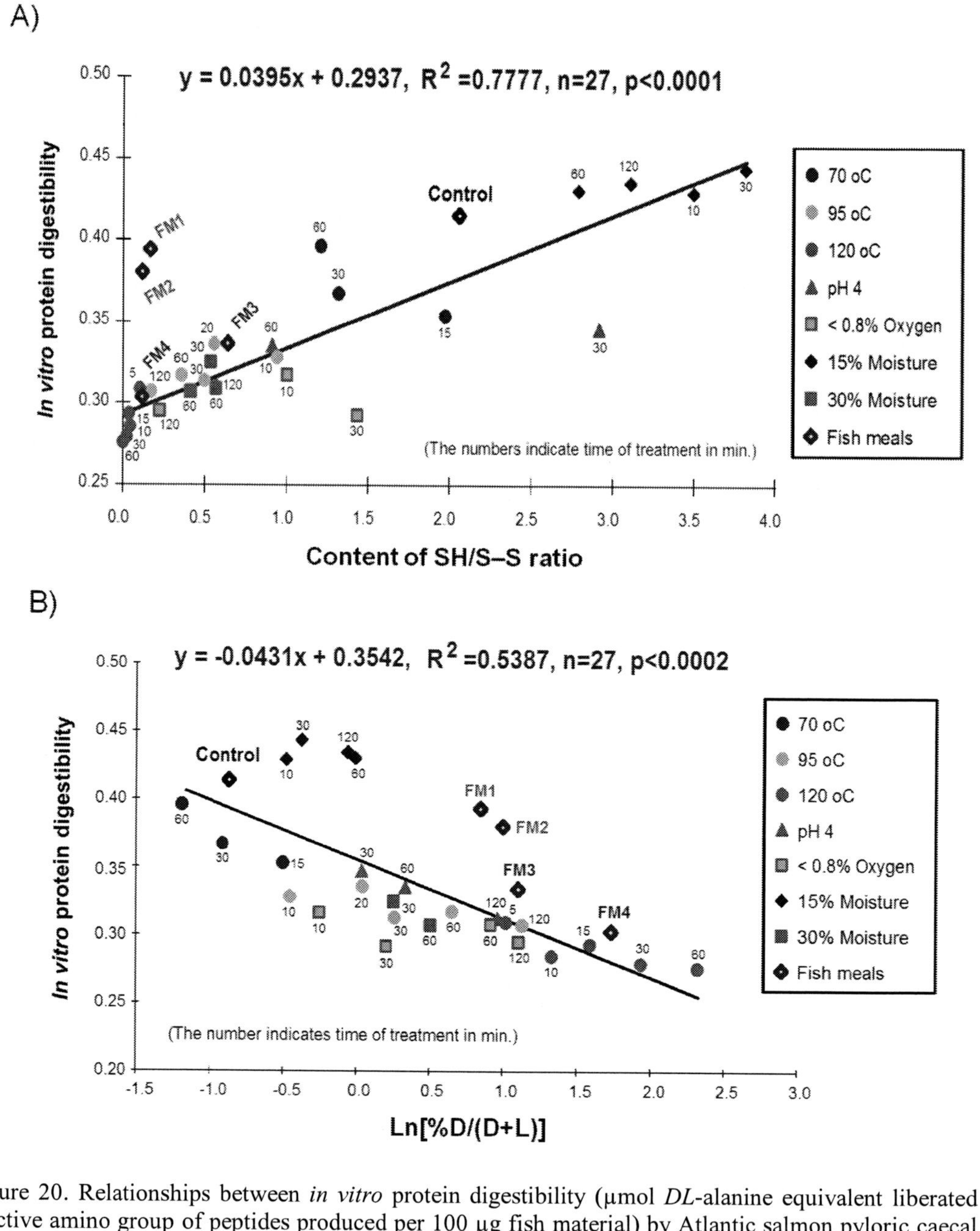

Figure 20. Relationships between *in vitro* protein digestibility (μmol *DL*-alanine equivalent liberated reactive amino group of peptides produced per 100 μg fish material) by Atlantic salmon pyloric caecal crude enzyme extract (A) with SH/S–S content ratio and (B) with *D*-Aspartic acid content, of 27 different fish materials produced under different processing conditions. The values of different fish meals (FM1–FM4) are also illustrated, but not included in the regressions. (From Rungruangsak-Torrissen et al. [55], with permission from John Wiley and Sons, Inc.).

The technique could differentiate the qualities of salmon filets showing a better protein digestibility with a better preserved protein structure (shown by 2D-electrophoresis) in the presence of the substance after heated for 45 min at 95 °C, dried overnight at 60 °C, and kept in the refrigerator for a week (Figure 21A). It has also been shown that the substance also showed a property of anti-protease activities even on ice at around zero °C (Figures 21B and

21C), and it could preserve protein by preventing autolysis of krill for months in the refrigerator (Figure 21D).

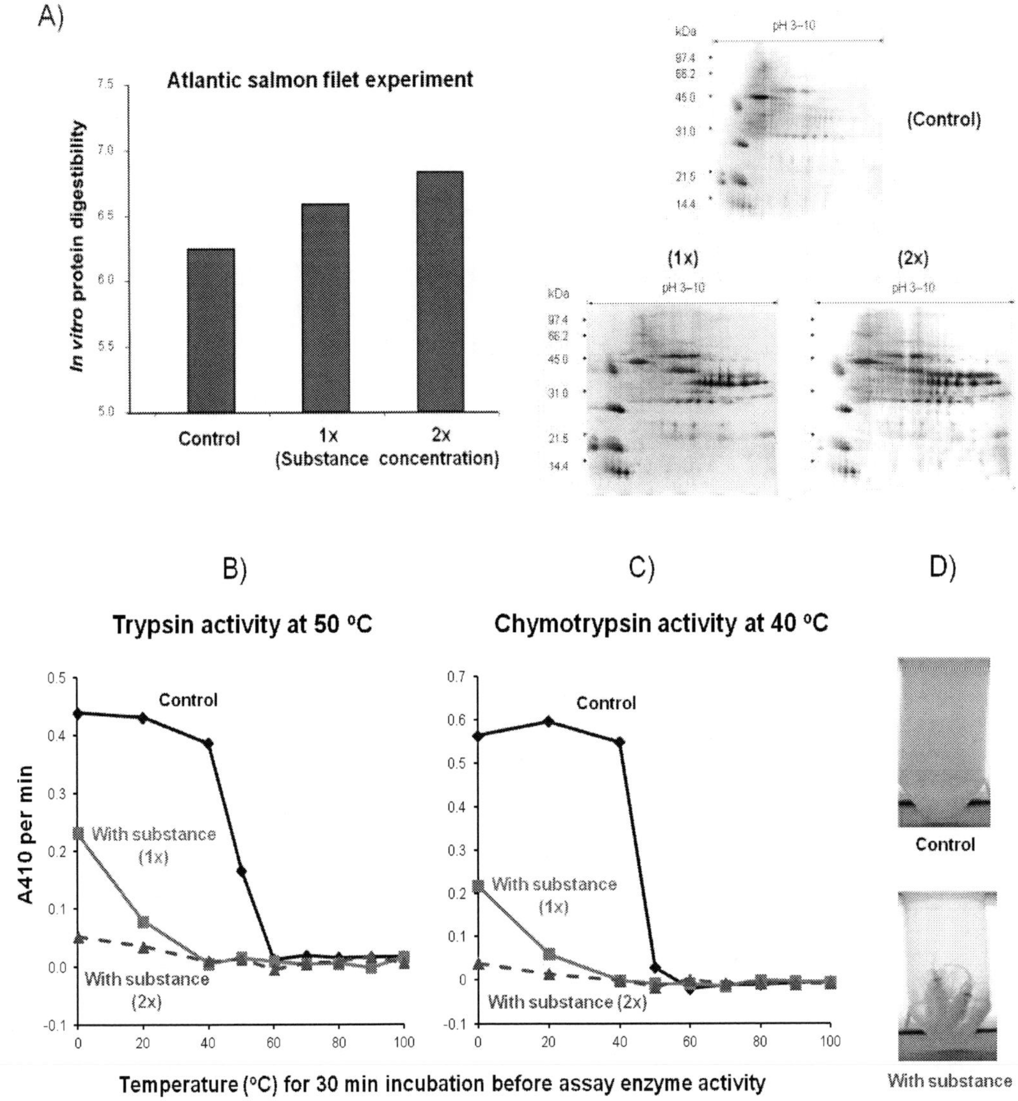

Figure 21. (A) An *in vitro* protein digestibility test of Atlantic salmon filet mixed with a non-toxic substance with anti-oxidant property at two different concentrations (1X and 2X) with 2D-electrophoresis showing an anti-autolysis of protein structure of the filets in the presence of the substance, and the effects of the substance on the activities of (B) trypsin and (C) chymotrypsin after 30 min incubation at different temperatures, and (D) preservation of krill showing an anti-autolysis of krill in the presence of the substance. The *in vitro* protein digestibility was expressed as μmol *DL*-alanine equivalent g filet^{-1}. The molecular weights (kDa) of the separated proteins are shown on the side of the gel pictures. The activities of trypsin and chymotrypsin were determined at 50 °C and 40 °C, using initial reaction rate with benzoyl-*L*-arginine-*p*-nitroanilide (BAPNA) and *N*-succinyl-Ala-Ala-Pro-Phe-*p*-nitroanilide (SAPNA) as specific substrates, respectively. (Rungruangsak-Torrissen [unpublished data], with the pictures of 2D-electrophoresis provided by M. Ruud and H.B. Jensen).

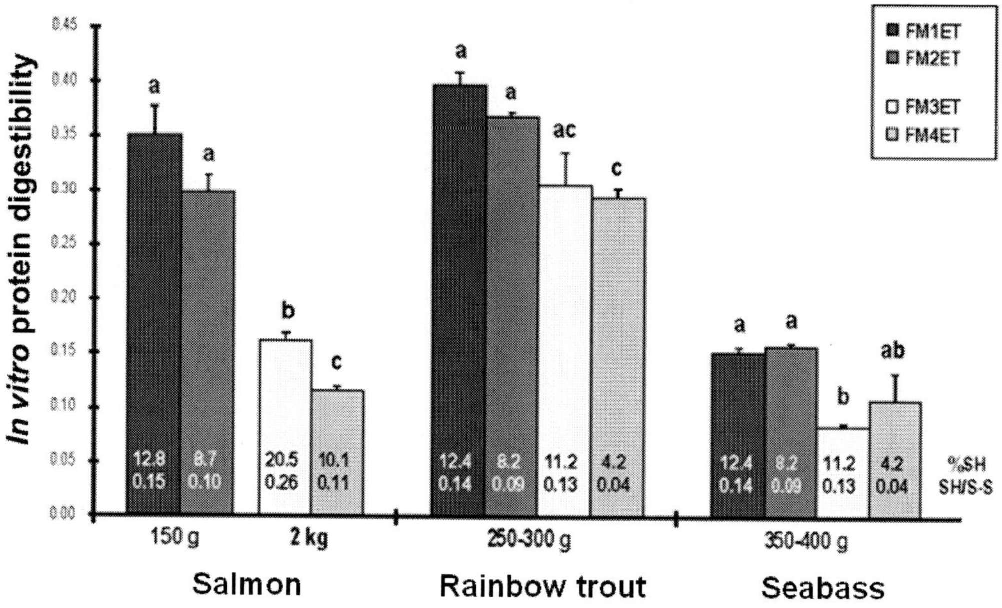

Figure 22. Association of SH content and SH/S–S content ratio of different experimental feeds with in vitro protein digestibility (μmol DL-alanine equivalent liberated reactive amino group of peptides produced per 100 μg fish material) by crude enzyme extracts from different fish species that had never been fed experimental feeds before. The same trypsin activity (454 μmol p-nitroaniline produced h^{-1} ml^{-1}) in the dialyzed crude enzyme extracts was used for all species. The bars with different superscripts are significantly different ($P < 0.05$). (From Rungruangsak-Torrissen et al. [55], with permission from John Wiley and Sons, Inc.).

By utilizing the techniques on *in vitro* protein digestibility and protease activities of trypsin and chymotrypsin, the properties of the substance in stabilizing protein structure and as anti-microbial agent could be indicated (Figure 21). This could be an advantage for food industry. The *in vitro* protein digestibility values are associated with the biochemical structure of the protein (Figures 19 and 20), and could be useful for studying and illustrating the quality of food raw materials.

In Vitro Protein Digestibility and Standardized by Trypsin Activity

In order to compare the *in vitro* protein digestibility values resulted from different crude enzyme extracts, the values have to be standardized by trypsin activity [40, 55]. Different fish species have different digestion ability to the same feed types (Figure 22), and the effective time for feed utilization and growth is dependent on fish sensitivity and the extent of differences in digestibility between the feeds consumed [55], whereas the sensitivity ranking of the enzymes to feed quality under a studied condition has been shown as Atlantic salmon > rainbow trout > European seabass, *Dicentrarchus labrax* L. (Figure 22).

By using crude enzyme extracts before feeding the experimental diets, significant differences in the *in vitro* protein digestibility between the experimental feeds could be observed whereby there would be differences in feed efficiency within 3 months of feeding [40, 55]. Not only feed quality but also fish age could affect the *in vitro* protein digestibility, as less fish meal replacement by krill meal (Figures 23A and 23B) and younger fish (Figure 23A) resulted in higher *in vitro* protein digestibility values. Younger fish also showed less sensitivity to feed quality than older fish (Figure 23A), indicating that younger fish can adapt to new feeds better than the older ones. Moreover, the technique could provide a decision for a maximum inclusion of krill meal at 60% replacement of fish meal for feed formulation (Figures 23A and 23B).

Relationships between the *in vitro* protein digestibilities of different feed qualities with various biochemical parameters in fish growth studies have been reported [40, 55]. The levels of *in vitro* protein digestibility of experimental feeds have been shown to positively correlate with fish weights (Figure 24A), feed conversion efficiency [40, 55], and the activity ratio of trypsin to chymotrypsin (T/C ratio) as shown in Figure 24B. This indicates that it would be practical, quick and reliable to determine the *in vitro* protein digestibility of the experimental diets, by using crude enzyme extract from the species of interest and standardized by trypsin activity, before starting up growth experiments that may not be necessary [40, 55].

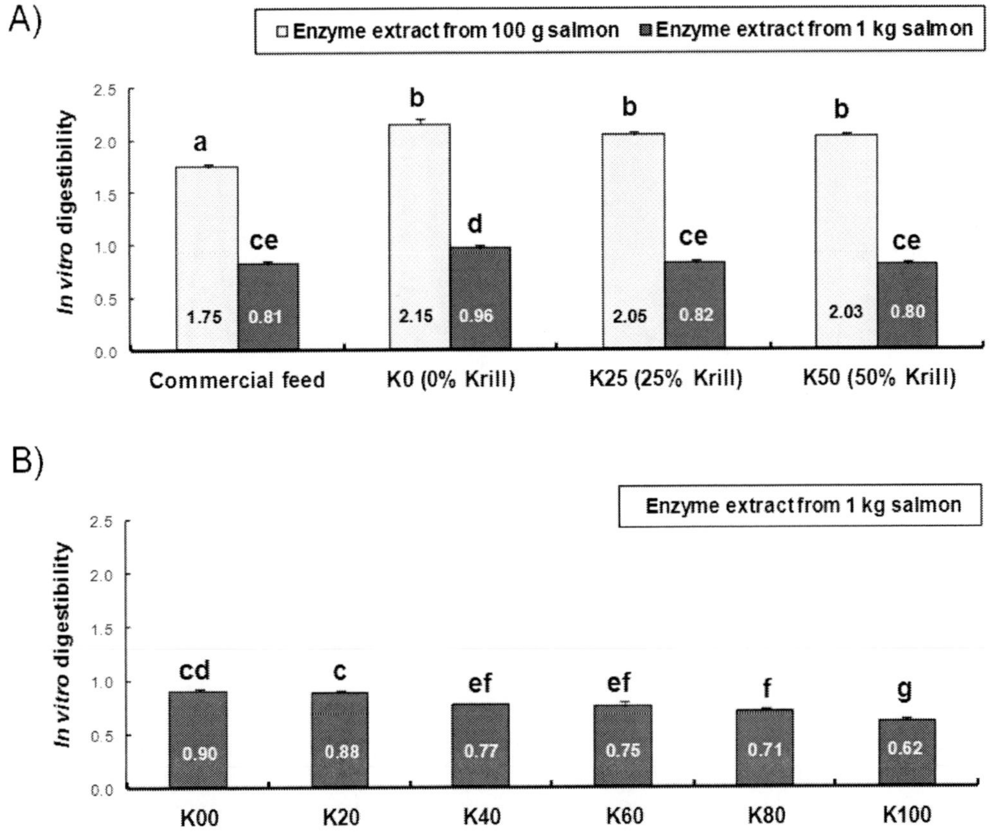

Figure 23. *In vitro* protein digestibility values (μmol *DL*-alanine equivalent mg feed^{-1}) of a commercial feed and of different experimental diets with fish meal replaced by krill meal at different levels (0–100%). The crude enzyme extracts were from 100 g and 1 kg Atlantic salmon, and standardized to trypsin activity level of 500 μmol *p*-nitroaniline produced h^{-1} ml^{-1}. The average *in vitro* protein digestibility value is indicated in each bar. The bars with different superscripts are significantly different ($P < 0.05$). (From Rungruangsak-Torrissen [40], with permission from John Wiley and Sons, Inc.).

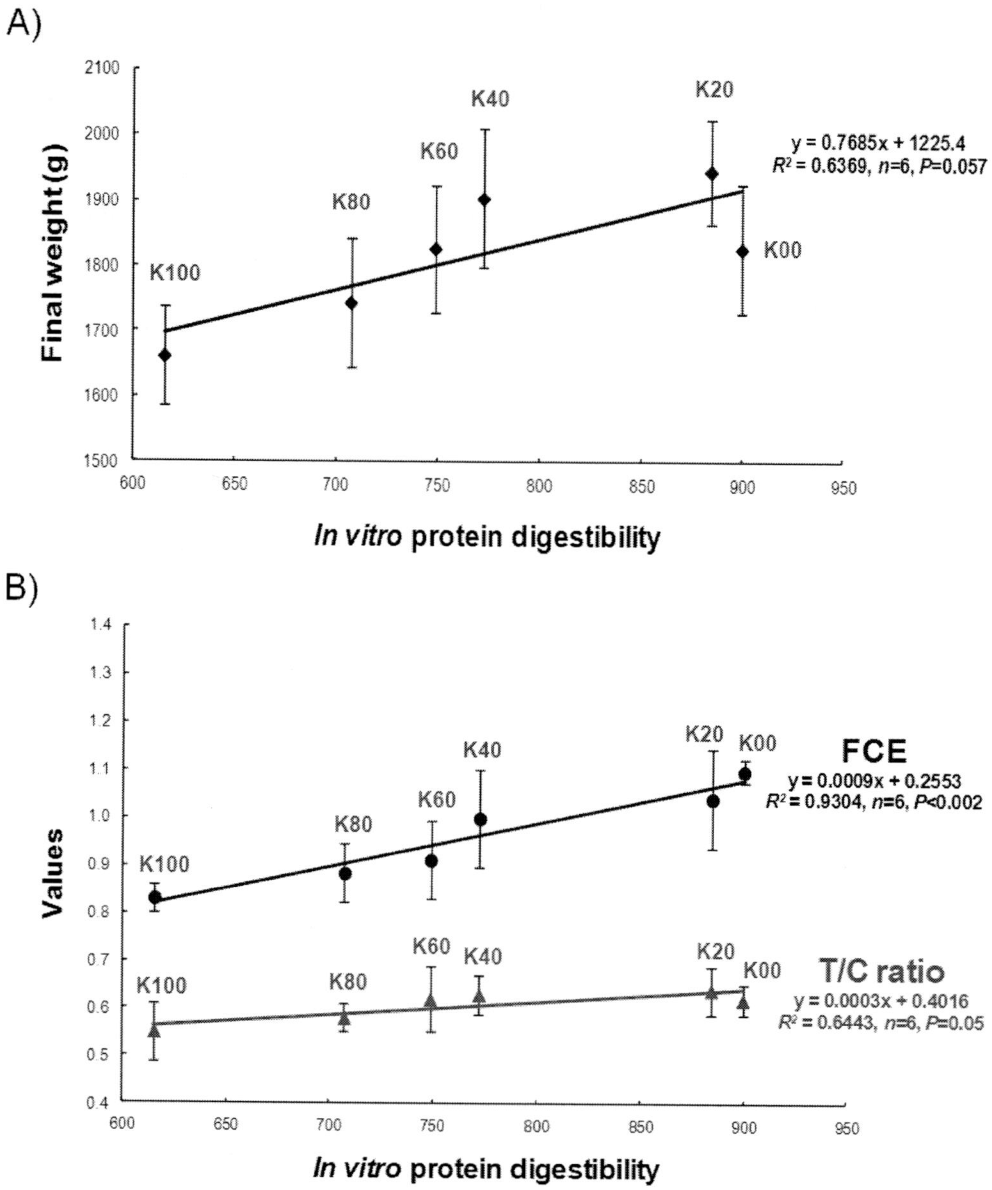

Figure 24. Relationships (A) between *in vitro* protein digestibility value (of formulated feeds with krill meal as a fish meal replacer at different levels of 0–100%) and final fish weight, and (B) between the *in vitro* protein digestibility value with feed conversion efficiency (FCE), and the protease activity ratio of trypsin to chymotrypsin (T/C ratio). The *in vitro* protein digestibility value was expressed as nmol *DL*-alanine equivalent mg feed^{-1}, FCE as kilogram weight gained kilogram dry feed consumed^{-1}, and the T/C ratio with protease specific activities expressed as μmol *p*-nitroaniline produced h^{-1} mg protein^{-1}. (Adapted from Rungruangsak-Torrissen [40], with permission from John Wiley and Sons, Inc.).

Dietary quality assessment by the *in vitro* protein digestibility, using intestinal crude enzyme extract from the species of interest, has been shown to relate with the dietary protein structure of raw materials (Figures 19, 20 and 21A) and correspond with growth studies [40, 55] as shown in Figure 24. Therefore, it is very practical to obtain the first information of diet quality by using this technique and standardized with respect to trypsin activity for a possibility of comparison if the crude enzyme extracts are from different sources.

Moreover, it is interesting to note that carnivorous fish, such as Atlantic salmon, rainbow trout and European seabass, would show higher *in vitro* protein digestibility for animal protein than plant protein. Contrastingly, omnivorous fish such as Nile tilapia would show higher *in vitro* protein digestibility for plant protein than animal protein, but increased animal protein in the diets would still increase fish growth performance quality [19] due to more balance of amino acids in animal protein than plant protein.

Therefore, if the crude enzyme extracts for *in vitro* protein digestibility study are from omnivorous fish (probably also herbivorous fish), the *in vitro* protein digestibility values should be compared among animal proteins or among plant proteins, and not between animal and plant proteins. In addition, *in vitro* digestibility of carbohydrate (the secondary factor after protein) could be necessary for studying the quality of dietary carbohydrate. In that case, the *in vitro* carbohydrate digestibility values should be standardized with respect to amylase activity for a possibility of comparison if the crude enzyme extracts are from different sources [77]. Thongprajukaew [77] has used the technique of standardized *in vitro* carbohydrate digestibility values for studying qualities of feeds with carbohydrate modification. The work of Thongprajukaew et al. on effects of different modified diets on fish growth performance quality quality using standardized *in vitro* digestibility techniques for both protein and carbohydrate has been recently published [78].

In Vitro Digestibility Study for Plankton Quality

The *in vitro* digestibility techniques for both protein and carbohydrate have been applicable for studying plankton quality for food formulation for freshwater pearl mussel, *Hyriopsis* (*Hyriopsis*) *bialatus* [73, 74]. Although carbohydrate digestibility is the secondary factor after protein digestibility, regardless of whether the animals are predominantly herbivorous or carnivorous [73, 74], it is still important especially for herbivorous and omnivorous species.

Different stages of the freshwater pearl mussel have shown variations in the *in vitro* digestibilities for protein and carbohydrate of different phytoplankton species [73, 74] and at different ages of phytoplankton [74], as shown in Figure 25. Juvenile mussels (Figure 25AB, 25DE) are more sensitive to variety and age of phytoplankton than adult mussels (Figure 25C, 25F), as variations in the *in vitro* digestibilities were observed among differences and ages of phytoplankton species. This has made a possibility to formulate suitable combinations of phytoplankton species with highly digestible and utilizable for optimum growth of the mussel, especially at juvenile stage (Figure 26).

Young animals prefer preys with easier utilizable protein, while older animals prefer older preys with higher protein content [74]. Moreover, it has also shown that both protein and carbohydrate qualities (not concentrations) in the phytoplankton are very important, as the digestibility values were not related to their levels in the phytoplankton mixtures [74].

The *in vitro* digestibility technique could be applicable for studying the quality of different plankton species in natural ecosystems, which may vary according to climate changes. By using crude enzyme extracts from different animal species in nature, the preference of plankton species for each predator would be known.

This could be a new approach in plankton research. Moreover, Rungruangsak-Torrissen et al. [20] have reported that phytoplankton that usually bloom during winter may provide energy for maturing females for gamete development. By utilizing the *in vitro* digestibility technique for both protein and carbohydrate, the information of phytoplankton species preference for maturation process in nature would probably be revealed.

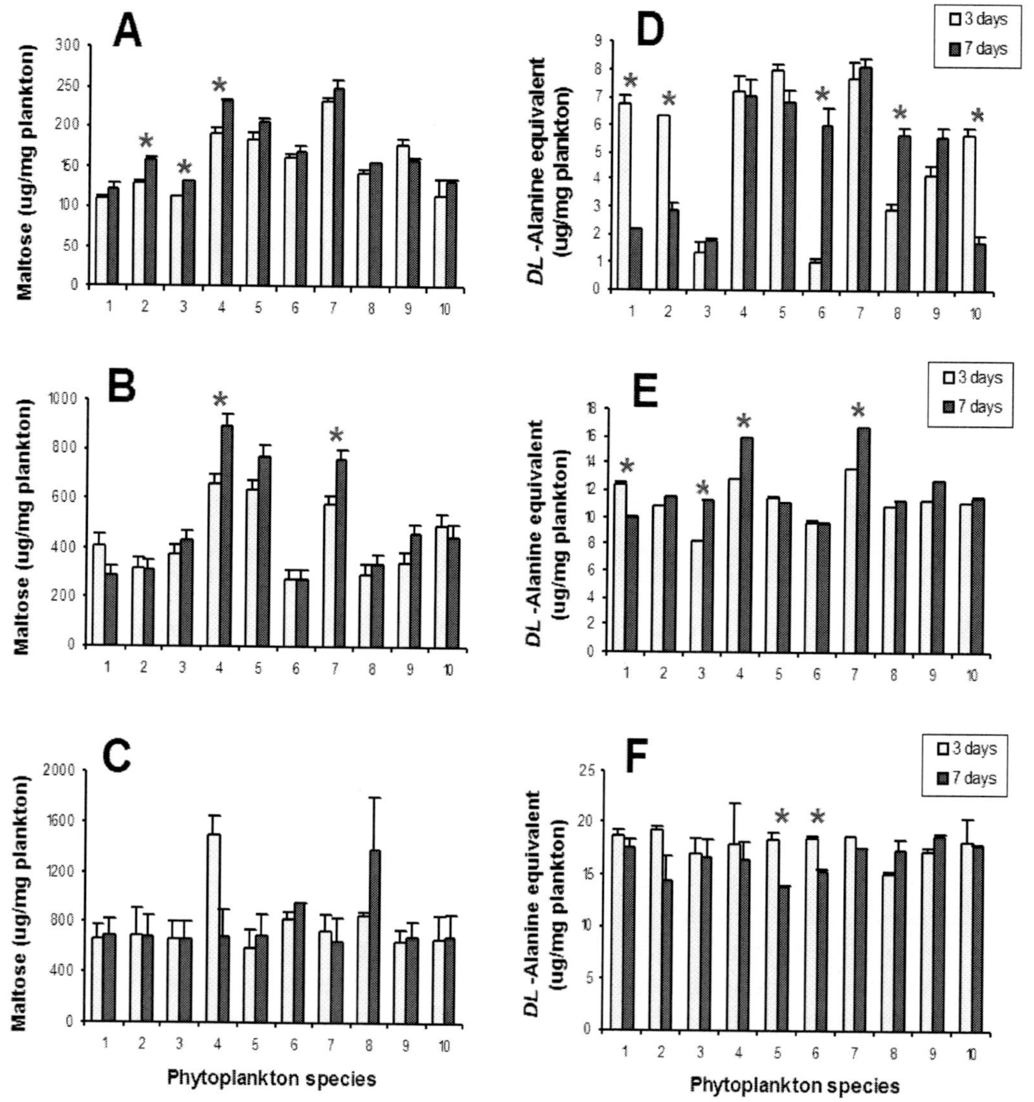

Figure 25. *In vitro* digestibility for carbohydrate (μg maltose mg plankton^{-1}) and protein (μg *DL*-alanine equivalent mg plankton^{-1}) of ten algal species at 3 and 7 day-old, using crude enzyme extracts from: (A and D) 30 day-old juveniles; (B and E) 130 day-old juveniles; (C and F) adult freshwater pearl mussel, *Hyriopsis* (*Hyriopsis*) *bialatus*. Phytoplankton species: (1) *Ankistrodesmus* sp.; (2) *Chlamydomonas* sp.; (3) *Chlorella* sp.1; (4) *Chlorella* sp.2; (5) *Chlorococcum* sp.; (6) *Coccomyxa* sp.; (7) *Kirchneriella incurvata*; (8) *Monoraphidium* sp.; (9) *Scenedesmus* sp.; (10) *Stichococcum* sp., and the bars with asterisk (*) indicate significant differences in the *in vitro* digestibility values between the 3 and 7 day-old phytoplanktons ($P < 0.05$). (From Supannapong et al. [74], with permission from Springer Corp.).

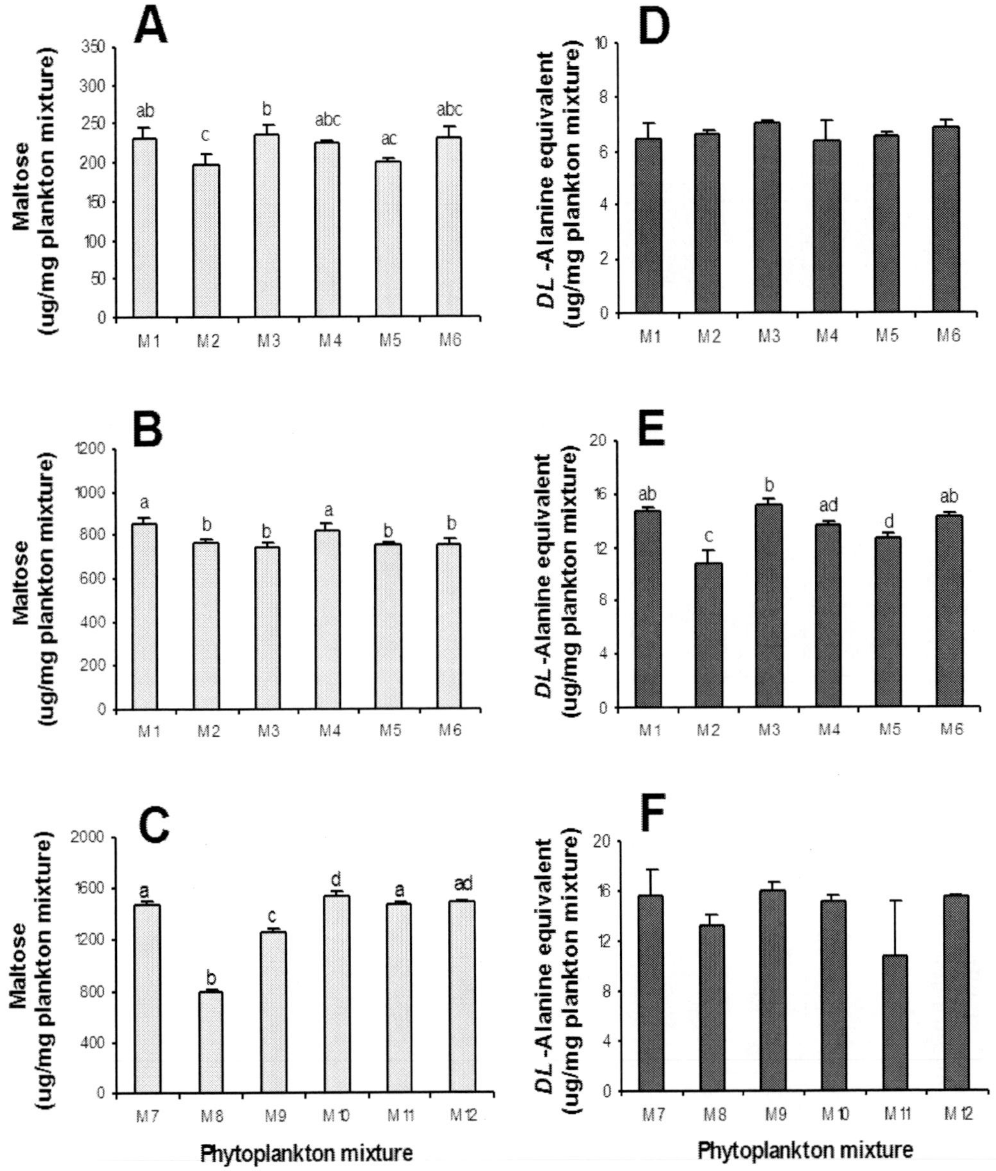

Figure 26. *In vitro* digestibility for carbohydrate (μg maltose mg plankton mixture^{-1}) and protein (μg *DL*-alanine equivalent mg plankton mixture^{-1}) of different phytoplankton mixtures (M1–M12), using crude enzyme extracts from: (A and D) 30 day-old juveniles; (B and E) 130 day-old juveniles; (C and F) adult freshwater pearl mussel, *H.* (*H.*) *bialatus*. The bars with different superscripts are significantly different ($P < 0.05$). (From Supannapong et al. [74], with permission from Springer Corp.).

Table 7. Correlation coefficient (*r*) between different parameters studied in Atlantic salmon with different feedings. The values with significant correlation are written in big bold numbers ($P < 0.05$). (Unpublished data calculated from Rungruangsak-Torrissen [40])

Parameters (n = 108)	W	L	CF	SGR	T	C	T/C	Faeces			White muscle (M)			Oocytes (O) (n = 59)		
								T	C	T/C	RNA	P	R/P	T	RNA	P
Weight (W)	1															
Length (L)	**0.92**	1														
Condition factor (CF)	**0.60**	**0.24**	1													
Specific growth rate (SGR)	**0.78**	**0.70**	**0.54**	1												
Trypsin (T)	**–0.26**	**–0.24**	–0.14	–0.18	1											
Chymotrypsin (C)	–0.13	–0.11	–0.06	–0.09	**0.84**	1										
T/C ratio	0.05	0.00	0.05	0.06	–0.19	**–0.60**	1									
Faecal trypsin (T)	–0.04	–0.00	–0.07	0.04	**0.24**	0.13	0.05	1								
Faecal chymotrypsin (C)	–0.00	0.03	–0.03	0.02	0.17	0.13	–0.02	**0.87**	1							
Faecal T/C ratio	–0.14	–0.12	–0.10	0.02	**0.25**	0.09	0.09	**0.58**	0.16	1						
M-RNA (R)	**–0.27**	**–0.22**	**–0.26**	**–0.35**	0.05	0.03	–0.09	0.03	0.04	–0.03	1					
M-Protein (P)	–0.05	–0.07	0.05	0.08	–0.03	–0.13	0.14	0.02	0.02	0.01	0.12	1				
M- RNA/Protein (R/P)	–0.07	–0.03	–0.15	**–0.20**	0.04	0.13	–0.19	–0.04	–0.03	–0.04	**0.36**	**–0.86**	1			
O-Trypsin-like (T)	**–0.25**	**–0.33**	–0.02	–0.16	–0.03	–0.01	0.01	–0.00	–0.06	0.07	0.08	–0.01	0.05	1		
O-RNA (R)	**–0.54**	**–0.46**	**–0.37**	**–0.29**	**0.39**	0.22	0.08	0.12	–0.10	**0.42**	0.05	0.09	–0.08	0.13	1	
O-Protein (P)	0.12	0.10	0.10	0.09	–0.02	0.00	–0.02	–0.15	0.01	**–0.29**	–0.12	0.00	–0.08	**–0.33**	–0.19	1
O-RNA/Protein (R/P)	**–0.45**	**–0.40**	**–0.29**	–0.18	**0.28**	0.16	0.04	0.18	–0.07	**0.46**	0.07	0.09	–0.06	**0.29**	**0.80**	**–0.71**

Condition factor (CF), calculated as $100xW/L^3$.

Table 8. Correlation coefficient (*r*) between different parameters studied in Atlantic mackerel with different feedings. The values with significant correlation are written in big bold numbers ($P < 0.05$). (Unpublished data calculated from Rungruangsak-Torrissen and Fosseidengen [41])

($n = 30$)	W	T	C	T/C	White muscle (M)							Oocytes (O) ($n = 11$)						
					EAA	NEAA	E/N	TFAA	RNA	P	R/P	T	EAA	NEAA	E/N	TFAA	RNA	P
W	1																	
T	–0.03	1																
C	0.28	**0.73**	1															
T/C ratio	**–0.53**	–0.01	**–0.65**	1														
M-EAA	0.27	0.10	0.22	–0.24	1													
M-NEAA	**0.45**	0.11	0.23	–0.29	**0.80**	1												
M-E/N	–0.30	–0.05	–0.06	0.13	**0.46**	–0.15	1											
M-TFAA	**0.39**	0.11	0.23	–0.28	**0.94**	**0.96**	0.14	1										
M-RNA	**–0.74**	0.03	**–0.36**	**0.53**	–0.25	–0.34	0.15	–0.31	1									
M-Protein	**–0.84**	–0.08	**–0.45**	**0.62**	–0.34	**–0.42**	0.13	**–0.40**	**0.81**	1								
M-R/P	**0.66**	0.01	**0.43**	**–0.62**	**0.46**	0.36	0.16	**0.43**	**–0.67**	**–0.84**	1							
O-T	0.56	–0.21	–0.17	–0.15	0.42	0.55	–0.39	0.51	0.11	–0.48	0.18	1						
O-EAA	0.58	0.12	0.47	–0.53	0.06	–0.01	0.02	0.02	–0.41	–0.55	0.46	0.09	1					
O-NEAA	0.52	0.15	0.55	–0.57	0.04	–0.09	0.13	–0.04	–0.50	–0.57	0.55	–0.06	**0.98**	1				
O-E/N	**0.66**	0.04	0.37	–0.52	0.12	0.07	–0.07	0.09	–0.36	–0.54	0.40	0.24	**0.97**	**0.90**	1			
O-TFAA	0.54	0.14	0.53	–0.56	0.05	–0.06	0.09	–0.02	–0.47	–0.57	0.53	–0.01	**0.99**	**1.00**	**0.93**	1		
O-RNA	**–0.82**	0.25	0.16	0.19	–0.43	–0.41	0.13	–0.42	0.17	0.50	–0.31	**–0.76**	–0.47	–0.32	–0.59	–0.37	1	
O-Protein	–0.25	–0.08	–0.14	0.17	–0.08	0.04	–0.26	–0.01	0.32	0.05	–0.09	0.25	–0.53	–0.47	–0.57	–0.49	0.14	1
O-R/P	**–0.69**	0.28	0.21	0.12	–0.38	–0.42	0.27	–0.41	0.06	0.48	–0.29	**–0.83**	–0.26	–0.15	–0.36	–0.18	**0.89**	–0.31

Weight (W), Trypsin (T), Chymotrypsin (C), Essential FAA (EAA), Non-EAA (NEAA), EAA/NEAA (E/N), Total FAA (TFAA), RNA (R), Protein (P), Oocyte trypsin-like (T).

Table 9. Correlation coefficient (*r*) between different parameters studied in Nile tilapia with different feedings. The values with significant correlation are written in big bold numbers ($P < 0.05$). (Unpublished data calculated from Rungruangsak-Torrissen et al. [19])

(*n* = 240)	W	L	SGR	FE	T	C	T/C	TP	A	L8	L10	White muscle (M)					Oocytes (O) (*n* = 22– 39)				
												RNA	P	R/P	L	P/L	T	RNA	P	R/P	L
W	1																				
L	**0.95**	1																			
SGR	**–0.74**	**–0.86**	1																		
FE	**–0.50**	**–0.53**	**0.70**	1																	
T	–0.11	**–0.23**	**0.22**	**–0.29**	1																
C	**0.16**	0.07	–0.11	**–0.54**	**0.78**	1															
T/C ratio	**–0.35**	**–0.41**	**0.49**	**0.41**	**0.41**	**–0.17**	1														
TP	**0.40**	**0.48**	**–0.54**	**–0.64**	**0.34**	**0.50**	**–0.20**	1													
A	**0.68**	**0.69**	**–0.64**	**–0.47**	0.06	**0.28**	**–0.25**	**0.49**	1												
L8	–0.17	**–0.23**	**0.23**	**–0.26**	**0.62**	**0.48**	**0.22**	**0.32**	0.02	1											
L10	–0.12	**–0.24**	**0.17**	**–0.35**	**0.68**	**0.72**	0.03	**0.21**	0.00	**0.56**	1										
M-RNA	0.01	–0.09	**0.14**	–0.00	**0.24**	**0.16**	**0.13**	–0.06	0.03	**0.26**	**0.25**	1									
M-Protein	–0.01	–0.04	0.02	**–0.18**	**0.34**	**0.23**	**0.16**	**0.27**	**0.16**	**0.50**	**0.15**	**0.23**	1								
M-R/P	**0.13**	**0.13**	**–0.15**	–0.02	–0.11	0.01	**–0.14**	**–0.16**	0.09	**–0.29**	0.01	**0.24**	**–0.43**	1							
M-L	0.03	–0.02	–0.00	–0.07	**0.18**	**0.21**	–0.02	–0.10	–0.01	0.02	**0.14**	0.01	–0.04	0.08	1						
M-P/L	**0.18**	**0.15**	–0.11	**–0.16**	0.04	0.01	0.02	**0.22**	**0.22**	**0.29**	–0.01	**0.29**	**0.59**	**–0.22**	**–0.48**	1					
O-T	0.06	0.05	–0.18	–0.23	0.15	–0.07	0.18	–0.27	0.02	–0.01	–0.09	0.03	0.07	–0.06	0.02	0.03	1				
O-RNA	–0.07	–0.08	0.21	0.05	–0.29	–0.13	–0.24	–0.10	–0.19	0.18	0.07	**0.33**	–0.11	–0.03	0.03	0.23	0.18	1			
O-Protein	**0.50**	**0.48**	–0.05	–0.04	–0.01	0.15	–0.16	0.04	0.30	–0.10	0.30	–0.01	–0.24	–0.08	–0.05	–0.01	–0.13	**0.47**	1		
O-R/P	–0.23	–0.24	0.23	0.03	–0.12	–0.05	–0.16	–0.13	**–0.34**	0.19	0.05	0.30	–0.00	–0.01	0.23	0.15	0.27	**0.78**	–0.13	1	
O-Lipid	0.13	0.14	0.04	–0.03	0.17	–0.23	0.36	**–0.54**	–0.01	–0.19	–0.14	–0.10	–0.04	–0.09	–0.05	–0.03	**0.64**	0.07	0.07	–0.02	1
O-P/L	0.21	0.18	0.34	**0.53**	–0.14	**0.46**	**–0.52**	0.40	0.29	0.08	0.18	–0.11	0.18	–0.30	–0.01	0.01	**–0.46**	–0.08	**0.71**	–0.36	**–0.53**

Weight (W), Length (L), Specific growth rate (SGR), Feed efficiency (FE), Trypsin (T), Chymotrypsin (C), Total protease (TP), Amylase (A), Lipase pH 8 (L8), Lipase pH 10 (L10), RNA (R), Protein (P), Lipid (L), Oocyte trypsin-like (T).

Table 10. Correlation coefficient (*r*) between different parameters studied in wild Northeast Arctic cod with different feedings in the Barents Sea. The values with significant correlation are written in big bold numbers ($P < 0.05$). (From Rungruangsak-Torrissen et al. [20])

($n = 107$)	W	L	CF	T	C	T/C	A	White muscle (M)					Oocytes (O) ($n = 60$)						
								RNA	P	R/P	L	P/L	T	C	T/C	RNA	P	R/P	L
Weight (W)	1																		
Length (L)	**0.91**	1																	
CF	**0.32**	**0.38**	1																
Trypsin (T)	0.12	0.08	–0.04	1															
Chymotrypsin (C)	0.12	0.15	–0.05	**0.82**	1														
T/C ratio	0.14	0.01	0.09	**0.58**	0.05	1													
Amylase (A)	**0.27**	0.20	**–0.25**	–0.05	–0.06	–0.06	1												
M-RNA (R)	0.06	0.10	–0.05	**0.39**	**0.35**	**0.34**	–0.16	1											
M-Protein (P)	–0.13	–0.13	**–0.29**	0.05	0.01	0.05	–0.00	–0.20	1										
M-R/P	0.12	0.16	0.19	0.08	0.11	0.07	–0.02	**0.62**	**–0.79**	1									
M-Lipid (L)	–0.11	–0.15	–0.19	–0.12	–0.14	–0.01	0.15	0.07	0.20	–0.14	1								
M-P/L ratio	–0.02	0.01	–0.06	0.14	0.11	0.09	–0.12	–0.18	**0.71**	**–0.57**	**–0.45**	1							
O-T	0.05	0.16	0.04	0.14	**0.43**	–0.34	–0.14	0.12	–0.05	0.10	0.12	–0.10	1						
O-C	0.10	0.18	0.06	0.19	0.42	–0.22	–0.19	–0.00	–0.04	0.05	0.10	–0.09	**0.96**	1					
O-T/C ratio	–0.28	–0.18	–0.05	–0.18	0.07	**–0.46**	0.16	0.37	–0.07	0.17	–0.05	–0.00	0.01	–0.28	1				
O-RNA (R)	–0.26	–0.06	**0.39**	–0.08	0.12	–0.27	–0.15	–0.12	0.11	0.02	**–0.43**	0.32	0.06	0.05	0.10	1			
O-Protein (P)	–0.28	**–0.39**	–0.32	–0.08	–0.34	0.32	0.15	0.06	0.20	–0.03	0.37	–0.10	–0.36	–0.22	–0.38	–0.09	1		
O-R/P	0.03	0.19	0.26	–0.04	0.22	–0.36	–0.14	–0.16	–0.03	–0.07	–0.37	0.19	0.20	0.11	0.36	**0.45**	**–0.87**	1	
O-Lipid (L)	0.09	0.03	–0.18	0.12	0.19	–0.16	0.21	0.10	–0.27	0.22	–0.24	–0.12	0.01	–0.09	0.38	–0.13	–0.08	–0.01	1
O-P/L ratio	–0.27	–0.32	–0.22	–0.12	**–0.44**	**0.47**	0.08	–0.10	0.23	–0.14	0.39	–0.05	–0.29	–0.11	**–0.62**	–0.05	**0.67**	**–0.54**	**–0.64**

Condition factor (CF), calculated as $100xW/L^3$.

Relationships of Different Biological Parameters

In order to be able to understand biological associations (directly and indirectly) among different parameters, the relationships among them have to be studied simultaneously in individual animals.

Very few researchers have performed this. Rungruangsak-Torrissen's research team has been studying some important biological parameters simultaneously in individuals, and their relationships have been reported [19, 20, 35, 36, 40, 41]. It is of interest to show various biological relationships in different species as shown for Atlantic salmon in Tables 6 and 7, Atlantic mackerel in Table 8, Nile tilapia in Table 9, and Northeast Arctic cod in Table 10.

Trypsin, Chymotrypsin, T/C Ratio, and Growth

The relationships among different biological parameters vary according to the growth status of the animals while being sampled. Specific activities of trypsin and chymotrypsin in the pyloric caeca are always highly correlated ($r > 0.7$, Tables 6–10) because trypsin directly activates chymotrypsinogen in the pancreatic acinar cells to become active chymotrypsin. During growing phase, trypsin specific activity and the activity ratio of trypsin to chymotrypsin (T/C ratio) are positively correlated with specific growth rate of the fish (Tables 6 and 9), while during steady growth or a reduction in growth rate, no such correlations would be observed (Table 7).

This has an advantage for predicting growth status of fishes in natural ecosystems where growth could not be directly measured. As shown in Table 8, there was no relationship between trypsin specific activity and T/C ratio in the Atlantic mackerel experiment indicating the fish were at a non-growing period, while the relationship was significant in the Northeast Arctic cod experiment indicating the fish were still at a growing phase (Table 10).

Surprisingly, a high relationship between trypsin and chymotrypsin specific activities was also observed in faeces where the levels of faecal trypsin and T/C ratio were correlated with pyloric caecal trypsin specific activity (Table 7). This suggests a possibility to study the two proteases in faeces for an indication of digestive efficiency (T/C ratio), but not for fish growth status [40]. It is interesting to note that among different studied pyloric caecal digestive enzymes (trypsin, chymotrypsin, total protease, amylase, and lipase), only the T/C ratio that showed a positive relationship with feed efficiency (Table 9).

Moreover, a high correlation between trypsin-like and chymotrypsin-like specific activities in the oocytes has also been observed [20, 77], as shown in Table 10. The proteases, trypsin-like and chymotrypsin-like, in the oocytes are not the same as the proteases observed in the digestive tract, as they have different characteristics under the same temperatures whereas the pyloric caecal proteases are more sensitive to higher temperatures than the oocyte proteases [20, 77]. The T/C ratios in the pyloric caeca and oocytes are negatively correlated due to decreasing somatic growth during increasing oocyte development for sexual maturation (Table 10). Since the *in vitro* protein digestibility correlates with the T/C ratio and feed efficiency (Figure 24), the observed inverse relationship between the *in vitro* protein digestibility and specific growth rate at maturity [42] also confirms that diet utilization during maturation is not for somatic growth but for gamete development.

Protein Mobilization during Maturation

The activity ratio of trypsin to chymotrypsin (T/C ratio) in the pyloric caeca has been shown to correlate negatively (Table 9) or positively (Table 10) with the level ratio of protein to lipid (P/L ratio) in the oocytes because of muscle protein deposition level (affected by protein digestion) influencing oocyte protein level. This indicates a mobilization of muscle protein to oocytes, as very low (Table 9) or no (Table 10) correlation between pyloric caecal T/C ratio and muscle protein level was observed, respectively. The negative relationship between oocyte T/C ratio and oocyte P/L ratio is due to protein hydrolysis in the oocytes during sexual maturation process (Table 10).

The T/C ratio levels in the pyloric caeca correlated with feed efficiency, and feed efficiency correlated with oocyte P/L ratio (Table 9), suggesting an important of protein digestive efficiency for oocyte quality. During growing phase, the levels of pyloric caecal T/C ratio could affect the levels of white muscle free amino acids (Table 6), but this was not observed during maturation when growth reduced (Table 8). The levels of white muscle free amino acids from nutrient transport could influence the levels of protein and protein turnover in the white muscle (Tables 6 and 8), but this was not observed in oocytes due to free amino acids in the oocytes were from the hydrolysis of the oocyte self-protein (Table 8).

Protein turnover process (indicated by the levels of free hydroxyproline and RNA/Protein ratio) in the white muscle could affect growth by both protein and lipid depositions, depending on the dietary quality and protein digestive efficiency (pyloric caecal T/C ratio) as well as the growth status of the fish. A reduced protein synthesis in the white muscle (white muscle RNA levels with mainly negative relationships with growth parameters) suggested a higher lipid deposition during growing phase as RNA levels related with RNA/protein ratio but not with protein levels in the white muscle (Tables 6 and 7), or more protein mobilization during maturing process as RNA levels related positively with protein levels but negatively with RNA/protein ratio (Table 8). On the other hand, an increased protein synthesis in the white muscle (white muscle RNA levels with mainly positive relationships with growth parameters) suggested a higher protein deposition or less protein mobilization during maturing process (Tables 9 and 10). These results suggest that the fishes studied in Tables 6–10 were under different growth statuses and had differences in growth performance quality including mobilization of white muscle protein. The knowledge of these relationships has provided more understanding on performance qualities of growth and maturation that would be varied under different environmental conditions and growth status of the fishes.

Moreover, the levels of trypsin-like specific activity in the oocytes were correlated with the levels of some oocyte free amino acids, such as leucine ($r = 0.77$), creatinine ($r = 0.71$), and glycine ($r = -0.69$) [unpublished data from 41]. Leucine (an essential amino acid) probably has an important role in the oocytes, as its levels in oocytes were also different between fish with different feedings (Table 5).

Creatinine may also have an important role in the oocytes. Glycine is the essential amino acid in collagen [68], and could be a precursor for synthesis as well as a catabolic product of connective tissues. The negative correlation between trypsin-like specific activity and glycine levels suggested a higher protein hydrolysis in the oocytes at higher maturing stage with lower trypsin-like specific activity. This is in accordance with the indications of lower protein levels with lower trypsin-like specific activity in eggs at higher maturing stage [20] shown in Figure 18.

Future Research

It is important that future research is emphasized on improvement for more understanding of the previous knowledge both theoretically and practically, and with more perspective to long-term consequences than to short-term outcomes. Scientific exploitation through industrial propaganda has to be governed wisely, as usually giving less benefit to the consumers. Rungruangsak-Torrissen and Fosseidengen [41] have reported that, based on muscle contributing 60% of the body weight, the slower growth mackerel of 294 ± 10 g produced 33.6 ± 1.8 g of muscle protein (19.0 ± 0.8 %), while the higher growth artificially fed mackerel of 487 ± 14 g produced only 27.5 ± 1.8 g of muscle protein (9.6 ± 0.7 %). This is common between slower and higher growth animals, whereas slower growth animals in nature have higher protein deposition than higher growth cultivated animals. Aquaculture products should have been the sources for high protein with high nutritional values, but feed industry has been producing new feeds resulting in opposite outcomes. This is one of the reasons why organic animal production is now preferred to artificial animal production.

Changes in environmental conditions (i.e. temperature, food) can influence gene expression of the fish at DNA, RNA and protein levels, regardless of the genetic expression of parents [79], and could affect reproduction processes [40, 41]. Genetic manipulated animals will never replace evolutional and naturally adaptive animals, as changes in biochemical processes are not the same between them, and genetic manipulated animals could cause environmental impact [79]. The work illustrated in this chapter has been mainly published in aquaculture related journals, and the knowledge should have been more utilized by the industry.

Recently, the techniques have also been successfully implemented for studying in natural ecosystem [20], as shown in Figure 27. Wild maturing Northeast Arctic cod has been studied during winter, and for the first time, the fish distributed in different areas in the Barents Sea showed differences in food utilization efficiency, protein mobilization and maturation rate (Figure 27), as well as in trypsin isozymes expressions whereas higher percentage of cod in areas A and B with higher food varieties had exogenous low molecular weight trypsin isozyme fragments from prey items (see Figure 3), compared to area C. Populations in areas A and C living in separate environments showed parallel regressions of pyloric caecal slope T/C ratio with higher elevations of trypsin specific activity in area A, similar to the observation in Figure 15B. It has been concluded that younger females (probably also males) living closer to coastal area with higher temperature and food varieties would reach sexual maturity faster than older cod and those living far from coastal area [20] (see Figure 27). The techniques are applicable for studying biochemical changes in food utilization for growth and maturation of animals under any conditions both in cultivation and natural ecosystem.

Moreover, the *in vitro* digestibility techniques for both protein and carbohydrate of different plankton species [73, 74], as shown in Figure 25, could be applicable for studying highly digestible and utilizable plankton species suitable for each species of interest in nature. This can provide new knowledge of interactions between different species from low to high food chain. Natural behaviour of fishes is usually dependent on feeding and food utilization. The effect of genetic variation in food utilization could influence the fishes to distribute in different areas (i.e. with different temperatures) suitable for optimizing digestive efficiency for growth [9, 21], as well as for reproduction and survival.

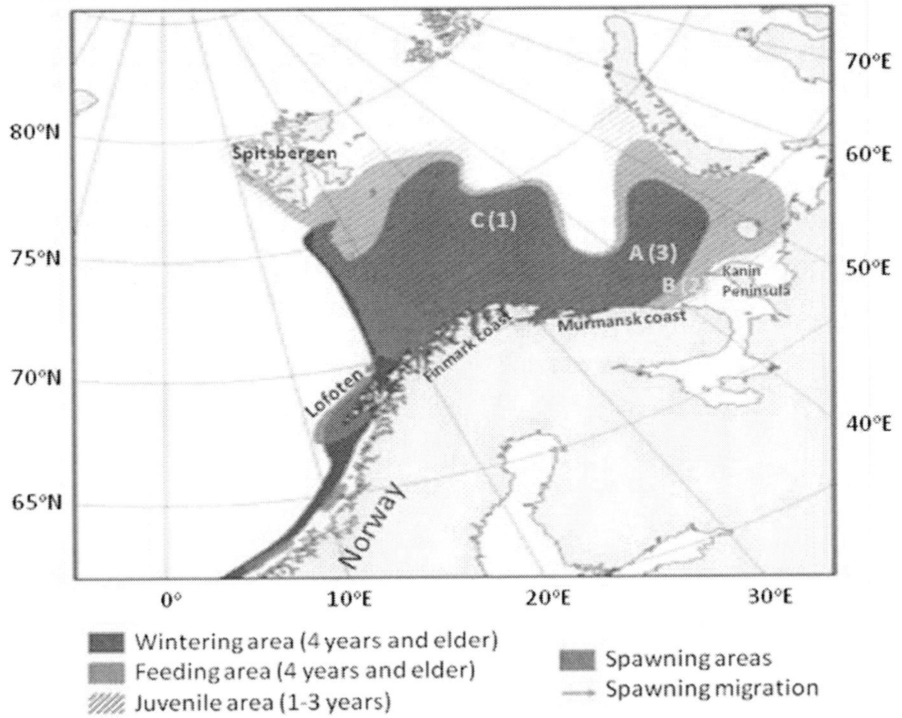

Regardless of sexes		Female oocytes	
Cod weight (0.97 ± 0.10 kg)	B* < C < A*	Maturation rate	B* > A* > C*
Cod length (42.77 ± 1.46 cm)	B < C < A		
(year age)	(3.23) (3.98) (4.09)	(Water temperature °C)	(3.45) (1.61) (1.69)
Pyloric caecal T/C ratio	B < C < A**	T/C ratio	B* > A > C*
Pyloric caecal trypsin	B* < C* < A*	Trypsin-like	B* < A* < C*
Pyloric caecal chymotrypsin	B* < C < A*	Chymotrypsin-like	B* < A* < C*
White muscle RNA	B < C* < A*	RNA	B > C > A
White muscle protein	B < C < A	Protein	B** > C > A
White muscle lipid	B > C > A	Lipid	B > C > A
Muscle Protein/Lipid ratio	B < C < A	RNA/Protein ratio	B** < C < A
Muscle RNA/Protein ratio	B > A > C	Protein/Lipid ratio	C > B > A
Pyloric caecal amylase	B > A > C		

Figure 27. Distribution areas of Northeast Arctic cod in the Barents Sea, with three main studied areas (A, B and C) illustrated, which covered six trawl stations in the area of 68–75°N 41–32°E. The area A was between North Kanin Bank and Eastern Basin, area B was Kanin Bank, and area C was Central Bank. The number of trawl station(s) studied in each area is shown in the bracket. Variations in the parameters studied among the different areas are shown where the areas with asterisk (*) are significantly different, and the area with double asterisk (**) is significantly different from the other two areas ($P < 0.05$). The relationships among these parameters are shown in Table 10. (Adapted from Rungruangsak-Torrissen et al. [20]).

Genetic differences in food utilization have been established at the early life period of fishes and could affect food utilization and growth during the whole life cycle [6, 9, 24].

Environmental changes (i.e. water temperature, pH, current) could impact the whole food chain, and change migration patterns as well as nutritional quality of living organisms. Variations in abundance, quality, and variety of food will affect genetic expression of offsprings, food utilization, growth, reproduction, and migration patterns of fishes. This means that the environmental condition has to be conserved in order to control the genetic structure of animals in the wild; otherwise, an incidence of the offsprings to change their gene expressions for adapting to new environment for growth and survival will be seen [9, 79]. Biochemical changes in food utilization and performance qualities of growth and maturation of fishes [20, 40–42] due to environmental impact are needed for improving knowledge of living organisms in nature for future advice. Most ecologists are not yet familiar with the techniques, and most climate change studies have been on physical changes. An integration of the work on biochemical changes in food utilization, growth and reproduction of living organisms due to environmental impact in climate change study should be practical, challenged and prioritized.

Conclusion

Trypsin, the key protease enzyme in the intestine, has been implemented as the key factor for consumption of food/feed and dietary protein in aquatic animals. The function of trypsin is related to increasing growth while the function of chymotrypsin (activated by trypsin) is related to limiting or decreasing growth. This has made the activity ratio of trypsin to chymotrypsin (T/C ratio) an important biological factor for diet utilization efficiency and growth without necessity of knowing consumption rate. Therefore, the T/C ratio is the useful biological factor for studying food utilization efficiency and growth of animals in natural ecosystems where food consumption rate cannot be measured. Regression levels of slope T/C ratio and the elevations of trypsin specific activity between regressions could indicate whether these populations have been living in distinct environments or overlapping environments and which populations having higher diet or protein consumption, respectively. Animals consuming higher levels of dietary protein would show a higher skeletal growth (body length) with higher protein deposition in body and white muscle. Different slope levels of regressions of trypsin specific activities and T/C ratio with different elevations of T/C ratio between regressions could indicate growth variations between populations and could suggest the differences in maturation rate of maturing females between the populations. Animals usually reduce somatic growth during maturing processes. Trypsin-like and chymotrypsin-like activities could be observed in female oocytes. The levels of the two enzymes specific activities and the T/C ratio in the oocytes could indicate the levels of maturation rate of maturing females between populations. Maturing females have higher capacity for protein synthesis in the oocytes than in the white muscle.

Protein has been found to be the primary key nutrient in diet utilization, followed by carbohydrate as the secondary nutrient. *In vitro* digestibility of dietary protein or carbohydrate has been studied using animal digestive extracts of specific species of interest. The *in vitro* digestibility of dietary protein or carbohydrate of the same diets could be comparable among different developmental stages and different species if the values are standardized by trypsin activity or amylase activity, respectively. This could indicate the dietary quality suitable for each growth stage and each species. Moreover, the *in vitro* protein digestibility values also associate with the composition and chemical structure of the dietary protein. The technique is more practical with less time consuming than the conventional growth experiment.

Expression of trypsin isozymes in the intestine is dependent on dietary quality and environmental condition as well as genetics of the animals themselves. Animals possessing different trypsin phenotypes have different abilities to digest the same diets and require different temperatures for optimal utilization of the diets. Dietary quality and environmental condition at the early life stage could affect animal trypsin phenotypes independent of the phenotypes of the parents. This could influence food utilization and growth of the animals under different environmental conditions during the whole life cycle. The implementations of trypsin together with chymotrypsin, as well as protein synthesis capacity, for studying growth, maturation, and dietary quality assessment are useful for deeper understanding of the biochemical processes. They could be practical standard techniques for studying changes in the biochemical processes in any living organisms under any environmental conditions.

References

[1] Rungruangsak Torrissen, K., and Male, R. (2000). Trypsin isozymes: development, digestion and structure. In N. F. Haard, and B. K. Simpson (Eds.), *Seafood Enzymes: Utilization and influence on postharvest seafood quality* (pp. 215–269). New York: Marcel Dekker, Inc., US.

[2] Torrissen, K. R. (1984). Characterization of proteases in the digestive tract of Atlantic salmon (*Salmo salar*) in comparison with rainbow trout (*Salmo gairdneri*). *Comp. Biochem. Physiol.*, 77B, 669–674.

[3] Torrissen, K. R., and Barnung, T. N. 1991. Genetic difference in trypsin-like isozyme pattern between two strains of Arctic charr (*Salvelinus alpinus*). *Aquaculture*, 96, 227–231.

[4] Torrissen, K. R., and Torrissen, O. J. (1985). Protease activities and carotenoid levels during the sexual maturation of Atlantic salmon (*Salmo salar*). *Aquaculture,* 50, 113–122.

[5] Torrissen, K. R. (1987). Genetic variation of trypsin-like isozymes correlated to fish size of Atlantic salmon (*Salmo salar*). *Aquaculture*, 62, 1–10.

[6] Torrissen, K. R. (1991). Genetic variation in growth rate of Atlantic salmon with different trypsin-like isozyme patterns. *Aquaculture*, 93, 299–312.

[7] Torrissen, K. R., and Shearer, K. D. (1992). Protein digestion, growth and food conversion in Atlantic salmon and Arctic charr with different trypsin-like isozyme patterns. *J. Fish Biol.*, 41, 409–415.

[8] Torrissen, K. R., Male, R., and Nævdal, G. (1993). Trypsin isozymes in Atlantic salmon, *Salmo salar* L.: studies of heredity, egg quality and effect on growth of three different populations. *Aquacult. Fish. Manage.*, 24, 407–415.

[9] Rungruangsak-Torrissen, K., Pringle, G. M., Moss, R., and Houlihan, D. F. (1998). Effects of varying rearing temperatures on expression of different trypsin isozymes, feed conversion efficiency and growth in Atlantic salmon (*Salmo salar* L.). *Fish Physiol. Biochem.*, 19, 247–255.

[10] Torrissen, K. R., Lied, E., and Espe, M. (1994). Differences in digestion and absorption of dietary protein in Atlantic salmon (*Salmo salar*) with genetically different trypsin isozymes. *J. Fish Biol.*, 45, 1087–1104.

[11] Bassompierre, M., Ostenfeld, T. H., McLean, E., and Torrissen, K. R. (1998). *In vitro* protein digestion, and growth of Atlantic salmon with different trypsin isozymes. *Aquacult. Int.*, 6, 47–56.

[12] Rungruangsak-Torrissen, K., Carter, C. G., Sundby, A., Berg, A., and Houlihan, D. F. (1999). Maintenance ration, protein synthesis capacity, plasma insulin and growth of Atlantic salmon (*Salmo salar* L.) with genetically different trypsin isozymes. *Fish Physiol. Biochem.*, 21, 223–233.

[13] Rungruangsak-Torrissen, K., Wergeland, H. I., Glette, J., and Waagbø, R. (1999). Disease resistance and immune parameters in Atlantic salmon (*Salmo salar* L.) with genetically different trypsin isozymes. *Fish and Shellfish Immunol.*, 9, 557–568.

[14] Male, R., Lorens, J. B., Smalås, A. O., and Torrissen, K. R. (1995). Molecular cloning and characterization of anionic and cationic variants of trypsin from Atlantic salmon. *Eur. J. Biochem.*, 232, 677–685.

[15] Sainz, J. C., Garcia-Carreno, F. L., and Hernandez-Cortes, P. (2004). *Penaeus vannamei* isotrypsins: purification and characterization. *Comp. Biochem. Physiol.*, 138B, 155–162.

[16] Sainz, J. C., Garcia-Carreno, F. L., Cordova-Murueta, J. H., and Cruz-hernandez, P. (2005). Whiteleg shrimp (*Litopenaeus vannamei*, Boone, 1931) isotrypsins: Their genotype and modulation. *J. Exp. Mar. Biol. Ecol.*, 326, 105–113.

[17] Hernandez, J. C. S., and Murueta, J. H. C. (2009). Activity of trypsin from *Litopenaeus vannamei*. *Aquaculture*, 290, 190–195.

[18] Perera, E., Moyano, F. J., Diaz, M., Perdomo-Morales, R., Montero-Alejo, V., Alonso, E., Carrillo, O., and Galich, G. S. (2008). Polymorphism and partial characterization of digestive enzymes in the spiny lobster *Panulirus argus*. *Comp. Biochem. Physiol.*, 150B, 247–254.

[19] Rungruangsak-Torrissen, K., Engkagul, A., Aeidnoie, Y., Kovitvadhi, S., Kovitvadhi, U., Siruntawineti, J., Choowongkomon, K., Unajak, S., Preprame, P., Trenet, E., Meeswad, P., and Sunthornchot, J. (2010). Development of suitable feed for commercial production of Nile tilapia, *Oreochromis niloticus*. *Kasetsart University Technical Report* 2010, 184 pp. Biochemical Research Unit for Feed Utilization Assessment, Kasetsart University, Bangkok, Thailand. [in Thai].

[20] Rungruangsak-Torrissen, K., Thongprajukaew, K., Sansuwan, K., Thapthimdaeng, P., Kovitvadhi, U., Seetaha, S., Choowongkomon, K., Beck, I. M., and Arnøy, O. O. Ecological effects on food utilization, trypsin isozymes, and performance qualities of growth and maturation in Northeast Arctic cod (*Gadus morhua* L.). *The Open Fish Science Journal,* (submitted).

[21] Rungruangsak-Torrissen, K., and Stensholt, B. K. (2001). Spatial distribution of Atlantic salmon post-smolts: Association between genetic differences in trypsin isozymes and environmental variables. In G. H. Kruse, N. Bez, A. Booth, M. W. Dorn, S. Hills, R. N. Lipcius, D. Pelletier, C. Roy, S. J. Smith, and D. Witherell (Eds.), *Spatial Processes and Management of Marine Populations* (pp. 415–429). Fairbanks: University of Alaska Sea Grant, AK-SG-01-02.

[22] Rungruangsak-Torrissen, K., and Sundby, A. (2000). Protease activities, plasma free amino acids and insulin at different ages of Atlantic salmon (*Salmo salar* L.) with genetically different trypsin isozymes. *Fish Physiol. Biochem.*, 22, 337–347.

[23] Torrissen, K. R., Lied, E., and Espe, M. (1995). Differences in utilization of dietary proteins with varying degrees of partial pre-hydrolysis in Atlantic salmon (*Salmo salar* L.) with genetically different trypsin isozymes. In J. Svasti, V. Rimphanitchayakit, A. Tassanakajorn, P. Pongsawasdi, B. Sonthayanon, K. Packdibamrung, S. Soontaros, T. Limpaseni, P. Wilairat, J. Boonjawat, and S. Kamolsiripichaiporn (Eds.), Biopolymers and Bioproducts: Structure, Function and Applications (pp. 432–442). *Proceedings of the 11th FAOBMB Symposium* (IUBMB Symposium No.239). Bangkok: Samakkhisan Public Company Limited, ISBN 974-632-655-4.

[24] Rungruangsak-Torrissen, K., Moss, R., Andresen, L. H., Berg, A., and Waagbø, R. (2006). Different expressions of trypsin and chymotrypsin in relation to growth in Atlantic salmon (*Salmo salar* L.). *Fish Physiol. Biochem.*, 32, 7–23.

[25] Perera, E., Moyano, F. J., Rodriguez-Viera, L., Cervantes, A., Martinez-Rodriguez, G., and Mancera, J. M. (2010). *In vitro* digestion of protein sources by crude enzyme extracts of the spiny lobster *Panulirus argus* (Latreille, 1804) hepatopancreas with different trypsin isoenzyme patterns. *Aquaculture*, 310, 178–185.

[26] Kishimura, H., Hayashi, K., Miyashita, Y., and Nonami, Y. (2005). Characteristics of two trypsin isozymes from the viscera of Japanese anchovy (*Engraulis japonica*). *J. Food Biochem.*, 29, 459–469.

[27] Kishimura, H., Tokuda, Y., Klomklao, S., Benjakul, S., and Ando, S. (2006). Enzymatic characteristics of trypsin from pyloric ceca of spotted mackerel (*Scomber australasicus*). *J. Food Biochem.*, 30, 466–477.

[28] Kishimura, H., Tokuda, Y., Klomklao, S., Benjakul, S., and Ando, S. (2006). Comparative study of enzymatic characteristics of trypsins from the pyloric ceca of yellow tail (*Seriola quinqueradiata*) and brown hakeling (*Physiculus japonicus*). *J. Food Biochem.*, 30, 521–534.

[29] Kishimura, H., Tokuda, Y., Yabe, M., Klomklao, S., Benjakul, S., and Ando, S. (2007). Trypsins from the pyloric ceca of jacopever (*Sebastes schlegelii*) and elkhorn sculpin (*Alcichthys alcicornis*): Isolation and characterization. *Food Chem.*, 100, 1490–1495.

[30] Kishimura, H., Klomklao, S., Benjakul, S., and Chun, B. S. (2008). Characteristics of trypsin from the pyloric ceca of walleye Pollock (*Theragra chalcogramma*). *Food Chem.*, 106, 194–199.

[31] Klomklao, S., Kishimura, H., Nonami, Y., and Benjakul, S. (2009). Biochemical properties of two isoforms of trypsin purified from the intestine of skipjack tuna (*Katsuwonus pelamis*). *Food Chem.*, 115, 155–162.

[32] Fuchise, T., Kishimura, H., Sekizaki, H., Nonami, Y., Kanno, G., Klomklao, S., Benjakul, S., and Chun, B. S. (2009). Purification and characteristics of trypsins from cold-zone fish, Pacific cod (*Gadus macrocephalus*) and saffron cod (*Eleginus gracilis*). *Food Chem.*, 116, 611–616.

[33] Kanno, G., Yamaguchi, T., Kishimura, H., Yamaha, E., and Saeki, H. (2010). Purification and characteristics of trypsin from masu salmon (*Oncorhynchus masou*) cultured in fresh-water. *Fish Physiol. Biochem.*, 36, 637–645.

[34] Klomklao, S., Kishimura, H., Benjakul, S., Simpson, B. K., and Visessanguan, W. (2010). Cationic trypsin: A predominant proteinase in Pacific saury (*Cololabis saira*) pyloric ceca. *J. Food Biochem.*, 34, 1105–1123.

[35] Sunde, J., Eiane, S. A., Rustad, A., Jensen, H. B., Opstvedt, J., Nygård, E., Venturini, G., and Rungruangsak-Torrissen, K. (2004). Effect of fish feed processing conditions on digestive protease activities, free amino acid pools, feed conversion efficiency and growth in Atlantic salmon (*Salmo salar L.*). *Aquacult. Nutr.*, 10, 261–277.

[36] Sunde, J., Taranger, G. L., and Rungruangsak-Torrissen, K. (2001). Digestive protease activities and free amino acids in white muscle as indicators for feed conversion efficiency and growth rate in Atlantic salmon (*Salmo salar* L.). *Fish Physiol. Biochem.*, 25, 335–345.

[37] Rungruangsak-Torrissen, K., Sunde, J., Berg, A. E., Nordgarden, U., Fjelldal, P. G., and Oppedal, F. (2009). Digestive efficiency, free amino acid pools and quality of growth performance in Atlantic salmon *(Salmo salar* L.) affected by light regimes and vaccine types. *Fish Physiol. Biochem.*, 35, 255–272.

[38] Lemieux, H., Blier, P. U., and Dutil, J-D. (1999). Do digestive enzymes set physiological limit on growth rate and food conversion efficiency in Atlantic cod (*Gadus morhua*)? *Fish Physiol. Biochem.*, 20, 293–303.

[39] Blier, P. U., Lemieux, H., and Devlin, R. H. (2002). Is the growth rate of fish set by digestive enzymes or metabolic capacity of tissues? Insight from transgenic coho salmon. *Aquaculture,* 209, 379–384.

[40] Rungruangsak-Torrissen, K. (2007). Digestive efficiency, growth and qualities of muscle and oocyte in Atlantic salmon (*Salmo salar* L.) fed on diets with krill meal as an alternative protein source. *J. Food Biochem.*, 31, 509–540.

[41] Rungruangsak-Torrissen, K., and Fosseidengen, J. E. (2007). Effect of artificial feeding on digestive efficiency, growth and qualities of muscle and oocyte of maturing Atlantic mackerel (*Scomber scombrus* L.). *J. Food Biochem.,* 31, 726–747.

[42] Rungruangsak-Torrissen, K., Stien, L. H., Daae, B. S., Vågseth, T., Thorsheim, G. B., Tobin, D., and Ritora, O. (2009). Different dietary levels of protein to lipid ratio affected digestive efficiency, skeletal growth, and muscle protein in rainbow trout families. *Scholarly Research Exchange*, vol. 2009, Article ID 709529, doi:10.3814/2009/709529.

[43] Nordgarden, U., Fjelldal, P. G., Hansen, T., Björnsson, B. T., Wargelius, A. (2006). Growth hormone and insulin-like growth factor-I act together and independently when regulating growth in vertebral and muscle tissue of Atlantic salmon postsmolts. *Gen. Comp. Endocrinol.*, 149, 253–260.

[44] Einarsson, S., Davies, P. S., and Talbot, C. (1996). The effect of feeding on the secretion of pepsin, trypsin and chymotrypsin in the Atlantic salmon, *Salmo salar* L. *Fish Physiol. Biochem.*, 15, 439–446.

[45] Muhlia-Almazan, A., and Garcia-Carreno, F. L. (2002). Influence of molting and starvation on the synthesis of proteolytic enzymes in the midgut gland of the white shrimp *Penaeus vannamei. Comp. Biochem. Physiol.*, 133B, 383–394.

[46] Comoglio, L. I., Gaxiola, G., Roque, A., Cuzon, G., and Amin, O. (2004). The effect of starvation on refeeding, digestive enzyme activity, oxygen consumption, and ammonia excretion in juvenile white shrimp *Litopenaeus vannamei. J. Shellfish*, 23, 243–249.

[47] Bolasina, S., Perez, A., and Yamashita, Y. (2006). Digestive enzymes activity during ontogenetic development and effect of starvation in Japanese flounder, *Paralichthys olivaceus*. *Aquaculture*, 252, 503–515.

[48] Chen, B. N., Qin, J. G., Carragher, J. F., Clarke, S. M., Kumar, M. S., and Hutchinson, W. G. (2007). Deleterious effects of food restrictions in yellowtail kingfish *Seriola lalandi* during early development. *Aquaculture*, 271, 326–335.

[49] Imani, A., Yazdanparast, R., Farhangi, M., Bakhtiyari, M., and Saljoghi, Z. S. (2009). Effect of different food deprivation periods on digestive enzyme activities of rainbow trout *Oncorhynchus mykiss*. *Aquaculture Europe* 09, August 14–17, 2009, Trondheim, Norway, pp. 191–192.

[50] Gisbert, E., Fernandez, I., and Alvarez-Gonzalez, C. A. (2011). Prolonged feed deprivation does not permanently compromise digestive function in migrating European glass ells *Anguilla Anguilla*. *J. Fish Biol.*, 78, 580–592.

[51] Applebaum, S. L., and Holt, G. J. (2003). The digestive protease, chymotrypsin, as an indicator of nutritional condition in larval red drum (*Sciaenops ocellatus*). *Mar. Biol.*, 142, 1159–1167.

[52] Gildberg, A. (2004). Digestive enzyme activities in starved pre-slaughter farmed and wild-captured, Atlantic cod (*Gadus morhua*). *Aquaculture*, 238, 343–353.

[53] Chan, C. R., Lee, D. N., Cheng, Y. H., Hsieh, D. J. Y., and Weng, C. F. (2008). Feed deprivation and re-feeding on alterations of proteases in tilapia *Oreochromis mossambicus*. *Zool. Stud.*, 47, 207–214.

[54] Imani, A., Farhangi, M., Yazdanparast, R., Bakhtiyari, M., Saljoghi, Z. S., and Amiri, B. M. (2009). Effect of different starvation and refeeding regimes on the compensatory growth and feed utilization indices of rainbow trout *Oncorhynchus mykiss*. *Aquaculture Europe* 09, August 14–17, 2009, Trondheim, Norway, pp. 275–276.

[55] Rungruangsak-Torrissen, K., Rustad, A., Sunde, J., Eiane, S. A., Jensen, H. B., Opstvedt, J., Nygård, E., Samuelsen, T. A., Mundheim, H., Luzzana, U., and Venturini, G. (2002). *In vitro* digestibility based on fish crude enzyme extract for prediction of feed quality in growth trials. *J. Sci. Food Agric.*, 82, 644–654.

[56] Yoneda, M., and Wright, P. J. (2005). Effects of varying temperature on food availability on growth and reproduction in first-time spawning female Atlantic cod. *J. Fish Biol.*, 67, 1225–1241.

[57] Craik, J. C. A., and Harvey, S. M. (1987). The causes of buoyancy in eggs of marine teleosts. *J. Mar. Biol. Ass.* U. K., 67, 169–182.

[58] Thorsen, A., Fyhn, H. J., and Wallace, R. A. (1993). Free amino acids as osmotic effectors for oocyte hydration in marine fishes. In B. T. Walther, and H. J. Fyhn (Eds.), *Physiological and Biochemical Aspects of Fish Development* (pp. 94–98). Bergen: University of Bergen, Norway.

[59] Thorsen, A., Kjesbu, O. S., Fyhn, H. J., and Solemdal, P. (1996). Physiological mechanisms of buoyancy in eggs from brackish water cod. *J. Fish Biol.*, 48, 457–477.

[60] Yoshikuni, M., Sagegami, R., and Nagahama, Y. (2003). Proteome analysis: a new approach to identify key proteins involved in acquisition of maturational competence and oocyte maturation of medaka oocytes. *Fish Physiol. Biochem.*, 28, 379–380.

[61] Von Schalburg, K. R., Rise, M. L., Brown, G. D., Davidson, W. S., and Koop, B. F. (2005). A comprehensive survey of the genes involved in maturation and development of the rainbow trout ovary. *Biol. Reprod.*, 72, 687–699.

[62] Le, T. Q., Kawachi, M., Yamada, H., Shiota, M., Okumura, Y., and Kido, H. (2006). Identification of trypsin I as a candidate for influenza A virus and Sendai virus envelope glycoprotein processing protease in rat brain. *Biol. Chem.*, 387, 467–475.

[63] Skern, R. (2005). Trypsin and trypsin-like peptidases from *Lepeophtheirus salmonis*, functional implications from molecular studies. *Ph.D. thesis*. Institute of Marine Research, Bergen, and Department of Molecular Biology, University of Bergen, Norway. ISBN 82–308–0058–8.

[64] Rowen, L., Koop, B. F., and Hood, L. (1996). The complete 685-kilobase DNA sequence of the human β T cell receptor locus. *Science,* 272, 1755–1762.

[65] Fabra, M., and Cerda, J. (2004). Ovarian cysteine proteinases in the teleost *Fundulus heteroclitus*: Molecular cloning and gene expression during vitellogenesis and oocyte maturation. *Mol. Reprod. Dev.*, 67, 282–294.

[66] LaFleur, G. J., Raldua, D., Fabra, M., Carnevali, O., Denslow, N., Wallace, R. A., and Cerda, J. (2005). Derivation of major yolk proteins from parental vitellogenins and alternative processing during oocyte maturation in *Fundulus heteroclitus*. *Biol. Reprod.*, 73, 815–824.

[67] Carnevali, O., Cionna, C., Tosti, L., Lubzens, E., and Maradonna, F. (2006). Role of cathepsins in ovarian follicle growth and maturation. *Gen. Comp. Endocrinol.*, 146, 195–203.

[68] Stryer, L. (1988). Connective-tissue proteins. In L. Stryer (Ed.), *Biochemistry* (pp. 261–281). New York: W. H. Freeman, USA.

[69] Shigemasa, K., Tanimoto, H., Sakata, K., Nagai, N., Parmley, T. H., Ohama, K., and O'Brien, T. J. (2000). Induction of matrix metalloprotease–7 is common in mucinous ovarian tumors including early stage disease. *Med. Oncol.,* 17, 52–58.

[70] Furuya, S., Sakamoto, K., and Takahashi, S. (1979). A new *in vitro* method for the estimation of digestibility using the intestinal fluid of the pig. *Br. J. Nutr.*, 41, 511–520.

[71] Dimes, L. E., Garcia-Carreno, F. L., and Haard, N. F. (1994). Estimation of protein digestibility–III. Studies on the digestive enzymes from the pyloric caeca of rainbow trout and salmon. *Comp. Biochem. Physiol.,* 109A, 349–360.

[72] Bassompierre, M., Børresen, T., Sandfeld, P., Rønsholdt, B., Zimmermann, W., and McLean, E. (1997). An evaluation of open and closed systems for *in vitro* protein digestion of fish meal. *Aquacult. Nutr.*, 3, 153–159.

[73] Areekijseree, M., Engkagul, A., Kovitvadhi, S., Kovitvadhi, U., Thongpan, A., and Rungruangsak-Torrissen, K. (2006). Development of digestive enzymes and *in vitro* digestibility of different species of phytoplankton for culture of early juveniles of the freshwater pearl mussel, *Hyriopsis* (*Hyriopsis*) *bialatus* Simpson, 1900. *Invert. Reprod. Develop.*, 49, 255–262.

[74] Supannapong, P., Pimsalee, T., A-komol, T., Engkagul, A., Kovitvadhi, U., Kovitvadhi, S., and Rungruangsak-Torrissen, K. (2008). Digestive enzymes and *in vitro* digestibility of different species of phytoplankton for culture of the freshwater pearl mussel, *Hyriopsis* (*Hyriopsis*) *bialatus*. *Aquacult. Int.*, 16, 437–453.

[75] Luzzana,U., Mentasti, T., Moretti, V. M., Albertini, A., and Valfre, F. (1996). Aspartic acid racemization in fish meal as induced by thermal treatment. *Aquacult. Nutr.*, 2, 95–99.

[76] Luzzana,U., Mentasti, T., Opstvedt, J., Nygård, E., Moretti, V. M., and Valfre, F. (1999). Racemization kinetics of aspartic acid in fish material under different conditions of moisture, pH and oxygen pressure. *J. Agric. Food Chem.*, 47, 2897–2884.

[77] Thongprajukaew, K. (2011). Feed development using digestive enzyme technology for successive growth in Siamese fighting fish (Betta splendens Regan, 1910). PhD Thesis (139 pp.). Kasetsart University, Department of Zoology, Bangkok, Thailand.

[78] Thongprajukaew, K., Kovitvadhi, U., Kovitvadhi, S., Somsueb, P., and Rungruangsak-Torrissen, K. (2011). Effects of different modified diets on growth, digestive enzyme activities and muscle compositions in juvenile Siamese fighting fish (*Betta splendens* Regan, 1910). *Aquaculture*, 322–323, 1–9.

[79] Rungruangsak-Torrissen, K. (2002). Wild salmon should not be threatened by healthy and non-genetically manipulated escapees. ICES CM 2002 Documents, ICES Conference, CM 2002/T:07, 16 pp., October 1–5, Copenhagen, Denmark.

In: Trypsin: Structure, Biosynthesis and Functions
Editors: Kirk Weaver and Clayton Kelley
ISBN 978-1-61942-319-0

Chapter II

Trypsins from Submammalian Vertebrates with Special Emphasis on Fish

T. B. Ng *** *and Jack H. Wong*** *****
School of Biomedical Sciences, Faculty of Medicine,
The Chinese University of Hong Kong, Hong Kong, China

Abstract

This article reviews trypsins from submammalian vertebrates including fish, amphibians and birds. A trypsin-like enzyme has been purified from ostrich skeletal muscle.The serine proteases in snake venoms are thrombins and affect platelet aggregation. The trypsins from amphibian sperms and oviducts play a role in fertilization and early development. Trypsins have been isolated from the pylric caeca and intestine of a number of fish species. Some of these trypsins resemble mammalian trypsin in structure.

Keywords: Trypsins, submammalian vertebrates, birds, snakes, amphibians, fish

Introduction

The enzymes trypsin and chymotrypsin are highly homologous. Their mechanisms are similar involving catalytic triads but the substrate specificities are different. Trypsin cleaves at the peptide bond after lysine and arginine whereas chymotrypsin cleaves at the peptide bond after amino acids with an aromatic or long nonpolar side chain like phenylalanine. Elastase is also related to trypsin and chymotrypsin. The purpose of this article is to review trypsins from submammalian vertebrates.

---

* Corresponding authors.

Anguilla Japonica (Eel)

A 26-kDa anionic trypsin 1, with an isoelectric point of 5.5 and an amino acid composition analogous to that of bovine cationic trypsin and anionic trypsins from other fish species, was isolated from *Anguilla japonica* pancreas. The enzyme was stable at pH 6 to 9 in the presence of calcium ions. Km and kcat values of the enzyme for N-tosyl-L-arginine methyl ester and N-tosyl-L-lysine methyl ester resembled those of catfish anionic and bovine cationic trypsins (Yoshinaka et al.,1985).

Two anionic enzymes, trypsins 1 and 2, with similar pH optima of near 8.3 for the hydrolysis of N-tosyl-L-arginine methyl ester, were purified from the eel pancreas. Trypsin 1 was stabilized in the presence of calcium ions but the stability of trypsin 2 was unaffected although both enzymes were inhibited by serine proteinase inhibitors (Yoshinaka et al.,1985).

Asterina Pectinifera (Starfish)

A 28-kDa trypsin with the N-terminal amino acid sequence IVGGHEF was purified from pyloric ceca of *A. pectinifera* by ammonium sulfate precipitation, gel filtration, and cation-exchange chromatography.Its optimum pH and temperature for hydrolysis of N(alpha)-p-tosyl-L-arginine methyl ester hydrochloride were approximately pH 8.0 and 55 degrees C, respectively. It was unstable at above 50 degrees C and below pH 5.0, and $Ca^{(2+)}$ ions did not activate the enzyme (Kishimura et al., 2002).

Boops Boops (Bogue)

A 23- kDa trypsin was isolated from Bogue viscera by ammonium sulphate precipitation, gel filtration on Sephadex G-100 and anion exchange chromatography,on Mono Q-Sepharose. The enzyme exhibited esterase-specific activity toward N-α-benzoyl-L-arginine ethyl ester and amidase activity toward N-α-benzoyl-DL-arginine-p-nitroanilide (BAPNA). Its optimum temperature and pH with BAPNA as substrate were 55°C and pH 9.0, respectively. Its Km, kcat, and kcat/Km on BAPNA were 0.13 mM and 1.56 $s^{(-1)}$, and 12 $s^{(-1)}$ $mM^{(-1)}$, respectively. The enzyme can be used as a possible biotechnological tool in fish processing and food industries (Barkia et al., 2010).

Coryphaenoides Pectoralis (Pectoral Rattail)

A 24- kDa trypsin with the N-terminal amino acid sequence IVGGYECQEHSQ was purified from the pyloric ceca of pectoral rattail *(Coryphaenoides pectoralis)* by using ammonium sulfate precipitation, and chromatography on Sephacryl S-200, DEAE-cellulose and Sephadex G-50. Its optimal pH and temperature, with N(alpha)-p-tosyl-l-arginine methyl ester hydrochloride as substrate were 45 degrees C and pH8.5, respectively. It was stable in the pH range of 6-11 but unstable at temperatures above 40 degrees C. Trypsin was stabilized by calcium ion. Its activity was inhibited by soybean trypsin inhibitor and TLCK and to a lesser extent by EDTA. Its K(m)' K(cat), and K(cat)/K(m)were 0.15 mM, 210 s(-1),and 1400 $s^{(-1)}$ $mM^{(-1)}$ respectively. (Klomklao et al., 2009).

Ctenopharyngodon Idellus (Grass Carp)

Two trypsin isoforms (GT-A and GT-B), with molecular masses of 30.74 kDa and 26.4 kDa, respectively, from the grass carp intestine. Enzyme activity was inhibited by three organic trypsin inhibitors but not by EDTA. Their optimal temperatures and optimal pH values with N-benzoyl-L: -arginine ethyl ester.HCl as substrate were 38.5 and 44.0 degrees C, and pH 8.0 and pH 8.5, respectively,

They lost 95.8 and 93.7% of their activities, respectively, after exposure to 65 degrees C for 20 min. Their thermal denaturation temperatures, were 66.3 and 67.3 degrees C, respectively. GT-A exhibited a K(m) value of 21.2 microM and a V(max) of 2.0 x 10(3) $min^{(-1)}$ whereas GT-B manifested a K(m) value of 31.7 microM and a V(max) of 3.3 x 10(3) $min^{(-1)}$. Their physiological efficiencies were 94.3 and 105.3 $microM^{(-1)}$ $min^{(-1)}$, respectively.

The Arrhenius activation energies of GT-A and GT-B were 4.16 and 4.38 kcal/mol, respectively. The activities of GT-A and GT-B were not activated by $Ca^{(2+)}$ ions, but their thermostability wasenhanced by $Ca^{(2+)}$ ions. Enzyme activity was attenuated by $Zn^{(2+)}$, $Cu^{(2+)}$, $Hg^{(2+)}$ and $Al^{(3+)}$ ions. Thermal stabilities of GT-A and GT-B were intermediate between Arctic and tropical fish species, and consistent with the wide range of water temperatures to which grass carp are exposed in most provinces of China (Liu et al., 2007).

Engraulis Encrasicholus (Anchovy)

Two trypsin-like enzymes, designated trypsin A and B, with a molecular wight of 27kDa and 28kDa and an isoelectric point of about 4.9 and 4.6, respectively,were purified from the pyloric caeca and intestine of anchovy by (NH4)2SO4 fractionation, affinity chromatography on Benzamidine-Sepharose-6B and ion exchange chromatography on DEAE-Sepharose. Both trypsins catalyzed the hydrolysis of N-benzoyl-DL-arginine p-nitroanilide (BAPNA), p-tosyl-L-arginine methyl ester (TAME), casein and myofibrillar protein and inhibited by trypsin-inhibitors. They had similar amino acid compositions. The enzymes had a pH optimum of 8-9 for the hydrolysis of BAPNA and of 9.5 for the digestion of casein and myofibrillar protein. Their activity and stability were affected by calcium ions. Trypsins A and B resemble other fish trypsins in molecular. Weight pI, kinetic properties and stability at low pH and bovine trypsin in dependence on Ca^{2+} ions for activity and stability (Martínez et al.,1988).

Engraulis Japonicus (Japanese Anchovy)

Two isoforms of anchovy trypsin (aT-I and aT-II) were purified from the visceral extracts by $(NH_4)_2SO_4$ fractionation, affinity chromatography, gel filtration, and ion-exchange chromatography. Both were completely inhibited by serine protease inhibitors as well as by specific trypsin inhibitors. The purified anchovy trypsins showed considerably higher catalytic efficiencies (kcat/Km) toward benzoyl-arginine p-nitroanilide and benzoyl-arginine ethyl ester than bovine trypsin at 25 degrees C; in particular, aT-II was 35 times more efficient than its mammalian counterpart.

This was attributed largely to a pronounced fall in Km values for anchovy trypsins, indicative of an evolutionary response toward increased substrate binding at suboptimal temperatures in the marine environment. (Ahsan and Watabe, 2001).

Gadus Morhua (Cod)

Chymotrypsin, trypsin and elastase, with a molecular weight of about 27 kDa and isoelectric points between 5 and 7. 6 have been isolated from cod pyloric caeca by affinity/hydrophobic chromatography on phenyl-butyl-amine substituted Sepharose. The enzymes are quickly inactivated at low pH's (Raae and Walther, 1989)

A trypsin was purified from the pyloric caeca of Atlantic cod (*Gadus morhua*), and separated by chromatofocusing into three forms with similar molecular mass (24.2 kDa) but with different charges (pI 6.6, 6.2 and 5.5). Their N-terminal amino acid sequences were homologous with dogfish and some mammalian trypsins. The apparent Km values determined at 25 degrees C for the predominant form towards p-tosyl-L-arginine methyl ester and N-benzoyl-L-arginine p-nitroanilide were 29 microM and 77 microM respectively, lower than those of bovine trypsin (46 microM and 650 microM respectively). The kcat values for Atlantic cold trypsins were consistently higher than that for bovine trypsin. The higher catalytic efficiency (kcat/Km) of Atlantic cod trypsin compared with bovine trypsin may reflect an evolutionary adaptation of the poikilothermic species to low environmental temperatures(Asgeirsson et al., 1989).

Atlantic cod trypsin I, a cold-adapted protease, demonstrates about 20 times higher catalytic efficiency (kcat/KM) than its mesophilic bovine counterpart for BAPNA. Cold-adapted proteases are sensitive to autolytic degradation, thermal inactivation and molecular aggregation, even at 18-25 degrees C which may account for the problems encountered during expression, activation, and purification. Jónsdóttir et al., (2004) describesd the expression, activation, and purification of recombinant cod trypsin I in the His-Patch ThioFusion *Escherichia coli* expression system. The *E. coli* pThioHis expression vector used facilitated formation of a fusion protein between a highly soluble fraction of HP-thioredoxin contained in the vector and the N-terminal end of the precursor form of cod trypsin I. The HP-thioredoxin part of the fusion protein binds to a metal-chelating ProBond column. The cod trypsin I part of the purified fusion protein was released by proteolysis, leadind to concurrent activation of the recombinant enzyme. The recombinant cod trypsin I was purified to homogeneity on a trypsin-specific benzamidine affinity column. There was a stepwise increase in the catalytic efficiency (k(cat)/K(m)) when substrates containing one to three amino acid residues were used. Its activity was maintained longer at 15 degrees C than at higher temperatures. Eleven autolytic cleavage sites were detected within the molecule. Unfolding experiments demonstrated that autolysis is a contributing factor in its stability.Cod trypsin I is less stable towards thermal unfolding than its mesophilic bovine analogue (Stefansson et al., 2010).

Gadus ogac (Greenland Cod)

A 23.5-kDa trypsin was isolated from pyloric ceca of Greenland cod catalyzed hydrolysis of N alpha-benzoyl-DL-arginine p-nitroanilide, tosyl arginine methyl ester and protein.The enzyme was inhibited by the serine protease inhibitor PMSF and other trypsin inhibitors.It was more stable at alkaline pH than at acid pH; and was thermolabile. Like other trypsins, the enzyme had a rich content of acidic amino acid residues but a low content of basic amino acid residues.(Simpson BK and Haard NF 1984).

Lithognathus Mormyrus (Striped Seabream)

A 27.5- kDa alkaline trypsin was purified from the intestine of striped seabream (*Lithognathus mormyrus*) by ammonium sulfate precipitation, gel filtration on Sephadex G-100 and cation-exchange chromatography on CM-Sephadex.It was highly active using N-alpha-benzoyl-dl-arginine-p-nitroanilide as substrate over a wide range of pH from 8.0 to 11.0, with an optimum at pH 10.0. The relative activities at pH 8.0, 11.0, and 12.0 were 73%, 67% and 50.4%, respectively.

The enzyme was extremely stable over a pH range of 5.0-12.0.Its optimum temperature was 50 degrees C. Th enzyme was strongly inhibited by soybean trypsin inhibitor). In addition,it displayed remarkable stability toward various surfactants and bleach agents and compatibility with some commercial solid and liquid detergents.Its Km kcat, and kcat/Km, on BAPNA, were 0.29 mM and 1.36 $s^{(-1)}$, respectively, while the catalytic efficiency was 4.68 $s^{(-1)}$ $mM^{(-1)}$.(El Hadj Ali et al., 2009).

Mustelus Mustelus (Smooth Hound)

A 24- kDa trypsin with the N-terminal amino acid sequence IVGGYECKPHSQ f was purified from the intestine of smooth hound (*Mustelus mustelus*) by ammonium sulfate fractionation, gel filtration on Sephadex G-75, and ion exchange chromatography on DEAE-cellulose,. The purified enzyme showed esterase-specific activity on N(alpha)-p-tosyl-L-arginine methyl ester hydrochloride (TAME) that was four times greater than its amidase-specific activity on Nalpha-benzoyl-DL-arginine-p-nitroanilide (BAPNA). Its optimum temperature and pH using TAME as a substrate were 50 degrees C and pH 8.5, respectively,. The enzyme was extremely stable in the pH range of 7.0-9.0 and highly stable up to 40 degrees C after 1 h of incubation.

The purified enzyme was strongly inhibited by soybean trypsin inhibitor and N-p-tosyl-1-lysine chloromethyl ketone.The trypsin showed higher proteolytic activity at high NaCl concentration, demonstrating its potential for protein hydrolysis at high salt content.It exhibited a (K(m)) and (K(cat)) of 0.387 +/- 0.02 mM and 2.62 +/- 0.11 $s^{(-1)}$, respectively, when BAPNA was used as a substrate. For the hydrolysis of TAME, K(m) and K(cat) were 0.156 +/- 0.01 mM and 59.15 +/- 2.2 $s^{(-1)}$, respectively.

Oncorhynchus sp. (Pacific Salmon)

A 22.5- kDa trypsin with an amino acid composition typical of anionic trypsins was purified from pyloric caeca of Pacific salmon by affinity chromatography on hexamethylenediamine- glycidylmethacrylate-cellulose. It differed from the cationic trypsins by a lower content of lysine residues.

The differences in properties caused by change of the enzyme molecule charge are similar to those observed in cationic trypsin when the lysine epsilon-amino groups of the latter are modified (change of pI, shift of the pH-optimum towards basic values, increase of stability to autolysis). An unusual interaction of the enzyme with the specific inhibitor N-L-tosyl-L-lysine chloromethyl ketone was observed. (Pivnenko et al., 1989).

Oncorhynchus Keta (Chum Salmon)

A 24 -kDa anionic trypsin from pyloric caeca of chum salmon (*Oncorhynchus keta*) was purified by ammonium sulfate and acetone fractionation, affinity chromatography, gel-filtration, and DEAE-anion exchange chromatography. The enzyme was moderately active toward esterase substrates such as tosyl-L-arginine methyl ester and tosyl-L-lysine methyl ester. Its amidase activity toward benzoyl-L-arginine p-nitroanilide was similar to those of bovine and *Streptomyces griseus* trypsins. (Sekizaki et al., 2000).

Oncorhynchus Masou (Masu Salmon)

A 24-k Da trypsin with the N-terminal amino acid sequence IVGGYECKAYSQPHQVSLNS was isolated from the pyloric ceca of masu salmon cultured in fresh wate. The purification procedure entailed gel filtration on Sephacryl S-200 and Sephadex G-50 and ion exchange chromatography on diethylaminoethyl cellulose.

The enzyme was strongly inhibited by phenylmethylsulfonyl fluoride, soybean trypsin inhibitor, and N (alpha)-p-tosyl-L: -lysine chloromethyl ketone, and stabilized by calcium ions. Its optimum pH was around pH 8.5, and was unstable below pH 5.0.Its optimum temperature was around 60 degrees C, and was stable below 50 degrees C, like trypsins from temperate-zone and tropical-zone fish (Kanno et al., 2010).

Oncorhynchus Tshawytscha (Chinook Salmon)

A 28- kDa trypsin fraction was isolated from the pyloric ceca of New Zealand farmed chinook salmon by ammonium sulfate fractionation, acetone precipitation and affinity chromatography. The enzyme hydrolyzedDL-BAPNA and was inhibited by phenyl methyl sulfonyl fluoride, and also by the specific trypsin inhibitors - soybean trypsin inhibitor and benzamidine. The enzyme was active over a broad pH range (from 7.5 to at least pH 10.0) at 25 degrees C and was stable from pH 4.0 to pH 10.0 at 20 degrees C, with a maximum at pH 8.0. Its optimum temperature was 60 degrees C, but was unstable at temperatures above 40 degrees C. (Kurtovic et al., 2006).

Oreochromis Niloticus x O.aureus (Hybrid Tilapia)

A 22-k Da trypsin was purified from the intestine of hybrid tilapiaby acetone precipitation, ammonium sulfate fractionation, gel filtration on Sephacryl S-200, and ion exchange chromatography on DEAE-sephacel. Its optimum temperature and pH for casein hydrolysis were 60 degrees C and 9.0, respectively. It was stable over a pH range from 7.0 to 12.0 at 30 degrees C, and inactive at temperatures above 50 degrees C.

Its Km was 0.46 mg/mL. It was inhibited by phenyl methyl sulphonyl fluoride and also N-p-tosyl-L-lysine chloromethyl ketone (TLCK) using Nalpha-CBZ-L-lysine p-nitrophenyl ester hydrochloride as a substrate. The protease was inhibited by the following ions in decreasing order: $Zn^{2+}>Fe^{3+}>Cu^{2+}>Al^{3+}>Co^{2+}=Pb^{2+}>Cd^{2+}>Mn^{2+}$. The ions Li^{+}, Na^{+}, K^{+}, Mg^{2+}, and Ba^{2+} had little effect on the enzyme, and Ca2+ can partially promote its activity at low concentration (Wang et al.,2010).

Pomatomus Saltatrix (Bluefish)

A 28- kDa trypsin with the N-terminal amino acid sequence IVGGYECKPKSAPVQVSLNL was purified from the pyloric caeca of bluefish (*Pomatomus saltatrix*) by ammonium sulfate precipitation, acetone precipitation and affinity chromatography on soybean trypsin inhibitor-Sepharose 4B. Its optima temperature and pH using benzoyl-dl-arginine-p-nitroanilide (BAPNA) as substrate were 55 degrees C and pH 9.5, respectively.

The enzyme was stable over a broad pH range (7 to 12), but was unstable at acidic pH, and at temperatures above 40 degrees C. The enzyme was inhibited by soybean trypsin inhibitor, N-p-tosyl-l-lysine chloromethyl ketone and phenylmethyl sulfonylfluoride. CaCl2 partially protected the enzyme against activity loss at 40 degrees C, but NaCl (0 to 30%) reduced the activity in a concentration- dependent manner. (Klomklao et al.,2007).

Protopterus Aethiopicus (African Lungfish)

Three pancreatic trypsinogens A1, A2, and A3, with the same amino-terminal amino acid sequence Leu-Pro-Leu-Glu-Asp-Asp-Lys-.were isolated from the African lungfish. They were activated by trypsin, enterokinase, acid protease from *Aspergillus oryzae*, and autoactivation. Their amino acid sequences differ from the homologous trypsinogen B signifying that trypsinogens A and B are products of different gene loci (de Haën et al.,1977).

Salmo Salar (Atlantic Salmon)

The crystal structure of cationic trypsin from the Atlantic salmon has been refined at 1.70 A resolution. The crystals are orthorhombic, belong to space group P212121, with lattice parameters a = 65.91, b = 83.11 and c = 154.79 A, and comprise four molecules per asymmetric unit. The structure was solved by molecular replacement with AMoRe and refined with X-PLOR to an R value of 17.4% and Rfree of 21.5% for reflections |F| > 3sigmaF between 8.0 and 1.7 A resolution. The four non-crystallographic symmetry related molecules in the asymmetric unit display r.m.s. deviations in the range 0.31-0.74 A for main-chain atoms, with the largest differences confined to two loops.

One of these is the calcium-binding loop where the electron-density indicates a calcium ion for only one of the four molecules. In order to find structural rationalizations for the observed difference in thermostability and catalytic efficiency of cationic trypsin, anionic salmon trypsin and bovine trypsin, the three structures have been extensively compared. The largest deviations for the superimposed structures occur in the surface loops and particularly in the so-called 'autolysis loop'. Both the salmon enzymes possess a high methionine content, lower overall hydrophobicity and enhanced surface hydrophilicity, compared with bovine trypsin. These properties have so far been correlated to cold-adaptation features, while in this work it is shown that the non-psychrophilic cationic salmon trypsin shares these features with the psychrophilic anionic salmon trypsin (Schrøder et al., 1998).

Sarda sarda (Atlantic Bonito)

A 29-kDa trypsin with an N-terminal amino acid sequence IVGGYECQAHSQPWQPVLNS was purified from the pyloric ceca of Atlantic bonito (*Sarda sarda*). Its optimal temperature and pH with BAPNA as substrate were 65 degrees C and pH 9. The enzyme was stable up to 50 degrees C and within the pH range of 7-12. It was stabilized by calcium ions, but its activity was strongly inhibited by soybean trypsin inhibitor, N-p-tosyl-L-lysine chloromethyl ketone, and phenyl methyl sulfonyl fluoride. The enzyme underwent a progressive decrement in activity when the NaCl concentrationwas elevated. (Klomklao et al., 2007).

Sardinops Sagax Caerulea (Monterey Sardine)

A 25- kDa trypsin from pyloric caeca of Monterey sardine was purified using a protocol that involved ammonium sulfate fractionation, gel filtration, affinity chromatography and ionic exchange. The enzyme displayed esterase-specific activity toward Nalpha-p-tosyl-L-arginine methyl ester (TAME) that was 4.5 times greater than amidase-specific activity toward N-benzoyl-L-arginine-p-nitroanilide. It was partially inhibited by the serine-protease inhibitor phenyl-methyl-sulfonyl fluoride and totallly inhibited by soybean trypsin inhibitor and benzamidine, but was not inhibited by the metallo-protease inactivator EDTA or the chymotrypsin inhibitor tosyl-L-phenylalanine chloromethyl-ketone. Its optimum pH was 8.0 and maximum stability was noted between pH 7 and 8. A pronounced decline in stability was noted below pH 4 and above pH 11. Its optimum temperature was 50 degrees C and. Its K(m), k(cat), and (k(cat)/K(m)) were 0.051 mM and 2.12 $s^{(-1)}$, and 41 $s^{(-1)}$ $mM^{(-1)}$, respectively. Monterey sardine trypsin generally resembles other fish trypsins, especially those from the anchovy *Engraulis japonica* and *Engraulis encrasicholus.*

Thunnus Tonggo (Tongol Tuna)

A 24-kDa trypsin with an N-terminal amino acid sequence IVGGYECQAHSQPHQVSLNA was purified from tongol tuna (*Thunnus tonggol*) spleens by ammonium sulfate precipitation and column chromatographic procedures. Its optimal temperature and pH were 65 degrees C and pH 8.5, respectively. It was stable in the pH range of 6-11 but unstable at temperatures above 50 degrees C. Calcium ions are crucial for thermostability. The activity was strongly inhibited by 1.0 g/L soybean trypsin inhibitor and 5 mM TLCK and to a lesser extent by 2 mM ethylenediaminetetraacetic acid. Activity was reduced as the NaCl concentration was increased. Its Km for Nalpha-p-tosyl-L-arginine methyl ester hydrochloride was 0.25 mM and Kcat was 200 s^{-1}. (Klomklao et al., 2006).

Xenopus Laevis

Three *Xenopus* cDNAs encoding trypsin-like serine proteases designated as *Xenopus* embryonic serine protease (Xesp)-1, Xesp-2, and XMT-SP1, a homolog of human MT-SP1, have been identified from *Xenopus laevis*. Xesp-1 is a secreted protein that functions in the extracellular space. Xesp-2 and XMP-SP1 are type II membrane proteases with multidomain structures. Xesp-2 displays eight low density lipoprotein receptor (LDLR) domains and one scavenger receptor cysteine-rich (SRCR) domain. XMT-SP1 exhibits four LDLR domains and two CUB domains. The temporal expressions of these genes have distinctive patterns during embryogenesis, and different distribution in adult tissues. Overexpression of Xesp-2 or XMT-SP1 but not Xesp-1 brought about defective gastrulation or apoptosis, suggesting that these proteases may play important roles during early development such as regulation of cell movement in gastrulae (Yamada, 2000).

The glycoprotein envelope around the *Xenopus laevis* egg is changed from an unfertilizable to a fertilizable form during passage through the pars recta portion of the oviduct envelope. The pars recta protease oviductin, which selectively hydrolyzes envelope glycoprotein gp43 to gp4, plays a role in the conversion. Dring post-translational proteolytic processing of the mosaic oviductin glycoprotein, the processed N-terminal protease domain is released coupled to two C-terminal CUB domains and constitutes the enzymatically active protease molecule. In functional studies, isolated coelomic egg envelopes treated with oviductin demonstrated a striking increase in sperm binding, proving the identity of oviductin as the oviductal factor for converting the egg envelope to a sperm-penetrable form, via an increase in sperm binding. Trypsin mimicked the effect of oviductin on envelope hydrolysis and sperm binding, demonstrating that gp43 processing is the only requirement for envelope conversion (Lindsay et al., 1999).

Egg activation in cross-fertilization between *Xenopus* eggs and *Cynops* sperm may be attributed to protease activity against Boc-Gly-Arg-Arg-MCA in the sperm acrosome. The tryptic protease was inhibited by trypsin inhibitors. The protease induces activation in *Xenopus* eggs and fertilization, most probably by taking part in egg activation (Mizote et al.,1999).

Bufo Arenarum (Toad)

When the jelly-less eggs collected from the most cephalic region of the toad oviduct were inseminated with a high concentration of sperms, fertilization often resulted. In contrast, control eggs taken from the pleuroperitoneal cavity (coelomic eggs) were not fertilized under the same conditions. However, fertilization was achieved when coelomic eggs were preincubated in the presence of the fluid secreted by the ovidutal epithelium or oviductal extract.The active principle contributing to this effect acts on the vitelline envelope of the egg, rendering it more susceptible to sperm lysine and more easily penetrable by sperms. The active factor was a 47-kDa trypsin-like enzyme inhibitable by trypsin inhibitors from soybean and lima-bean. Its secretion is dependent on the pituitary and its activity is not influenced by pH 6.0--8.4 (Miceli et al., 1978)

Bothrops Atrox (Snake)

A 33-kDa serine protease from *Bothrops atrox* (Peruvian specimen's venom) was isolated bygel filtration and reverse phase-HPLC. It exhibited a pI of 5.06, a Km of 0.2 x $10^{(-1)}$ M and a V (máx) of 4.1 x $10^{(-1)}$ nmoles p-NA/lt/min on the synthetic substrate BapNA. It was also capable of coagulating bovine fibrinogen. Soybean trypsin inhibitor inhibited the serine protease. Its primary structure possessed His(44), Asp(94) and Ser(193) residues in the positions corresponding to the catalytic triad established in serine proteases. It had 293 amino acid residues and the primary structure was VIGGDECDIN EHPFLAFMYY SPRYFCGMTL INQEWVLTAA HCRYFCGMTL IHLGVHRESE KANYDEVRRF PKEKYFIFCD NNFTDDEVDK DIMLIRLDKP VSNSEHIAPL SLPSNPPSVG SVCRIMGWGQ TTTSPIDVLS PDEPHCANIN LFDNTVCHTA HPQVANTRTS TDTLCAGDLQ GGRDTCNGDS GGPLICNEQL HGILSWGGDP CAQPNKPAFY TKVYYFDHPW IKSIIAGNKK TVNFTCPPLR SDAKDDSTTY INQEWDWVLT AEHCDRTHMR NSFYDYSSIN SDS (Ponce-Soto et al., 2007).

Bothrops Jararaca (Snake)

A 30-kDa platelet-aggregating enzyme was isolated from the venom. It catalyzed the hydrolysis of several p-nitroanilide peptide substrates containing Arg or Lys at the scissile bond; among these the most sensitive were the thrombin substrates D-Phe-Pip-Arg-pNA and Tos-Gly-Pro-Arg-pNA. The platelet-aggregating and amidolytic activities of PA-BJ were destroyed by phenylmethanesulfonyl fluoride and the amidolytic activity by benzamidine derivatives which competitively inhibit trypsin-like serine proteinases. Among the compounds tested, the thrombin inhibitor NAPAP [N alpha-[(2-naphthylsulfonyl)-glycyl]-4-amidinophenylalanine piperidide] displayed the most potent inhibitory activity. PA-BJ is composed of 232 amino acid residues and contains one N- and one O-glycosidically linked carbohydrate moiety at amino acid residues Asn20 and Ser23. Sequence comparison with other venom serine proteinases disclosed homology in regions around the catalytic triad and conserved cysteine residues (Serrano et al., 1995).

Struthio Camelus (Ostrich)

A 21-kDa myofibril-bound tryptic-like serine protease was purified from ostrich (*Struthio camelus*) skeletal muscle. The protease was dissociated from the myofibrillar fraction by ethylene glycol treatment at pH 8.5, followed by purification on Toyopearl Super Q 650 S and p-aminobenzamidine column. Its optima temperature and pH were 40 degrees C and pH 8, respectively.The protease cleaved synthetic fluorogenic substrates at the carboxyl side of arginine residues. Ostrich MBSP exhibited low sequence identity to bovine trypsin (44%), myofibril-bound serine protease from lizard fish skeletal muscle (33%) and trypsinogen from ostrich pancreas (22%) (Tshidino et al., 2009).

Discussion

From the foregoing account it can be seen that the bulk of information on submammalian trypsins is derived from fish gastrointestinal trypsins and that there is much less information available about trypsins from amphibians and birds which were isolated from the oviduct/sperms and skeletal muscle, respectively. The snake serine proteases are related to thrombin. Some of the fish trypsins differ in molecular weight,optimum pH, optimum temperature, Km and Kcat while others exhibit homology in N-terminal sequence. It is envisaged that trypsin will be reported from more organisms in the future and an insight into the chemical structures and physiological significance of these enzymes will be gained.

References

Ahsan MN, Watabe S. Kinetic and structural properties of two isoforms of trypsin isolated from the viscera of Japanese anchovy, *Engraulis japonicus*. *J Protein Chem.* 2001;20: 49-58.

Asgeirsson B, Fox JW, Bjarnason JB. Purification and characterization of trypsin from the poikilotherm *Gadus morhua*. *Eur J Biochem.* 1989 1;180:85-94.

Barkia A, Bougatef A, Nasri R, Fetoui E, Balti R, Nasri M. Trypsin from the viscera of Bogue (*Boops boops*): isolation and characterisation. *Fish Physiol Biochem.* 2010;36:893-902.

Bougatef A, Balti R, Nasri R, Jellouli K, Souissi N, Nasri M. Biochemical properties of anionic trypsin acting at high concentration of NaCl purified from the intestine of a carnivorous fish: smooth hound (*Mustelus mustelus*).*J Agric Food Chem.* 2010;58: 5763-9.

Castillo-Yáñez FJ, Pacheco-Aguilar R, García-Carreño FL, Navarrete-Del Toro Mde L. Isolation and characterization of trypsin from pyloric caeca of Monterey sardine *Sardinops sagax caerulea. Comp Biochem Physiol B Biochem Mol Biol.* 2005;140:91-8.

de Haën C, Walsh KA, Neurath H. Isolation and amino-terminal sequence analysis of a new pancreatic trypsinogen of the African lungfish *Protopterus protopterus. Biochemistry.* 1977;16:4421-5.

El Hadj Ali N, Hmidet N, Bougatef A, Nasri R, Nasri M. A laundry detergent-stable alkaline trypsin from striped seabream (*Lithognathus mormyrus*) viscera: purification and characterization. *J Agric Food Chem.* 2009 25;57:10943-50.

Jónsdóttir G, Bjarnason JB, Gudmundsdóttir A. Recombinant cold-adapted trypsin I from Atlantic cod-expression, purification, and identification. *Protein Expr Purif.* 2004;33:110-22.

Kanno G, Yamaguchi T, Kishimura H, Yamaha E, Saeki H. Purification and characteristics of trypsin from masu salmon (*Oncorhynchus masou*) cultured in fresh-water. *Fish Physiol Biochem.* 2010;36:637-45.

Klomklao S, Benjakul S, Visessanguan W, Kishimura H, Simpson BK. Trypsin from the pyloric caeca of bluefish (*Pomatomus saltatrix*). *Comp Biochem Physiol B Biochem Mol Biol. 2007;148:382-9.*

Klomklao S, Kishimura H, Benjakul S. Trypsin from the pyloric ceca of pectoral rattail (*Coryphaenoides pectoralis*): purification and characterization. *J Agric Food Chem.* 2009 Aug 12;57(15):7097-103.

Klomklao S, Benjakul S, Visessanguan W, Kishimura H, Simpson BK. 29 kDa Trypsin from the pyloric ceca of Atlantic Bonito (Sarda sarda): recovery and characterization. *J Agric Food Chem.* 2007 May 30;55(11):4548-53.

Klomklao S, Benjakul S, Visessanguan W, Kishimura H, Simpson BK. *Purification and characterization of trypsin from the spleen of tongol tuna (Thunnus tonggol). J Agric Food Chem.* 2006 Jul 26;54(15):5617-22.

Kishimura H, Hayashi K. Isolation and characteristics of trypsin from pyloric ceca of the starfish *Asterina pectinifera. Comp Biochem Physiol B Biochem Mol Biol.* 2002 Jun;132(2):485-90.

Kurtovic I, Marshall SN, Simpson BK. Isolation and characterization of a trypsin fraction from the pyloric ceca of chinook salmon (Oncorhynchus *tshawytscha). Comp Biochem Physiol B Biochem Mol Biol.* 2006 Apr;143(4):432-40.

Liu ZY, Wang Z, Xu SY, Xu LN. Two trypsin isoforms from the intestine of the grass carp (*Ctenopharyngodon idellus). J Comp Physiol* B. 2007 Aug;177(6):655-66.

Martínez A, Olsen RL, Serra JL. Purification and characterization of two trypsin-like enzymes from the digestive tract of anchovy *Engraulis encrasicholus. Comp Biochem Physiol B.* 1988;91(4):677-84.

Lindsay LL, Wieduwilt MJ, Hedrick JL. Oviductin, the *Xenopus laevis* oviductal protease that processes egg envelope glycoprotein gp43, increases sperm binding to envelopes, and is translated as part of an unusual mosaic protein composed of two protease and several CUB domains. *Biol Reprod.* 1999 Apr;60(4):989-95.

Miceli DC, Fernández SN, Raisman JS, Barbieri FD. A trypsin-like oviducal proteinase involved in *Bufo arenarum* fertilization. *J Embryol Exp Morphol.* 1978 Dec;48:79-91.

Mizote A, Okamoto S, Iwao Y. Activation of *Xenopus* eggs by proteases: possible involvement of a sperm protease in fertilization. *Dev Biol.* 1999 Apr 1;208(1):79-92.

Ponce-Soto LA, Bonfim VL, Novello JC, Navarro Oviedo R, Yarlequé Chocas A, Marangoni S. Isolation and characterization of a serine protease, Ba III-4, from Peruvian *Bothrops atrox* venom. *Protein J.* 2007 ;26:387-94.

Pivnenko TN, Epshteĭn LM, Kolodzeĭskaia MV, Kudinov SA Preparation and properties of trypsin from the pyloric caeca of Pacific Ocean salmon. *Prikl Biokhim Mikrobiol.* 1989 Jul-Aug;25(4):490-7.

Raae AJ, Walther BT. Purification and characterization of chymotrypsin, trypsin and elastase like proteinases from cod (*Gadus morhua L.*). *Comp Biochem Physiol B.* 1989;93(2): 317-24.

Schrøder HK, Willassen NP, Smalås AO. Structure of a non-psychrophilic trypsin from a cold-adapted fish species. *Acta Crystallogr D Biol Crystallogr.* 1998 Sep 1;54(Pt 5): 780-98.

Sekizaki H, Itoh K, Murakami M, Toyota E, Tanizawa K. Anionic trypsin from chum salmon: activity with p-amidinophenyl ester and comparison with bovine and *Streptomyces griseus* trypsins. *Comp Biochem Physiol B Biochem Mol Biol.* 2000 Nov;127(3):337-46.

Serrano SM, Mentele R, Sampaio CA, Fink E. Purification, characterization, and amino acid sequence of a serine proteinase, PA-BJ, with platelet-aggregating activity from the venom of *Bothrops jararaca*. *Biochemistry.* 1995;34:7186-93.

Simpson BK, Haard NF. Trypsin from Greenland cod, *Gadus ogac*. Isolation and comparative properties. *Comp Biochem Physiol B.* 1984;79(4):613-22.

Stefansson B, Helgadóttir L, Olafsdottir S, Gudmundsdottir A, Bjarnason JB. Characterization of cold-adapted Atlantic cod (*Gadus morhua*) trypsin I--kinetic parameters, autolysis and thermal stability. *Comp Biochem Physiol B Biochem Mol Biol.* 2010 Feb;155(2):186-94.

Tshidino SC, Krause J, Adebiyi AP, Muramoto K, Naudé RJ. Purification and partial characterization of a myofibril-bound serine protease from ostrich skeletal muscle. *Comp Biochem Physiol B Biochem Mol Biol.* 2009 Oct;154(2):229-34.

Wang Q, Gao ZX, Zhang N, Shi Y, Xie XL, Chen QX. Purification and characterization of trypsin from the intestine of hybrid tilapia (*Oreochromis niloticusxO.aureus*). *J Agric Food Chem.* 2010 Jan 13;58(1):655-9.

Yamada K, Takabatake T, Takeshima K. Isolation and characterization of three novel serine protease genes from Xenopus laevis. *Gene.* 2000 Jul 11;252(1-2):209-16.

Yoshinaka R, Sato M, Suzuki T, Ikeda S. Characterization of an anionic trypsin from the eel (*Anguilla japonica*). *Comp Biochem Physiol B.* 1985;80(1):11-4.

Yoshinaka R, Sato M, Suzuki T, Ikeda S. Purification and some properties of two anionic trypsins from the eel (*Anguilla japonica*). *Comp Biochem Physiol B.* 1985;80(1):5-9.

In: Trypsin: Structure, Biosynthesis and Functions
Editors: Kirk Weaver and Clayton Kelley
ISBN 978-1-61942-319-0

Chapter III

Functions/Applications of Trypsin in Food Processing and Food Science Research

Jianmei Yu * ***and Mohamed Ahmedna*** ‡
Department of Family and Consumer Science,
North Carolina AandT State University, Greensboro, USA
Center of Excellence in Post Harvest Technologies,
North Carolina AandT State University, Kannapolis, USA

Abstract

Trypsin is a serine protease in the digestive system of human and animals. The main function of this enzyme is to hydrolyze proteins into smaller peptides or even amino acids. Trypsin and other digestive proteases such as chymotrypsin are responsible for the digestion of food protein in the small intestine. This proteolytic function of trypsin has been widely used in protein chemistry, proteomics and nutrition research. This function is influenced by the sources of enzyme, and environmental factors such as pH, temperature, and the presence of trypsin inhibitors in the enzymatic reaction medium. In food processing, trypsin or a trypsin preparation which usually contains other enzymes has been used to improve both the functional and nutritional quality of food proteins. This chapter provides a review of the sources of trypsin preparation for food processing and the applications trypsin in food processing to 1) improve the functional properties such as solubility, emulsification, foaming and gelling properties of food proteins, 2) improve the digestibility of vegetable and seed proteins, 3) produce protein hydrolysates and bioactive peptides that are used in infant formulas and for people with special health problems such as hypertension, and 4) reduce the concentration of allergens in some foods. The applications of trypsin in food science research including food protein sequencing, *in*

* Department of Family and Consumer Science, North Carolina A&T State University, 1601 East market Street, Greensboro, NC 27411. Phone: 336-334-7963, Fax: 336-334-7239, Email: jyu@ncat.edu
‡ Center of Excellence in Post Harvest Technologies, North Carolina A&T State University, 500 Laureate Way, Suite 4222, Kannapolis, NC 28081. Phone: 704-250-5700, Fax: 704-2505709, Email: Ahmedna@ncat.edu

vitro determination of food protein digestibility, and evaluating the impacts of food processing methods on the activity of trypsin inhibitors are also covered in this chapter.

1. Introduction

Trypsin is a serine protease in the digestive system of human and animals. The enzyme is excreted by the pancreas. Trypsin and other digestive proteases such as chymotrypsin are responsible for the digestion of food protein in the small intestine. Trypsin cleaves peptides on the C-terminal side of lysine and arginine amino acid residues (Whitaker et al., 2003). Trypsin has been used in the development of cell and tissue culture protocols (Soleimani *et al.* 2009, Banumathi *et al.* 2009, and Yang *et al.* 2009), as well as protein identification through peptide sequencing techniques (Schuchert *et al.* 2009). Trypsin is also one of the most widely used enzymes that are used either alone or with other enzyme preparations in food processing. Proteases are produced naturally by many microbes; they also occur in many animals and plants. Many foodstuffs (meat, cheese, fish, fruits) also contain proteases.

Food proteins not only play critical roles in human and animal nutrition, but are also extremely important to the sensory quality of processed foods. In the past 20 years, the use of plant proteins from beans, peas and seeds in food product development has increased remarkably due to the absence of cholesterol and low cost compared to the proteins of animal origin. However, many plant proteins have lower nutritional quality (Krajcovicova-Kudlackova et al., 2005) and poor functionality compared to animal proteins (Damodaran, 2005; Drago and Conzález, 2001). Moreever, some proteins of plant origin cause allergic reactions in certain populations (Sicherer and Sampson, 2010). These disadvantages have limited the use of plant proteins in food and feed products. Therefore, numerous research efforts have attempted to improve their nutritional, functional and safety properties in order to make better use of plant proteins as food ingredients. In addition, milk proteins (caseins and whey proteins) have also been physically, chemically or enzymatically modified to produce bioactive peptides. Among different protein modification methods, enzymatic modifications using commercially available protease preparations or specific enzymes are the most widely used in food processing due to the economic and nutritional safety considerations (Damodaran, 2005; Kunst, 2003).

2. Sources of Trypsin Preparation for Food Applications

Traditionally food enzymes have been obtained from a number of different sources, for example by extraction from plant or animal tissues. Trypsin is often extracted and purified from animal pancreas such as porcine, bovine and ovine pancreases. Recently, considerable attention has been given to trypsin production from pyloric cecum of Atlantic cod, an economically important fish species in Iceland and elsewhere in the Northern hemisphere (Gudmundsdóttir and Pálsdóttir, 2005).The pyloric cecum, a digestive organ in the Atlantic cod, is a by-product of the fishing industry that is rich in digestive enzymes such as serine proteases (Ásgeirsson et al., 1989), particularly, trypsin. So far, the best characterized Atlantic cod adapted trypsins are the classic trypsin I (Stefansson et al., 2009) and recombinant trypsin Y (Spilliaert and Gudmundsdóttir, 1999). Trypsins from the Atlantic cod and other fish adapted to cold environments differ somewhat from their mammalian analogues in that they have higher catalytic efficiencies, especially at low temperatures (Ásgeirsson *et al.*, 1989; Gudmundsdóttir and Pálsdóttir, 2005). These enzymes are also more sensitive to inactivation by heat, low pH and autolysis than their mesophilic analogues (Ásgeirsson *et al.*, 1989). Some commercial trypsin containing protease preparations produced from animal tissues are Corolase PP, porcine pancreatin, PEM 2500s (porcinehovine), PEM *800s* (bovine), PEM 2700s (bovine), and PTN 3.0s (porcine) (McDonagh and FitzGeral, 1998; Mullally et al., 1994). However, enzyme production based on extraction from plant or animal sources suffers from a number of drawbacks, particularly: the limitations of raw material supplies and the low enzyme content in the raw material. A specialized process for each enzyme product is required. In many cases the raw material itself raises serious safety concerns of the enzyme product (Hjort, 2007).

A different way of producing food enzymes is through microbial fermentation. Microbial fermentation processes and the raw materials used can be much better controlled than in the case of protease extraction from plants and animal organs. Microbial enzymes used in food processing are sold as *enzyme preparations* that typically contain not only a desired enzyme activity but also other enzymes and metabolites of the production strain, as well as added materials such as preservatives and stabilizers (Pariza and Johnson, 2001; Olempska-Beer et al., 2006). Commercial microbial enzyme preparations that contain trypsin activity include but are not limited to Alcalase (a *Bacillus licheniformis* protease preparation commercialized by Novozymes), Protamex (a Bacillus protease complex developed by DSM Nutritional products Inc.), and Pronase (produced by Roche Applied Science), Fungal Protease, and Debitrase DBP.20 (*Lactococcus lactis, Aspergillus oryzae*, Imperial Biotechnology Ltd., London, U.K) (McDonagh and FitzGeral, 1998; Mullally et al., 1994). Microbials generally used to produce food protease preparations are *Penicillium* spp., *Aspergillus* spp., *Rhizopus* spp., *Rhizomucor* spp., *Mucor* spp. or *Candida* spp., *Bacillus* and *Lactococcus lactis* (Kilcawley et al., 2002).

The safety, particularly the toxigenic potential of the enzyme producing strain remains the primary consideration in evaluating enzyme safety in food applications. Thoroughly characterized nonpathogenic, nontoxigenic microbial strains, particularly those with a history of safe use in food enzyme manufacture, are logical candidates for generating a safe strain lineage, through which improved strains may be derived via genetic modification by using either traditional/classical methods or rDNA strain improvement strategies (Pariza and Johnson, 2001). In addition, all added materials for food grade enzyme preparation must be food grade and meet applicable regulatory standards. For more details about the evaluation of the safety of microbial enzymes, readers are referred to the extensive literature reviews written by Pariza and Johnson (2001) and Olempska-Beer et al. (2006).

Many enzymes currently used in food processing are derived from recombinant microorganisms. Such enzymes often originate from microorganisms that cannot be easily cultured under laboratory or industrial conditions. By judicious selection of host microorganisms, recombinant production strains can be constructed to allow efficient production of enzymes that are substantially free of undesirable enzymes or other microbial metabolites. *B. subtilis* and *B. licheniformis, Escherichia coli* K-12, *P. fuorescens, A. oryzae, A. niger,* and *F. venenatum,* are some of the host microorganisms for the recombinant production of food enzymes (Olempska-Beer et al.2006). In 1990, bovine chymosin, a milk-clotting enzyme (also known as rennin), expressed in *Escherichia coli* K-12 became the first recombinant enzyme approved for use in food by the US Food and Drug Administration (FDA) (Olempska-Beer et al., 2006).

Trypsin meets the general requirements and additional requirements for enzyme preparations in the Food Chemicals Codex, and is affirmed as GRAS (Generally Recognized as Safe) by the United States Food and Drug Administration (FDA) under 21 CFR 184.1914. In Canada, trypsin is approved as a "Food additive that may be used as food enzymes" (Item Code T.1, and added 14-12-89) permitted in or upon "hydrolyzed animal, milk or vegetable proteins." In the European Union and other parts of the world, trypsin was evaluated in 1971 by JECFA (Joint Expert Committee on Food Additives) as animal enzyme preparation for baking, tenderizing of meat and production of protein hydrolysates (*www.neovatech.com/pdfs/pancreatic/pancreatic_food.pdf*).

3. The Applications of Trypsin to Improve Functional Properties of Food Proteins

3.1. Functional Properties of Food Ingredients/Components

Functional properties of proteins were defined as those physical and chemical properties that affect the behavior of proteins in food systems during processing, storage, preparation, and consumption (Kinsella 1982), including hydration properties (solubility, water absorption and water binding), emulsification, foaming, gelation, elasticity, viscosity, fat absorption and binding, and flavor binding (deMan, 1999). These properties are affected by the intrinsic factors of protein such as molecular structure and size, and many environmental factors including the method of protein separation/production, pH, ionic strength, and the presence of other components in the food system (Damodaran, 2006). The importance of these properties varies with the type of food products in which the protein is used. For example, gelation is important in comminuted meats, while emulsification and foaming are important in coffee creamers and dessert toppings, respectively. Plant storage proteins such as legume proteins and oil seed proteins are globular proteins characterized with secondary and tertiary structures involving disulfide linkages and hydrophobic interactions between amino acid residues within the same molecule or between molecules. They usually have low solubility at acidic and neutral pH. Enzymatic hydrolysis of proteins is accompanied by three distinct effects: decrease in molecular weight, increase in the number of ionizable groups, and the exposure of hydrophobic groups hitherto concealed (Panyam and Kilara, 1996). Limited hydrolysis using protease preparations is so far the most studied and widely used technology for protein functionality modification.

Trypsin and protease preparations containing trypsin have been used by the food industry to modify and control the functional properties such as viscosity, elasticity, cohesion, emulsification, foam stability and whipability, and to achieve other purposes including flavor development, texture modification, nutritional quality, solubility and digestibility. Enzymatic processes have also been used to enhance the extractability of many food proteins such as milk proteins (casein and whey proteins), egg white protein, legume proteins (bean and pea proteins), oil seed proteins (soybean, peanut, canola seed, flax seed and rape seed proteins), cereal proteins (wheat gluten, corn protein, rice and oat bran protein), and protein in by-products of meat and fishery industry (collagen and gelatin proteins). The most frequently used enzymes in limited food protein hydrolysis include trypsin, chymotrypsin, pepsin, papain, bromelain, thermolysin and proteolytic preparations of microbial origin, such as Alcalase, Neutrase, Pronase and Protamex. Protein modification by enzymes yields products with improved nutritional, functional and organoleptic properties, and aids in a variety of processing operations.

3.2. Limited Hydrolysis of Food Proteins Using Trypsin for Functional Properties Improvement

Limited hydrolysis is restricted to the cleavage of single or a few peptide bonds, located mostly on the protein molecule surface and thus easily available to an enzyme. The functional properties of protein hydrolysates are closely associated with the type of enzyme used and the degree of hydrolysis (DH) of protein. The DH was defined as percentage of peptide bonds hydrolyzed (h) to the total number of peptide bonds in the substrate studied (htot, mM/g) (Adler-Nissen, 1986). Several methods exist for the determination of DH. The most commonly used of these include the pH-stat, trinitrobenzenesulfonic acid (TNBS), o-phthaldialdehyde (OPA), trichloroacetic acid soluble nitrogen (SN-TCA), and formol titration methods (Rutherfurd, 2010). The pH-stat method, the most widely used method in food industry, is based on the number of protons released during hydrolysis. With this method, the DH is calculated in each case from the amount of base added to keep the pH constant during the hydrolysis as follows (Adler-Nissen, 1986):

$$\text{DH}\ (\%) = (h/h\text{tot}) \times 100 = (BN\text{b}/M\text{p}) \times (1/\alpha) \times (1/h\text{tot}) \times 100$$

where B (mL) is the amount of base consumed to keep the pH constant during the reaction, Nb is the normality of the base, Mp(g) is the mass of protein (N × 6.25) and α is the average degree of dissociation of the α-NH2 groups released during hydrolysis. The α values at different pH and temperatures and h_{tot} value of some common proteins (including casein, whey protein meat, gelatin, soy protein, wheat gluten, maize protein isolate and fish protein isolate) are listed in the book *Enzymic Hydrolysis of Food Proteins* by Adler-Nissen (1986). The h_{tot} of a specific protein is dependent on the amino acid composition of the protein. The htot of egg yolk protein is 8.0 (Wang and Wang, 2009), while rice bran protein and oat bran protein have h_{tot} of 8.4 (Silpradit et al., 2010) and 7.31 (Guan et al., 2007), respectively.

The desired degree of hydrolysis (DH) varies considerably with the different food processing operations. Some proteolytic processes, such as soy sauce from soy protein or fish sauce from whole fish, require a DH close to 100%, some need extensive hydrolysis such as protein hydrolysate for infant formulas, while others require only limited hydrolysis. The combination of limited hydrolysis and cross-linking is sometimes needed to achieve some desirable functionalities such as viscosity and gel forming properties. Examples of limited hydrolysis to improve the functionality of food proteins are discussed below.

Milk Proteins: Milk proteins are highly nutritive and are rich source of biologically active peptides. Milk proteins consist of caseins (αs1-, αs2-, β- and κ-) and whey proteins that are differ in their physiological and biological properties. The casein content of milk represents about 80% of milk proteins. The caseins are quite small proteins, with a molecular mass of 20-25 kDa, which probably contributes significantly to their remarkably high stability. The caseins are relatively hydrophobic and, in particular, have a high surface hydrophobicity owing to their open structures which confers caseins good foaming and emulsifying properties but low solubility in water (Fox and Kelly, 2004). Tryptic hydrolysis of casein to the DH of 4.3, 8.0 and 9.9% greatly increased the solubility of casein at near isoelectric point (pH4.0-5.0).

The proteins appearing in the supernatant of milk after precipitation at pH 4.6 are collectively called whey proteins. Whey is typically a by-product of cheese making. Native whey proteins have good gelling and whipping properties, and good solubility in water over a wide range of pH values. Denaturation at low pH during cheese making or casein precipitation leads to aggregation and insolubility. Spray drying during the production of whey protein concentrate/isolate also alters the functional properties of whey protein (Kilara, 2004). Tryptic hydrolysis of whey proteins to between 2.3 and 6.7% degree of hydrolysis prevented gelation at pH 3.0 and 7.0, whereas hydrolysis to 2.3% DH with a Bacillus subtilis protease dramatically increased the gelling ability and gel strength at neutral pH (Ju et al., 1995). Ttrypic hydrolysis of whey protein concentrate to DH of 2.5, 3.9 and 5.3% resulted in significantly increased protein solubility at all pHs and better emulsion capacities than the unhydrolyzed control (Chobert et al., 1988). Extensive hydrolysis (to a degree of 18%) of whey protein isolate with Alcalase 2.4L caused the formation of strong elastic gels, similar to, but more stable over a wide range of temperature (10–65 °C) than heat-induced gels (Doucet *et al.*, 2001)

Some food proteins such as whey protein and casein have been enzymatically modified to produce protein-based fat replacer for low-fat diet recommended by dietitians for maintenance of health. The enzymatic modification of a protein for use as a fat replacer is carried out almost exclusively using proteases and transglutaminase. The important functional properties for a protein or modified protein to serve as a good fat-replacer are its gel-forming ability which is determined by the solubility, water binding, surface activities (emulsification and foaming) and viscoelasticity of the modified molecules (Leman, 2007).

Egg Proteins: Egg white protein is a highly nutritional protein for its amino acid composition resembles human bodies. Egg white is a widely used as ingredient in the food industry due to its multifunctional properties such as gelling, foaming and emulsifying characteristics, in addition to their high nutritional quality. However, its food applications are limited due to it's heat instability and high viscosity (Van der Plancken et al., 2007). The properties of protein in egg white can be improved by enzymatic hydrolysis and thus its application could be widen, for example, the decline of viscosity is beneficial to fluid transporting process (Chi et al., 2006).

Soy Proteins: Soybean is a dominant oilseed worldwide and a large amount of defatted soybean meals rich in protein are produced after extraction of oil. Defatted soybean meal is primarily used for animal feed and only a small portion is further processed into various types of soy protein products for human consumption (Johnson *et al.*, 1992). Soybean proteins possess good nutritional quality but less than desirable functional properties which traditionally limited their use in food industry (Kinsella, 1979). Although native soy protein has good gel forming ability and emulsification (Hettiarachchy and Kalapathy, 1997), soy protein isolate (SPI) has very low solubility and emulsion stability due to the effect of processing condition during protein isolation. Limited hydrolysis using trypsin or alcalase significantly increased the solubility and emulsification capacity of SPI, particularly, the solubility at isoelectric point (Kim et al., 1990). Partial hydrolysis of a commercial SPI with trypsin was reported to improve the solubility at pH 7.0 and 4.5, enhanced the ability to undergo thermal aggregation, and increased gel viscosity but caused a slight diminution of the water holding capacity (Iordan et al., 2008**).** It is also reported that limited hydrolysis with trypsin to 1-2% DH improved the emulsifying capacity of SPI, but higher DH impaired this functional property although the protein solubility increased (Zhao and Hou, 2009). Enzymatically modified soy protein products have been used in different types of food systems including bakery products as milk replacer, breakfast cereal products as protein enhancer, dairy-type products (such as yoghurt, ice cream and soy milk), minced meat products (sausage, hamburger, meat analog, etc) and pet foods etc (Endres, 2001). Functional properties of proteolytic hydrolysates is also influenced by the enzyme or enzyme preparation used. For example, when commercial defatted soy flour (DSF) were hydrolyzed using three different proteases (Flavourzyme 1000 L, Novozym FM 2.0 L and Alcalase 2.4 L FG), the highest degree of hydrolysis (DH 39.5) was observed in the presence of protease Flavourzyme. Treatment with Flavourzyme improved foaming and gelation properties of DSF proteins. In contrast, foaming stability was low in the presence of Novozym (Hrčková et al., 2002).

Cereal proteins: Wheat gluten hydrolysis results in peptide mixtures with high solubility and altered foaming and emulsifying characteristics, depending on the degree of hydrolysis (DH). Up to 5% of DH, wheat gluten hydrolyzed with trypsin and Alcalase had excellent solubility (>60%) over a pH range of 2–12 and remarkably higher emulsifying and foaming properties compared to the original gluten, but extensive hydrolysis resulted in significant reduction of emulsifying and foaming properties (Kong et al., 2007). Tryptic treatment of oat bran to degrees of hydrolysis of 4.1%, 6.4% and 8.3% increased the solubility, water-holding capacity, emulsifying activity and foaming ability of the hydrolysates gradually with the increase in DH. However, the oil-holding capacity, emulsifying stability and foaming stability of the hydrolysates reduced to a certain extent following enzymatic hydrolysis (Guan et al., 2007). Corn germ is a by-product of corn milling industry. Although rich in protein, corn germ protein's functional properties are poor. Partial hydrolysis of corn germ protein isolate with trypsin improved water absorption and foaming properties but decreased emulsifying capacity and nitrogen solubility of corn protein isolate. Treatment of partially hydrolyzed corn germ protein isolate with succinic anhydride improved water and oil absorption, nitrogen solubility, and foaming capacity but decreased emulsifying capacity with limited effect on foam stability (Messinger et al., 1987).

Fish Protein: The use of fish waste has been of increasing interest in the past years as the biomass of marine origin is considered a safe material and provides proteins with high nutritional properties and a good pattern of essential amino acids (Guerard, et al., 2001). Traditionally, fish wastes have been used as fish meal for animal feeding. Proteins extracted from fish processing byproducts can be modified to improve the quality and functional characteristics by enzymatic hydrolysis (Kristinsson and Rasco, 2000). Production of fish protein concentrate is a means of recovering valuable protein from underutilized fish species, such as sharks, and consequently obtaining a new-source protein ingredient for incorporation into foods (Tsumura et al., 2005).

In addition to the modification of functional properties, enzymatic hydrolysis of food proteins frequently results in bitter taste due to the formation of low molecular weight peptides composed of mainly hydrophobic amino acids (Saha and Hayashi, 2001). The bitterness of the protein hydrolysates depends on the enzyme used and the degree of hydrolysis (DH). One study tested the bitterness of soy protein hydrolysates produced by limited hydrolysis of a commercial soy protein isolated using commercial protease preparations (flavourzyme, alcalase, neutrase, protamex, papain, and bromelain) at E/S ratios of 0.5%, 1%, and 2%. The results show that the bitterness of the soy protein hydrolysates increased with the increase of DH. Alcalase showed the highest bitterness, followed by neutrase at same DH, and Flavourzyme showed the lowest TD factor at the entire DH ranges (Seo et al., 2008). Another study on the bitterness of hydrolysates produced by limited hydrolysis of a commercial pea protein with Flavourzyme, papain, alcalase, trypsin and α-chymotrypsin found similar results (Humiski and Aluko, 2007). Many methods have been proposed for debittering of protein hydrolysates.

These methods include selective separation such as treatment with activated carbon, extraction with alcohol, isoeletric precipitation, chromatography on silica gel, hydrophobic interaction chromatography, masking bitterness, further hydrolysis of bitter peptides with special enzymes, condensation of bitter peptides with using protease and use of Lactobacillus as a debittering starter adjunct. These methods were extensively reviewed by Saha and Hayashi (2001).

In summary, controlled enzymatic hydrolysis may enhance some functional properties and simultaneously be detrimental to others. The extent of proteolytic degradation of food proteins affects the functional properties of the hydrolysates as a consequence of reduced molecular size of the peptide units (Panyam and Kilara, 1996). A general beneficial effect of proteolytic hydrolysis of food proteins is the increased solubility. Other functional properties such as emulsifying and foaming, viscosity and gel forming properties change depending on the degree of hydrolysis and types of enzyme preparations used in the hydrolysis. Therefore, depending on the desired functional properties, it is critical to select the right protease preparation and carefully monitor the DH as to minimize the undesirable impacts of enzymatic hydrolysis of food protein and to produce a right ingredient with desirable functional, nutritional, and sensory properties.

4. Application of Trypsin for the Production of Food-Derived Bioactive Peptides

Food derived bioavtive peptides are different peptides of animal or plant origins that are biologically active and have regulatory functions in humans beyond normal and adequate nutrition. Different health benefits have been attributed to food-derived peptides, including antimicrobial properties, blood pressure-lowering (ACE inhibitory) effects, cholesterol-lowering ability, antithrombotic and antioxidant activities, enhancement of mineral absorption and/or bioavailability, cyto- or immunomodulatory effects, and opioid activities (Hartmann and Meisel, 2007).

Bioactive peptides from milk proteins have been intensively studied in the past 2-3 decades and the biological activities, health benefits and the applications of food- derived bioactive peptides were extensively reviewed by many scholars (Nagpal et al., 2011; Hartmann and Meisel, 2007; Korhonen and Pihlanto, 2003; Meisel and FitzGerald, 2003; Xu 2008; Tirelli et al., 1997). Recently, many attentions have been given to the bioactive peptides derived from plant materials such as soybean, chick pea, wheat, corn, rice, barley, buckwheat, and sunflower (Gibbs et al., 2004). However, not all bioactive peptides have positive effects on health. Beta-casomorphin-7, an opioid peptided released from milk protein beta-casein with sequence Tyr^{60}-Pro^{61}-Phe^{62}-Pro^{63}-Gly^{64}-Pro^{65}-Ile^{66}, has been suspected of contributing to an increased risk for certain non-communicable diseases, such as autism, cardiovascular diseases and type I diabetes (De Noni et al. 2009).

There are a number of methods to produce bioactive peptides from precursor proteins. The common methods include (a) enzymatic hydrolysis with digestive enzymes, (b) microbial fermentation and (c) hydrolysis of protein using bacterial enzymes derived from proteolytic micro-organisms such as lactic acid bacteria.

The production of bioactive peptides from milk proteins by different methods was reviewed by Korhonen and Pihlanto (2003). The main approach used to produce peptides is by enzymatic hydrolysis. These peptides are then further isolated by either ultrafiltration or by cationic exchange resins. Thus, peptides with different amino acid sequences that possess various biological activities can be obtained. The biological activities of the peptides depend on the initial protein source, enzyme used, and processing conditions. As shown in the Table 1, when different enzymes hydrolyze soy protein, it yields either antioxidant peptides (Chen, 1995), peptides with anticancer properties (Kim et al., 2000), or peptides with hypotensive activity (Wu and Ding 2001).

Soy protein and soy peptides have attracted considerable attention because of their potentially beneficial biological properties, including hypocholesterolemic, anticarcinogenic, hypotensive, immunostimulating and/or antioxidant effects (Kong et al., 2008; Fukushima, 2004). Soy crude peptide (SCP)-LD3, prepared by hydrolyze of soy protein isolate with endo-type protease showed hypolipidemic effects in HepG2 cells and OLETF rats and 3 di-peptides, Lys-Ala, Val-Lys, and Ser-Tyr separated from the soy crude peptide reduced TG synthesis, and Ser-Tyr additionally reduced apoB secretion in HepG2 cells (Inoue et al., 2011). Chen et al. (1995) isolated six antioxidative peptides (containing 5-19 amino acids) against peroxidation of linoleic acid from the protease hydrolysates of soybean beta-conglycinin. Yokomizo et al. (2002) also isolated four antioxidative peptides from the protease hydrolysates of the water-insoluble residues of soybeans; each peptide contains 2-3 amino acids. Lower molecular weight and positively charged peptides released from soy protein during Alcalase hydrolysis were effective in stimulating immunomodulating activity as evaluated by measuring their effect on in vitro proliferation of murine spleen lymphocytes and phagocytic activity of peritoneal macrophages. (Kong et al., 2008).

Fermented soybean products are a good source of ACE inhibitory bioactive peptides. ACE inhibitory peptides have also been found in many traditional Asian fermented soy foods, such as soybean paste (His-His-Leu) (Okamoto et al., 1995), soy sauce (Gibbes et al., 2004), natto and tempeh (Potter, 1995). Fermentation of milk with certain lactobacilli releases two interesting tripeptides Ile-Pro-Pro and Val-Pro-Pro from casein to the final product. These lactotripeptides have shown properties that attenuate the development of hypertension in several animal models and lower blood pressure in clinical studies. They inhibit ACE *in vitro* at micromolar concentrations, protect endothelial function *in vitro* and reduce arterial stiffness in humans (Jäkälä and Vapaatalo, 2010).

Table 1. Bioactive peptides produced by the hydrolysis of various animal and plant proteins using trypsin or the combined trypsin with other proteolytic enzymes

Protein source	Peptides	Activity	Reference
Casein	Phe-Phe-Val-Ala-Pro Gly-Leu-Phe	ACE-inhibition Immunomodulation	Migliore-Samour et al., 1988 Fait et al., 1993
Lactoglobulin	Ile-pro-Ala-Val-Phe-Lys	Bactericidal	Pellehrini, 2003
Rice albumin	Gly-Tyr-Pro-Met-Tyr-Pro-Leu-Pro-Arg	Immunostimulation	Takahashi et al., 1996
Peanut protein isolate (PPI)	Mixture of hydrolyzed PPI	Antioxidant ACE inhibition	Jamdar et al., 2010
Soy protein	Soy crude peptide (SCD-LD3)	Hypolipidemic effect	Inoue et al., 2011
Soy protein concentrate	Peptides with different molecular weights	Antioxidants	Chen et al., 1995
Soy protein isolate	X-Met-Leu-Pro-Ser-Tye-Ser-Pro-Tyr.	Anticancer	Kim, et al., 2000
Defatted soy flour	Soluble hydrolyzed sample fractionated on cationic exchange resin	Hypotensive (anti-ACE activity)	Wu and Ding, 2001
GM soy protein	LLPHH; RPLKPW	Antioxidative, antihypertensive	Korhonen and Pihlanto, 2003.
Whey protein	Freeze dried hydrolysates	Antigenicity	Zheng et al., 2008
α and α' fractions of β-conglycinin	Mixture of hydrolysates	Anticancer	Mora-Escobedo et al., 2009.
Legumes	Mixtures of *in vitro* gastrointestinal digestion	ACE-inhibition	Akıllıoğlu and Karakaya
Oat flour protein	2-10 kDa	Antioxidative	Tsopmo et al., 2010

The study using a macrophage cell line, RAW 264.7 (Oseguera-Toledo et al.,2011) shows that alcalase hydrolysates of the common beans (Pinto Durango and Negro 8025) inhibited cyclooxygenase-2 expression, prostaglandin E2 production, inducible nitric oxide synthase expression and nitric oxide production (the biomarkers used for inflammation measurement). These hydrolysates also significantly inhibited the transactivation of NF-κB and the nuclear translocation of the NF-κB p65 subunit. The study concluded that hydrolysates from the common beans can be used to combat inflammatory and oxidative-associated chronic diseases such as diabetes and cancer (Libby, 2007; Oberyszyn, 2007).

Enzymatic hydrolysis of chick pea and yellow pea proteins resulted in hydrolysates rich in small peptides with MWs under 4 kDa. The hydrolysates showed different degree of ACE inhibitory activities depending on the enzyme used. Papain hydrolysed yellow pea proteins showed the highest ACE inhibitory activity. In addition, chickpea desi proteins hydrolysed by *in vitro* gastrointestinal simulation showed higher ACE inhibition compared to its digests obtained by alcalase/flavourzyme or papain and compared to chickpea kabuli hydrolysed by gastrointestinal simulation (Barbana and Boye, 2010). Oat protein hydrolysates produced by hydrolysis of oat protein isolate using trypsin and alcalase were reported to have free radical scavenging and metal chelating properties, and ability to significantly inhibit the autoxidation of linoleic acid, a dominant fatty acid in vegetable and seed oil (Tsopmo et al., 2010).

Peptides from Flavourzyme hydrolyzed defatted corn exhibited significantly ($p < 0.05$) stronger bile acid binding capacity than all others hydrolysates tested. The bile acid binding capacity of Flavourzyme hydrolysate was almost preserved after gastrointestinal proteases digestion. The molecular weights of peptides in Flavourzyme hydrolysate were found between 500–180 Da. The results showed that Flavourzyme hydrolysate may be used as a potential cholesterol-reducing agent (Kongo-Dia-Moukala et al., 2011)

After proteolytic hydrolysis, the functional or bioactive peptides are typically present in the complex matrix containing a large number of hydrolyzed protein fractions, hence their separation and purification are required. The reported methods for fractionation and enrichment of bioactive peptides, such as casein phosphate peptides (CPPs), include selective precipitation, ultralfiltration and chromatography (Korhonen and Pihlanto, 2003). The first two methods are cost effective but produce products of low purity. The third method is the most selective, produces high purity product, but has fairly low CPP yield and high cost. Membrane processes and devices for separation of bioactive peptides have been developed. These processes include conventional pressure-driven ultrafiltration and nanofiltration, pressure driven-membrane separation assisted by electrical field and electrodialysis with ultrafiltration membrane (Bazinet and Firdaous, 2009).

5. Enzymatic Modifications for Reducing Allergenicity of Food Proteins

Food allergy is the adverse immune responses to foods, which affects approximately 5% of young children and 3% to 4% of adults in westernized countries and appear to have increased in prevalence over the past decade. Food-induced allergic reactions are responsible for a variety of symptoms and disorders involving the skin, gastrointestinal track and respiratory tract, and can be attributed to IgE-mediated and non–IgE-mediated (cellular) mechanisms (Sicherer and Sampson, 2010). Peanuts, tree nuts, wheat and soy, cow's milk, egg, fish and shellfish are responsible for the majority of food-induced allergic reactions (Mills and Breiteneder, 2005). Most food allergenic proteins bind IgE and cause cross-linking on the surface of mast cells which results in downstream cascades leading to the allergic response (Burks, 1988; Sicherer and Sampson, 2010). Portions of a protein that bind IgE are referred to as epitopes. Eggs, fish, shellfish, milk, peanuts, soy, tree nuts, and wheat are the eight of common sources of food allergens with those of milk, eggs and soy being the best characterized food allergens (Sicherer and Sampson, 2010). Some of these commodities are discussed below.

Milk: Allergy to cow milk is a serious problem to infants. About 2.5% of children below 3 years of age are allergic to cow milk and the major allergens from cow's milk are casein and beta-lactoglobulin (El-Ghaish et al., 2011). Therefore, milk proteins may create serious allergic reaction if fed to an infant allergic to cow milk. Different attempts have been made to reduce the allergenicity of dairy proteins. Extensive hydrolysis of milk with protease and fermentation with lactic acid bacterial are two major processing methods that have been applied to produce hypoallergenic dairy products. Hypoallergenic infant formulas are produced from caseins or whey proteins by means of heat denaturation and enzymatic hydrolysis which are sometimes combined with ultrafiltration (Besler, 2001). For a formula to be considered hypoallergenic, it should be well tolerated by at least 90% of individuals who are allergic to the parent protein from which the formula has been derived. Extensively hydrolyzed formulas (EHFs), derived from bovine casein or whey, are tolerated by approximately 95% of individuals with cow's milk allergic (Bahna, 2008).

Soybean and other legumes: According to the National Institute of Allergy and Infectious Diseases, soy allergies are particularly common in infants and young children. It's difficult to avoid eating soy products because of its wide use in many processed foods, including infant formula, cereals, and salad dressings. A total of 16 antigens recognized by IgE were identified in soybean by an immunoblotting technique (Daniel, 2004). Among these, Gly m Bd 68K, Gly m Bd 30K and Gly m Bd 28K were shown to be the major soybean allergens. These proteins were found to occur in the 7S-globulin fraction of soybean proteins (Ogawa et al., 1991). Some of the most allergenic fractions appear to be the Kunitz and Bowman–Birk trypsin inhibitors (Burk et al., 1988; Ogawa et al., 1991). Soybean lectin, another antinutrient has also been identified as an allergen (Barnett and Howden, 1987). However, miso, soy sauce and natto, the traditional fermented soy bean products commonly consumed in Asia contain almost no Gly m Bd 30K, and are considered to be hypoallergenic and have antiallergenic properties (Tsuji et al., 2001; Kobayashi, 2005). Soybean protein treated with digestive enzymes through two successive gastric fluid hydrolyses (pepsin) and duodenal fluid hydrolysis (trypsin, chymotrypsin and intestinal peptidase) resulted in a 10-fold decrease of IgE-binding in comparison to the native soybean protein (Burk et al., 1992). Hydrolysis of pea globulins (legumin and vicilin) with trypsin to DH 12% at 50°C was reported to reduce the immunoreactivities of legumin and vicilin by 98% and 97%, respectively (Szymkiewicz, 2005).

Wheat: Wheat is the most important crop worldwide and contains more than 10% gluten, the protein that is essential for baking. Wheat proteins can be either ingested or inhaled in the form of raw flour, which can lead to adverse reactions including wheat gluten enteropathy (celiac disease), T-cell-mediated intestinal inflammation, dermatitis herpetiformis, a blistering skin eruption, and respiratory allergy (Battais et al., 2008). Wheat allergy refers to adverse reactions involving immunoglobulin E (IgE) antibodies to one or more proteins found in wheat. The allergic reaction caused by gluten is known as coeliac disease, a sequence of immune related reactions leading to damage of the intestine and related malabsorption symptoms (Hamer,2005). Both gliadin and glutenin were reported to be allergenic, but the allergenicity of glutenin was much weaker than gliadin (Wieser, 1996). The most common allergenic peptide of gliadin has the structure Pro-Ser-Gln-Gln-, and -Gln-Gln-Gln-Pro, while the wheat glutenin IgE-binding epitope has the structure Gln-X-Y-Pro-Pro, where X and Y are replaceable amino acid residues (Watanabe et al., 1995). Complete acid hydrolysis of gliadin removed allergenicity, but peptic/tryptic digestion did not (Hamer, 2005). However, Bromelain, a mixture of sulfhydryl proteases, from plant extract, was found to effectively degrade the allergenic peptides in gluten and was used to produce wheat flour for hypoallergenic bread (Tanabe et al., 1996).

Rice: Rice is the most important crop that not only provides carbohydrate but also protein in Asian countries. However, rice is considered to be one of the representative allergic foods in Japan, Among rice proteins, a 16-kDa protein was found to be one of the major allergens in rice grains. This protein was also found to inhibit serum IgE-binding to other cereal grain extracts including wheat, maize and millet (Urisu, et al., 1991). Watanabe et al. (1993)

developed a unique process for producing hypoallergenic rice grain. The process enabled almost complete removal of the major allergenic proteins by proteolysis while retaining more than half the principal rice seed protein, glutelin. In clinical tests, this hypoallergenic rice dramatically improved rice-associated atopic dermatitis. The hypoallergenic rice has been industrially produced and supplied in Japan.

Peanuts: Among food allergies, peanut allergy is relatively common, typically permanent, often severe, and sometimes lethal. Peanut is a ubiquitous food. Sensitive patients, who often react to small doses (Sicherer and Sampson, 2007) are safe only with complete avoidance of contact with peanut proteins. So far, 11 allergenic peanut proteins have been identified, with Ara h 1 and Ara h 2 being the dominant allergens. More than 95% of peanut allergic individuals in the U.S. have specific IgE to Ara h 1 and Ara h 2 (Scurlock and Burks, 2004). Ara h 3 and 4 are recognized by at least 50% of the allergic population (Sampson et al., 2004). The sensitizing rate of Ara h5, Ara h6, and Ara h7 are estimated to be 13, 38, and 44%, respectively (Wen et al., 2007).

A study by Hong et al (1999) found that extensive digestion of peanut protein with pepsin at enzyme to substrate ratio of 1:3 for 24 or 48 hours completely destroyed the IgE-binding sites but maintained T-cell reactivity. These authors concluded that pepsin-digested peanut may be useful in peanut immunotherapy because pepsin digestion eliminates IgE reactivity. A recent study in our laboratory also found that soaking roasted peanut kernels in trypsin or chymotrypsin solutions for 1-3 hours at 37°C significantly reduced the detectable Ara h 1 and Ara h 2 in the peanuts (Yu et al., 2011). Other examples of enzyme treatment to remove allergens include producing hypoallergenic whey protein hydrolysate (Jost et al., 1991) and psyllium seed husk (Nielsen, 1993) using proteases such as trypsin and chymotrypsin.

6. Applications of Trypsin in Food Research

Digestibility is an important factor in the determination of the nutritive quality of a protein, because of its link to the bioavailability of amino acids in the native protein. Several biological and chemical assays exist for evaluation of the in vivo digestibility of proteins. However, these methods are often too expensive and time-consuming for application in the food industry. Therefore, faster and less costly *in vitro* methods have been developed (Hur et al., 2011). In the *in vitro* models, digestion of food protein is usually conducted under simulated gastrointestinal conditions that involve pepsin, trypsin and chymotrypsin. Trypsin is also used to identify antinutritional factors such as trypsin inhibitor and to evaluate the effects of food processing methods on the digestibility of proteins.

Legume seeds such as soybean, peanuts and kidney beans are good sources of proteins. However, legumes usually contain antinutritional factors such as phytates, condensed tannins and trypsin inhibitors. Many traditional and novel foods processing methods such as germination and roasting have shown to reduce/destroy these antinutritional factors, thus improving the digestibility of the proteins (Ejigui et al., 2005; Urbano et al., 2005). A study conducted by Ikeda et al (1995) found that the protein of *yuba* (soy protein-lipid film) was more digestible by protease, but the protein of *kinako* (roasted soy meal) was less digestible. The study also revealed that the trypsin inhibitory activities of processed soybean products were 21-612 folds lower than the raw soybean meal.

Van Der Plancken et al (2003) evaluated the effect of heating on the digestibility of egg white protein by an *in vitro* assay using α-chymotrypsin and trypsin from porcine pancreas. They found that the ovalbumin and albumen (the major proteins in chicken egg white) in their native form were resistant to digestion by trypsin. However, heat induced denaturation between temperature 75-85°C increased the susceptibility of these proteins to tryptic hydrolysis. Other studies reported that a multienzyme digestion system consisting of trypsin, chymotrypsin and peptidase improved protein digestibility of maize flour to which blood protein concentrate was added (Oshodi et al., 1997).

Conclusion

Trypsin has wide applications in food science and technology. In many situations, the combination of trypsin and other enzymes such as exopeptidases and transglutominase is required to produce the desirable end product, enhance the desired properties, or remove the undesirable properties of food proteins. When trypsin is used to modify functional properties of dietary proteins, the degree of hydrolysis has to be carefully controlled to minimize bitterness and other undesirable effects on the final product. To reduce the allergenicity of food proteins, a mixture of trypsin with other specific peptidase or non-specific peptidases is often needed, and extensive hydrolysis is required. Many technical aspects needs to be considered when considering the use of trypsin to produce bioactive peptides, particularly, the type of reactor, reaction conditions, and the type of downstream processing.

References

Adler-Nissen, J. (1986). A review of food hydrolysis specific areas. In J. Adler-Nissen (Ed), *Enzymic Hydrolysis of Food Proteins* (pp. 57–109). Elsevier Applied Science Publisher, London.

Akıllıoğlu, H.G. and Karakaya,S. (2009). Effects of heat treatment and in vitro digestion on the Angiotensin converting enzyme inhibitory activity of some legume species. *European Food Research Technology*, 229, 915–921.

Asgeirsson, B., Fox, J. W. and Bjarnason, J. B. (1989). Purification and characterization of trypsin from the poikilotherm Gadus morhua. *European Journal of Biochemistry*, 180, 85–94.

Bahna, S.L. (2008). Hypoallergenic formulas: optimal choices for treatment (Review Article). *Annals of Allergy, Asthma and Immunology, 101, 453-459.*

Banumathi, E., Haribalaganesh, R., Babu, S., Kumar, N. and Sangiliyandi, G. (2009). High-yielding enzymatic method for isolation. *Microvascular Research, 77*, 377-381.

Barbana, C. and Boye, J.I. (2010). Angiotensin I-converting enzyme inhibitory activity of chickpea and pea protein hydrolysates. *Food Research International*, 43, 1642–1649.

Barnett, D. and Howden, M.E. (1987). Lectins and the radioallergosorbent test. *Journal Allergy Clinical Immunology*, 80, 558-561.

Battais, F., Richard, C., Jacquenet, S., Denery-Papini, S.and Moneret-Vautrin, D.A.(2008). *Wheat grain allergies: an update on wheat allergens. European Annals of Allergy and Clinical Immunology*, 40, 67-76.

Bazinet, L. and Firdaous, L. (2009). Membrance processes and devices for separation of bioactive peptides. *Recent Patents and Biotechnology*, 3, 61-72.

Besler, M., Steinhart, H. and Paschke, A. (2001). Stability of food allergens and allergenicity of processed foods. *Journal of Chromatography B*, 756, 207–228.

Burks, A.W., Brooks, J.R. and Sampson, H.A. (1988). Allergenicity of major component proteins of soybean determined by enzyme-linked immunosorbent assay (ELISA) and immunoblotting in children with atopic dermatitis and positive soy challenges. *Journal of Allergy Clinical Immunology*, 81, 111135-1142.

Burks, A.W., Williams, L.W., Thresher, W., Connaughton, C., Cockrell, G. and Helm R.M. (1992). Allergenicity of peanut and soybean extracts altered by chemical or thermal denaturation in patients with atopic dermatitis and positive food challenges (Abstract). *Journal of Allergy Clinical Immunology*, 90, 889-897.

Chen, H. M., Muramoto, K. and Yamauchi, F. (1995). Structural analysis of antioxidative peptides from soybean beta-conglycinin, *Journal of Agricultural and Food Chemistry*, 43, 574-578.

Chi Y., Tian, B., Sun B. and Guo M. (2006). Enzymatic hydrolysis condition of egg white proteins. *Bulletin of the Faculty of Agriculture, Niigata University*, 582: 143-146.

Chobert, J.M., Bertrand-Harb,C. and Nicolas,M.G.(1988). Solubility and Emulsifying Properties of Caseins and Whey Proteins Modified Enzymatically by Trypsin. *Journal of Agricultural and Food Chemistry*, 36, 83-892.

Daniel, K.T. (2004). The hidden dangers of soy allergens. *Nexus Magazine*, 11. http://www.nexusmagazine.com/articles/Soy%20Allergens.html

Damodaran, S. (2005). Protein stabilization of emulsions and foams. *Journal of Food Science*, 70, R54-R66.

Damodaran, S. (2006). Amino acids, peptides and proteins. In S. Damodaran, K.L.Parkin, O.R. Fennema (Eds), Food Chemistry (4th Edition, pp: 219-329), CRC Press, Taylor and Francis Group. Boca Raton, FL.

deMan, J.M. (1999). *Principles of Food Chemistry*, (3rd Edition, pp: 134-138). Aspen Publishers, Inc. Gaithersburg, Maryland.

De Noni, I., FitzGerald, R.J., Korhonen, H.J.T, Le Roux, Y., Livesey, C.T., Thorsdottir, I., Tomé, D. and Witkamp R. (2009). Review of the potential health impact of beta-casomorphins and related peptides. *EFSA (European Food Safety Authoority) Scientific Report,* 231, 1-107.

Doucet, D., Gauthier, S. F. and Foegeding, E. A. (2001). Rheological characterization of a gel formed during extensive enzymatic hydrolysis. *Journal of Food Science.* 66, 711-715.

Drago, S.R. and Conzález, R.J. (2001). Foaming properties of enzymatically hydrolyzed wheat gluten. *Innovative Food Science and Engineering Technologies*, 1, 269-73.

Ejigui, J., Savoie, L., Marin, J. and Desrosiers, T. (2005). Influence of traditional processing methods on the nutritional composition and antinutritional factors of red peanuts (Arachis hypogeal) and small red kidney beans (Phaseolus vulgaris). *Journal of biological Science*, 5, 597-605.

El-Ghaish, S., Ahmadova A., Hadji-Sfaxi, I., Mecherfi, K.E.E., Bazukyan I. et al (2011). Potential use of lactic acid bacteria for reduction of allergenicity and for longer conservation of fermented foods. Trends in Food Science and Technology, doi:10.1016/j.tifs.2011.05.003.

Endres, J.G. (2001). Soy protein, characteristics, nutritional aspects and utilization. Missing editors (pp 26-30). Champaign, Illinois AOCS Press, Champaign, Illinois.

Fiat, A.M., Migliore-Samour, D., Jollés. P., Drouet, L., Collier, C. and Caen, J. (1993). Biologically active peptides from milk proteins with emphasis on two examples concerning antithrombotic and immunomodulating activities. *Journal of Dairy Science*, 76, 301.

Fernando, L., García-Carreño, Haejung, An and Norman, F. Haard. Protease Inhibitors in Food Processing. In D. Michaud (Ed), *Recombinant Protease Inhibitors in Plants*. Land BioScience, Austin, TX.

Fox, P.F. and Kelly, A.L. (2004). The Caseins. In R.Y. Yada (Ed.), *Proteins in Food Processing* (pp:29-71). CRC Press LLC. Boca Raton, FL.

Fukushima, D. (2004). Soy proteins. In R.Y. Yada (Ed.), *Proteins in Food Processing* (pp: 123-145). CRC Press LLC, Boca Raton, FL.

Gibbs, B.F., Zougman, A., Masse, R. and Mulligan, C. (2004). Production and characterization of bioactive peptides from soy hydrolysate and soy-fermented foods. *Food and Research International,* 37,123-131.

Guan, X., Yao, J., Chen, Z., Shan, L. and Zhang, M. (2007). Some Functional Properties of Oat Bran Protein Concentrate Modified by Trypsin. *Food Chemistry*, 101, 163-170.

Gudmundsdóttir, A. and Pálsdóttir, H.M. (2005). Atlantic Cod Trypsins: From Basic Research to Practical Applications. Mar. Biotechnol, 7, 77–88.

Guérard, F., Dufossé, L., De La Broise, D. and Binet, A. (2001). Enzymatic hydrolysis of proteins from yellowfin tuna (*Thunnus albacares*) wastes using Alcalase. *Journal of Molecular Catalysis B: Enzymatic*, 11, 1051–1059.

Hamer, R.J. (2005). Coeliac disease: background and biochemical aspects. *Biotechnology Advances*, 23, 401-408.

Hartmann, R. and Meisel, H. (2007). Food-Derived peptides with Biological Activity: from Research to Food Applications. *Current Opinion Biotechnology,* 18, 163-169.

Hettiarachchy, N. S. and Kalapathy U. (1998). Functional Properties of Soy Proteins. In J. R. Whitaker, F. Shahidi, A.L. Munguia, R. Y. Yada and G. Fuller (Eds.), Functional Properties of Proteins and Lipids (pp: 80-95). American Chemical Society, Washington D.C.

Hong, S.J., Michael, J.G., Fehringer, A. and Leung, D.Y. (1999). Pepsin-digested peanut contains T-cell epitopes but no IgE epitopes. *Journal of American Clinical Immunology*, 104, 473-477.

Hjort, C. (2007). Industrial enzyme production for food application. In R. Rastal, (Ed.), Novel Enzyme Technologies for Food Applications (pp 43-59). CRC Press LLC, Boca Raton, FL.

Hrčková, M., Rusňáková, M., and Zemanovič J. (2002). Enzymatic hydrolysis of defatted soy flour by three different proteases and their effect on the functional properties of resulting protein hydrolysates. *Czech Journal of Food Science*, 20, 7–14.

Humiski, L.M. and Aluko, R.E. (2007). Physicochemical and Bitterness Properties of Enzymatic Pea Protein Hydrolysates. *Journal of Food Science*, 72, S605-S611.

Hur, S.J., Lim, B.O., Eric, Decker A. and McClements, D.J. (2011). In Vitro Human Digestion Models for Applications. *Food Chemistry*, 125, 1-12.

Ikeda, K., Matsuda, A., Katsumaru, A., Teranishi, M., Yamamoto, T. and Kishida, M. (1995). Factors affecting protein digestibility in soybean foods. *Cereal Chemistry*, 72, 401-405.

Inoue, N., Nagao, K., Sakata, K., Yamano, N., Gunawardena, P.E.R., Han, S.Y., Matsui, T., Nakamori, T., Furuta, H., Takamatsu, K. and Yanagita, T. (2011). Screening of soy protein-derived hypotriglyceridemic di-peptides in vitro and in vivo. *Lipids in Health and Disease*, 10, 85-94.

Iordan. M., Nour, V., Stoica, A. and Barascu, E. (2008). Study concerning the effects of the proteolysis on some soy protein isolate functional properties. Bulletin UASVM *Agriculture*, 65, 253-256.

Jäkälä, P. and Vapaatalo, H. (2010). Antihypertensive Peptides from Milk Proteins. *Pharmaceuticals*, 3, 251-272.

Jamdar, S.N., Rajalakshmi, V., Pednekar, M.D., Juan, F., Yardi, V. and Sharma, A. (2010). Influence of degree of hydrolysis on functiona properties, antioxidant activity and ACE inhibitory activity of peanut protein hydrolysis. *Food Chemistry*, 121, 178-184.

Johnson, L.A., Myer, D.J. and Burden, D.J. (1992). Soy proteins history, prospects in food, feed. *INFORM*, 3, 429-444.

Jost, R., Meister, N. and Monti, J.C. (1991). Preparation of a hypoallergenic whey protein hydrolyzate and foods. US patent: 5039532.

Ju., Z.Y., Otte, J., Madsen, J.S. and Qvist, K.B. (1995). Effects of limited proteolysis on gelation and gel properties of whey protein isolate. *Journal of Dairy Science*, 78, 119-2128.

Kinsella, J.E. (1979). Functional properties of soybean protein. *Journal of the American Oil Chemists' Society*, 56, 242-252.

Kilcawley, K.N., Wilkinson , M.G.and Fox, P.F. (2002). Determination of key enzyme activities in commercial peptidase and lipase preparations from microbial or animal sources. *Enzyme and Microbial Technology*, 31, 310–320.

Kim, S.Y., Park, P.S.W., and Rhee, K.C. (1990). Functional properties of proteolytic enzyme modified soy protein isolate. *Journal of Agricultural and Food Chemistry, 38,* 651-656.

Kim, S.E., Kim, H.H., Kim, J.Y., Kang, Y.I., Woo, H.J. and Lee, H.J. 2000. Anticancer activity of hydrophobic peptides from soy proteins. *BioFactors* 12(1–4):151–5.

Kilara, A. (2004). Whey proteins. In R.Y. Yada (Ed.), *Proteins in Food Processing* (pp: 72-99). CRC Press LLC. Boca Raton, FL, US.

Kinsella, J.E. (1982). Relationship between structure and functional properties of food proteins. In P.F. Fox and J.J. Condon (Eds.), *Food Proteins (pp: 51-104).* Elsevier Science Publishing Co. Inc., New York, New York.

Kobayashi, M. (2005). Immunological functions of soy sauce: hypoallergenicity and antiallergic activity of soy sauce. Journal *of Bioscience and Bioengineering*, 100, 144–151.

Kong, X.Z., Guo, M.M., Hua, Y.F., Cao, D. and Zhang, C.M. (2008). Enzymatic preparation of immunomodulating hydrolysates from soy proteins. *Bioresource Techno*logy, 99, 8873–8879.

Kong, X.Z., Zhou, H. and Qian, H. (2007). Enzymatic preparation and functional properties of wheat gluten hydrolysates. *Food Chemistry*, 101, 615–620.

Korhonen, H. and Pihlanto, A. (2003). Food-Derived Bioactive Peptides –Opportunities for Designing Future Foods. *Current Pharmaceutical Design*, 9, 1297-1308.

Kongo-Dia-Moukala, J.U., Zhang, H. and Irakoze, P.C. (2011). *In Vitro* Binding capacity of bile acids by defatted corn protein hydrolysate. *International Journal of Molecular Science, 12*, 1066-1080.

Krajcovicova-Kudlackova, M., Babinska, K. and Valachovicova, M. (2005). Health benefits and risks of plant proteins. *Bratisl Lek Listy*, 106, 231-4.

Kristinsson, H. G. and Rasco, B. A. (2000). Fish protein hydrolysates: Production, biochemical and functional properties. *Critical Reviews in Food Science and Nutrition*, 40, 43–81.

Kunst, T. (2003). Protein modification to optimize functionality: protein hydrolysates. In J.R. Whitaker, A.G.J. Voragen and D.W.S. Wong (Eds.), *Handbook of Food Enzymology* (pp: 221-236). Marcel Dekker, Inc., New York, New York.

Leman, J. (2007). Enzymatically modified whey protein and other protein-based fat replacers. In Rastall R. (Ed.), *Novel Enzyme Technology for Food Applications*, CRC Press LLC., Boca Raton, US.

Libby, P. (2007). Inflammatory mechanisms: The molecular basis of inflammation and disease. *Nutrition Reviews*, 65, S140–S146.

McDonagh, D. and FitzGeral, R.J. (1998). Production of caseinophosphopeptides (cpps) from sodium caseinate using a range of commercial protease preparations. *International Dairy Journal, 8,* 39-45.

Meisel, H. and FitzGerald, R.J. (2003). Biofunctional peptides from milk proteins: mineral binding and cytomodulatory effects. *Current Pharmaceutical*, 9, 1289-1295.

Messinger, J.K., Rupnow, J.H., Zeece, M.G. and Anderson, R.L. (1987). Effect of partial proteolysis and succinylation on functionality of corn germ protein isolate. *Journal of Food Science*, 52. 1620-1624.

Mills, E.N.C. and Breitenederb, H. (2005). Food allergy and its relevance to industrial food proteins. *Biotechnology Advances*, 23, 409–414.

Migliore-Samour D. and Jolles P. (1988) Casein, a prohormone with an immunomodulating role for the newborn? *Experientia 44,* 188-193.

Mora-Escobedo, R., Robles-Ramírez, M.C., Ramón-Gallegos, E. and Reza-Alemán, R.l (2009). Effect of protein hydrolysates from germinated soybean on cancerous cells of the human cervix: an in vitro study. *Plant Foods and Human Nutrition*, 64, 271–278.

Mullally, M.M. O'Callaghan, D.M. FitzGerald, R.J. Donnelly. W.J. and Dalton, J.P. (1994). Proteolytic and peptidolytic activities in commercial pancreatic protease preparations and their relationship to some whey protein hydrolysate characteristics. *Journal of Agricultural and Food Chemistry, 42,* 2973-2981.

Nagpal, R., Behare, P., Rana, R., Kumar, A., Kumar, M., Arora, S., Morotta, F., Jaing, S. and Yadav, H. (2011). Bioactive peptides derived from milk proteins and their health beneficial potentials: an update. *Food and Function*, 2, 18–27.

Nielsen, S. (1993). Method fod decreasing the allergenicity of psyllium seed husk by enzyme treatment. US Patent: 5266473.

Oberyszyn, T. M. (2007). Inflammation and wound healing. *Frontier Biosciences*, 12, 2993–2999.

Ogawa, T. and Bando, N. et al. (1991). Investigation of the IgE–binding proteins in soybeans by immunoblotting with the sera of the soybean-sensitive patients with atopic dermatitis. *Journal Nutritional Science and Vitaminology*, 37, 555-565.

Okamoto, A., Hanagata, H., Matsumoto, E., Kawamura, Y. Koizumi, Y., Yanadiga, F. and Angiotensin, I. (1995). Converting enzyme inhibitory activities of various fermented foods. *Bioscience, Biotechnology, and Biochemistry,* 59,1147-1149.

Olempska-Beer, Z. S., Merker, R. I., Ditto, M. D., and DiNovi, M.J. (2006). Food-processing enzymes from recombinant microorganisms—a review. *Regulatory Toxicology and Pharmacology*, 45, 144–158.

Oseguera-Toledo, M.E., de Mejia, E.G., Dia, V.P. and Amaya-Llano, S. L. (2011). Common bean *(Phaseolus vulgaris L.)* hydrolysates inhibit inflammation in LPS-induced macrophages through suppression of NF-κB pathways. *Food Chemistry*, 127, 1175-1185.

Oshodi, A. A., Beames, R. M. and Nakai, S. (1997). In vitro protein digestibility, amino acid profile and available iron of infant-weaning food prepared from maize flour and bovine blood. *Food Research International,* 30, 193-197.

Panyam, D. and Kilara, A. (1996). Enhancing the functionality of food proteins by enzymatic modification. *Trends in Food Scienceand Technology*, 7, 120-125.

Pariza, M.W. and Johnson, E.A. (2001). Evaluating the safety of microbial enzyme preparations used in food processing: update for a new century. *Regulatory Toxicology and Pharmacology* ,33, 173–186.

Pellegrini, A. (2003). Antimicrobial Peptides from Food Proteins. *Current Pharmaceutical Design*, 9, 1225-1238.

Pihlanto-Leppälä A, Koskinen P, Piilola K, Tupasela T, Korhonen H. (2000). Angiotensin I-converting enzyme inhibitory properties of whey protein digests: concentration and characterization of active peptides. *Journal of Dairy Research*, 67, 53-64.

Potter, S.M. (1995). Overview of proposed mechanisms for the hypocholesterolemic effect of soy. *Journal of Nutrition,* 125, 606S.

Rutherfurd, S.M. (2010). Methodology for determining degree of hydrolysis of proteins in hydrolysates: a review. *Journal of AOAC International*, 93, 1515-22.

Saha, B. and Hayashi, K. (2001). Debittering of protein hydrolyzates. *Biotechnology Advances*, 19, 355-370.

Sampson, H.A. (2004). Update on food allergy. *Journal of Allergy Clinical Immunology*, 113, 805-819.

Schuchert-Shi, A. and Hauser, P.C. (2009). *Peptic and tryptic digestion Analytical Biochemistry, 387*, 202-7.

Scurlock, A.M. and Burks, A.W. (2004). Peanut allergenicity. *Annals of Allergy, Asthma, and Immunology*, 93, S12-8.

Seo, W.H., Lee, H.G. and Baek, H.H. (2008). Evaluation of bitterness in enzymatic hydrolysates of soy protein isolate by taste dilution analysis. *Journal of Food Science*, 73, S41-S46.

Sicherer, S.H. and Sampson, H.A. (2010). Food Allergy. *Journal of Allergy Clinical Immunology*, 125, S116-25.

Sicherer, S.H. and Sampson, H.A. (2007). Peanut Allergy: Emerging concepts and approaches for an apparent epidemic. *Journal of Allergy and Clinical Immunology*, 120,491-503.

Silpradit, K., Tadakittasarn, S., Rimkeeree, H., Winitchai, S. and Haruthaithanasan, V. (2010). Optimization of rice bran protein hydrolysate production using Alcalase. *Asian Journal of Food Agro-Industry,* 3, 221-231.

Soleimani, M. and Nadri, S. (2009). A protocol for isolation. *Nature Protocols*, *4*, 102.

Spilliaert, R. and Gudmundsdóttir, A. (1999). Atlantic cod trypsin Y- member of a novel trypsin group. *Journal of Marine Biotechnology*, 1, 598–607.

Satterlee, L. D. Marshall, H. F. and Tennyson, J. M. (1979). Measuring protein quality. *Journal of the American Oil Chemistry Society*, *56*, 103-109.

Stefansson, B. Helgadóttir, Olafsdottir, S. Gudmundsdottir, Á. and Bjarnason, J. (2009). Characterization of cold-adapted Atlantic cod (Gadus morhua) trypsin I — Kinetic parameters, autolysis and thermal stability. *Comparative Biochemistry and Physiology, Part B* 155, 186–194.

Szymkiewicz, A. and Jedrychowski, L.(2005). Reduction of immunoreactive properties of pea globulins as the result of enzymatic modification. *Acta Alimentaria*, 34, 295-306.

Takahashi, M., Moriguchi, S., Ikeno, M., Kono, S., Ohata, K., Usui, H., Usui, H., Kurahashi .K., Sasaki R. and Yoshikawa M. (1996). Studies on the ileum-contracting mechanisms and identification as a complement C3a receptor agonist of oryzatensin, a bioactive peptide derived from rice albumin. *Peptides*, 17: 5-12.

Tanabe, S., Arai, S. and Watanabe, M. (1996). Modification of wheat flour with bromelain and baking hypoallergenic bread with added ingredients. *Bioscience, Biotechnology, and Biochemistry*, **60**, 1269–1272.

Tirelli, A., DeNoni, I. and Resmini, P. (1997). Bioactive peptides in milk products. *Italian Journal of Food Science*, 9, 91-98.

Tsopmo, A. Cooper, A. and Jodayree, S. (2010). Enzymatic hydrolysis of oat flour protein isolates to enhance antioxidative properties. *Advance Journal of Food Science and Technology*, 2, 206-212.

Tsumura, K., Saito, T., Tsugea, K., Ashida, H., Kugimiya, W. and Inouye,K. (2005). Functional properties of soy protein hydrolysates obtained by selective proteolysis. *Lebensmittel-Wissenschaft und-Technologie*, 38, 255–261.

Tsuji, H., Kimoto, M. and Natori, Y. (2001). Allergens in major crops. *Nutrition Research*, 21, 925–934.

21 CFR 184.1914 – Trypsin. http://cfr.vlex.com/vid/184-1914-trypsin. Retrieved on July 29, 2011.

Urbano, G., López-Jurado, M., Frejnagel, S., Gómez-Villalva E., Porres, J. M. and Frías J., Vidal-Valverde, C. and Aranda, P. (2005). Nutritional assessment of raw and germinated pea (Pisum sativum L.) protein and carbohydrate by in vitro and in vivo techniques. *Nutrition*, 21, 230-239.

Urisu, A., Yamada, Y., Masuda, S., Komada, H., Wada, E., Kondo, Y., Horiba, F., Tsuruta, M., Yasaki, T., Yamada, M., Torii, S. and Nakamura, R. (1991). 16-kDa rice protein is one of the major allergens in rice grain extract and responsible for cross-allergenicity between cereal grains in the *Poaceae* family. *International Archives Allergy Applied Immunology*, 96, 244-52.

Van Der Plancken, I. Van Remoortere, M. Indrawati, Van Loey A. and Hendrickx, M.E. (2003). Heat-induced changes in the susceptibility of egg white proteins to enzymatic hydrolysis: a kinetic study. *Journal of Agricultural and Food Chemistry, 51,* 3819-3823.

Van der Plancken, I., Van Loey, A. and Hendrickx, M. E. G. (2007). Kinetic study on the combined effect of high pressure and temperature on the physico-chemical properties of egg white proteins. *Journal of Food Engineering*, 78,206–216.

Watanabe, M. Tanabe, S. Suzuki, T. Ikezawa, Z. and Arai, S. (1995). Primary structure of an allergenic peptide occurring in the chymotryptic hydrolysate of gluten. *Bioscience, Biotechnology, and Biochemistry*, 59, 1596–1597.

Watanabe, M. (1993). Hypoallergenic rice as a physiologically functional food. *Trends in Food Science and Technology*, 4, 125-128.

Wang, J.S. Zhao, M.M. Zhao, Q., Bao, Y. and Jiang, Y.M. (2007). Characterization of hydrolysates derived from enzymatic hydrolysis of wheat gluten. Journal of Food Science, 72, C103-107.

Wang, G. and Wang, T. (2009). Egg yolk protein modification by controlled enzymatic hydrolysis for imporoved functionalities. *International Journal of Food Science and Technology*, 44, 763-769.

Wen, H.W. Wysocki, W.B. Decory, T.R. and Durst, R.A. (2007). Peanut allergy, peanut allergens and methods for the detection of peanut contamination in food products. *Comprehensive Review in Food Science and Food Safety*, 6, 47-58.

Wieser, H. (1996). Relation between gliadin structure and celiac toxicity. *Acta Paediatrica Supplement*, 412, 3-9.

Whitaker, J.R. (2003). Proteolytic enzymes. In J.R. Whitaker, A.G.J. Voragen and D.W.S. Wong (Eds), *Handbook of Food Enzymology* (pp: 993-1018). Marcel Dekker, Inc., New York, New York.

Wu, J. and Ding, X. (2001). Hypotensive and physiological effect of angiotensin converting enzyme inhibitory peptides derived from soy protein on spontaneously hypertensive rats. *Journal of Agriculture Food Chemistry*, 49, 501–6.

Xu, R.J (2008). Bioactive peptides in milk and their biological and health implications. *Food Reveiws International*, 14, 1-16.

Yang, M., Chen, C. ,Wang, X., Zhu, Y. and Gu, Y. (2009). Favorable effects of the detergent and enzyme. *Journal of Biomedical Materials Res*earch, *91*, 354-361.

Yokomizo , A., Takenaka, Y., and Takenaka, T. (2002). Antioxidative activity of peptides prepared from okara protein. *Food Science and Technology Research*, 8, 357-359.

Yu, J., Ahmedna, M., Goktepe ,I., Cheng. H., and Maleki, S. (2011). Enzymatic treatment of peanut kernels to reduce allergen levels. *Food Chemistry*, 127, 1014-1022.

Zhang, G. L. T., Wand Q., Chen, L., Lei, J., Luo, J., Ma, G., and Su, Z. (2009). Mass Spectrometic detection of maker peptides in tryptic digests of gelation: A new method to differerntiate between bovine and porcine gelatin. *Food Hydrocolloids,* 23, 2001-2007.

Zhao X. and Hou, Y. (2009). Limited hydrolysis of soybean protein concentrate and isolate with two proteases and the impact on emulsifying activity index of hydrolysates. *African Journal of Biotechnology*, 8, 3314-3319.

Zheng, H., Shen, X., Bu, G., and Luo, Y. (2008). Effect of pH, temperature and enzyme-to-substrate ratio on the antigenicy of whey protein hydrolysates prepared by Alcalase. *International Dairy Journal*, 18, 1028-1033.

In: Trypsin: Structure, Biosynthesis and Functions
Editors: Kirk Weaver and Clayton Kelley
ISBN 978-1-61942-319-0

Chapter IV

Trypsin-Treated Erythrocytes Competition with Lectin-Specific Carbohydrates: Mushroom Lectins Select a Winner

Olga M. Tsivileva ***and Valentina E. Nikitina***
Laboratory of Microbiology,
Institute of Biochemistry and Physiology of Plants and Microorganisms,
Russian Academy of Sciences, Saratov, Russia

Abstract

The polyfunctional properties of carbohydrate-binding proteins, lectins, allow their application to various biological and medical studies as specific agglutinins in blood typing; in synthesis of affine stationary phases for fractionation and analysis of polysaccharides, glycolipids, or glycoproteins; and in cytochemical and histochemical studies of glycoconjugates of tissues and cell surfaces. The hemagglutination reaction, based on specific lectin binding to carbohydrates on erythrocyte surface, is the most common and appropriate test system for the determination of lectin activity and carbohydrate specificity. Treatment with trypsin interferes the pattern of erythrocyte binding by lectins and, therefore, the analytical characteristics of the test-system used for disclosing their carbohydrate-binding properties. Erythrocytes obtained from different organisms differ in carbohydrate determinants, the trypsin-treatment being capable of enzymatic constructing the optimal receptor sites on their surface.

Then we turn our attention to the results that our group has obtained over the last ten years. Trypsin-stimulated agglutination of animal (rabbit, horse, ram, bovine) erythrocytes was observed to be appropriate semi-qualitative analytical method for studying the lectin activity and carbohydrate specificity of the agglutinins of basidial mushrooms at the dikaryotic mycelium step. The difference in taxonomic characteristics and in the medium composition on growing the fungal cultures – representatives of

* E-mail: tsivileva@ibppm.sgu.ru

xylotrophic basidiomycetes – influenced the hemagglutinating activity to a much lesser extent, as compared with the aggregate state of nutrient medium and the type of erythrocytes in hemagglutination reaction.

Hemagglutinating activity of *Lentinula edodes* intracellular lectins at different morphogenesis steps was explored depending upon the type of erythrocytes, the growth medium, and the grade of proteins purity. The lectin activity under a solid-phase cultivation was appeared to depend on the type of erythrocytes used in a hemagglutination reaction, including the trypsin-treatment of erythrocytes, to a great extent. The sensitivity of the lectins towards trypsin-treated rabbit erythrocytes was no less than a hundredfold higher than towards any other erythrocyte type studied.

The culture of *L. edodes* F-249 occured to synthesize two extracellular lectins. We have isolated those from fungal culture liquid and purified to electrophoretic homogeneity. The lectins differ in physicochemical properties, composition, carbohydrate specificity, and ability for agglutination of erythrocytes of various types. The purified extracellular lectins of *L. edodes* are highly selective at recognition of definite structures on the surface of trypsinized rabbit erythrocytes and do not react with the erythrocytes of other animals and humans.

At the same time, a preferable agglutination of human trypsinized erythrocytes compared to untreated ones was not observed under any experimental conditions when exploring the blood-group specificity of the lectins of basidial xylotrophs from different systematic groups. The extent of manifestation of the hemagglutinating activity in respect to human erythrocytes had the peculiarities general for all the cultures along with somewhat differences caused obviously by the individual characteristics of each basidiomycete. The maximal values of hemagglutination titers for all the fungi were on the agar media. Judging from the results of solid-phase cultivation, the agglutinins of *Armillariella mellea* 1346 should be considered to be *H*(*O*) blood-group specific.

Trypsin-treated erythrocytes appeared to be worse test-system for agglutinating ability of mushroom mycelial hemagglutinin, a dimeric membrane-bound 68 kDa-lectin, which we isolated from the surface of dikaryotic mycelium of xylotrophic basidiomycete *Grifola frondosa*. The lectin exhibited high affinity to native rabbit erythrocytes and to human erythrocytes of the *O* blood group, but not to trypsin-treated ones. Only 13.9 μg/ml of the homogeneous preparation of a polysaccharide, a linear D-rhamnan with the definite structure of the repeated component, blocked hemagglutination completely. The lectins specific toward glycoconjugate, but not to any monosaccharide, presumably oppose a trypsin-assisted revision of the erythrocytes surface. Enzymatically lost complex carbohydrate-containing molecules – more or less perfect sites of endolectins binding with erythrocytes – results in poor agglutination and, may be, inadequate conclusions on lectins properties.

1. Introduction

According to current notions, lectins are nonimmunoglobulin proteins, which can recognize and reversibly bind carbohydrate portions of glycoconjugates without disrupting the covalent structures of any of the recognized glycosyl ligands.

To this very day hemagglutination is most commonly been used to reveal the presence of a lectin in a biological source [Lis and Sharon, 1986]. The hemagglutinating activity of extracts and other liquid samples is commonly determined in the hemagglutination reaction with free erythrocyte sedimentation, with 2% suspensions of trypsin-treated and intact animal erythrocytes, as well as four human blood types in a series of dilutions in standard immunoplates. Hemagglutination titers are expressed as the maximum lectin dilution at which erythrocyte agglutination is still recorded [Lutsik *et al.*, 1981].

The extent of complementarity of given biomolecules' spatial moieties manages their affinity in a biological sense, accompanied by the expected cellular response. The factors providing such affinity are spatial topology ("geometry") of the potential bonding groups and conformational dynamics both of the receptor and ligand molecules [Sacchettini *et al.*, 2001]. Direct contact therewith is realized via the principal kinds of intermolecular interactions, i.e. hydrogen bonds, van der Waals forces, hydrophobic effect [Quiocho *et al.*, 1991]. The functioning of some metabolic systems is possible due to the realization of a biospecific carbohydrate-protein interaction. These interactions are realized mainly via lectins/lectin-like substances capable of recognizing the specific carbohydrate determinants in the cellular structures [Lis and Sharon, 1998].

All the aforesaid explains a growing interest in investigating the structure and functions of both the lectins and glycoreceptors.

Carbohydrate-protein complexes are formed in the initial steps of a large number of physiological and pathological processes, which range from cell-pathogen interaction, to cell-cell recognition, to tumor metastasis, *etc*. Interference with these recognition events could be used to modulate or alter signal transmission, or to prevent the onset of diseases.

Molecular recognition by specific targets is at the heart of the drug discovery process. The synthesis of functional sugar mimics capable of antagonizing oligosaccharides at the protein receptor level has attracted a great deal of attention as a way to develop drugs with good stability and synthetic availability [Bernardi *et al.*, 2003; Mari *et al.*, 2005].

The study of the role of the lectins and lectin-like receptors in the immune system is a topic of current interest [Mari *et al.*, 2005]. The immunity-related reactions are known to be controlled in their early stages by the interaction of proteins with oligosaccharides, often in the form of glycoconjugates [Paul, 1984; Roitt, 1988; Ignatov, 2002; Bernardi *et al.*, 2004]. These interactions are realized mainly *via* lectins or lectin-like substances capable of recognizing the specific carbohydrate determinants in the cellular structures. Organelles self-assembling process is accompanied by the above interactions, too [Gendreau, 2004].

Lectins have been isolated from fruit bodies and mycelium of many macromycete species. Use of fungal lectins in biological and medical research is possible due to their biological activity [Batterbury *et al.*, 2002; Kent *et al.*, 2003; Wang *et al.*, 2004]. Recently works on the antitumor activity of fungal lectins have appeared [Mahajan *et al.*, 2002; Wasser, 2002; Ngai and Ng , 2004; Han *et al.*, 2005; Miyazaki *et al.* 2007; Li *et al.*, 2008]. Immobilized lectins have been extensively used for glycoproteomic research for the capture of glycoproteins [Zhou *et al.*, 2009].

Although lectins have been found widely in mushrooms, however, fungi examined for their lectins make up only a small proportion of the total number of higher fungi described. The vast majority of studies to locate lectins have focused on the basidiome, but *in vitro* mycelium cultures of certain species have shown that lectins are not produced solely by fruit bodies. Artificially grown spawn have been also refered to [Banerjee *et al.*, 1982; Ticha *et al.*, 1985, Musilek *et al.*, 1990; Giollant, 1991; Richard, 1995].

The higher cultivated basidiomycetes attract attention of the scientific community as sources of a number of biologically active substances. Morphology, life cycles and genetics of the basidiomycete *Lentinula edodes* (Berk.) Pegler [syn.: *Lentinus edodes* (Berk.) Sing.] (shiitake) have come under scrutiny of science only in the last three decades and laid the scientific foundations of current methods of the selection and cultivation of this mushroom [Przybylowicz and Donoghue, 1991]. Nevertheless, essential gaps in studying the biochemical aspects of *L. edodes* development and cultivation, especially in liquid media, exist to the present day.

Representatives of the order of *Aphyllophorales*, or polypores, belonging to the ecological group of wood destructors, hold a particular position. The pioneering works of Japanese researchers [Ikekawa *et al.*, 1969] have shown that aphyllophore basidial xylotrophs are sources of active antitumor substances. For example, about 30 biologically active substances, mostly polysaccharides with immunomodulating and antitumor properties, have been isolated by now from the fruit bodies and mycelium of the polypore *Grifola frondosa* (Fr.) S.F. Gray, or maitake mushrooms [Mizuno and Zhuang, 1995; Wasser, 2002].

2. Trypsin-stimulated Agglutination of Animal Erythrocytes

The early work of our group with mushroom lectins was aimed at finding and studying the hemagglutinating activity of culture liquid and submerged mycelium of *L. edodes*; at establishing the carbohydrate-binding specificity of the hemagglutinins revealed, and exploring the lectin activity in relation to selected physicochemical factors of cultivation [Tsivileva *et al.*, 2000, 2001].

At a start point of our Laboratory research in 2000, occasional facts on shiitake's fruit body lectins have been reported [Jeune *et al.*, 1990; Wang *et al.*, 1999]. In both studies, the results of lectin isolation from fruiting bodies are considered. It was of special interest to investigate the activity of intracellular lectins at various morphogenetic stages depending on the purification factor of lectin preparations, and types of erythrocytes used in the hemagglutination reaction. Studies [Jeune *et al.*, 1990; Wang *et al.*, 1999] did not concern these problems. For these purposes, the hemagglutinating activity of intracellular lectins from two *L. edodes* strains at various conditions mentioned above was investigated. The following morphogenetic stages were identified in shiitake cultures: nonpigmented mycelium, slightly pigmented mycelium, brown mycelial film, primordia, and fruiting body. Fruiting bodies formed in Petri dishes with wort agar 50–60 days after inoculation [Stamets, 1993].

Like all biomembranes, erythrocyte membranes contain proteins, lipids, glycolipids, and receptor proteins, glycoproteins [Kirichuk, 2002]. We used agglutination of different erythrocyte preparations, whose surfaces bore different sets of binding determinants, to characterize the specificity of shiitake lectins. The receptors of human erythrocyte membranes contain β-D-galactose moieties and certain amounts of N-acetyl-D-glucosamine, N-acetyl-neuraminic acid, N-acetyl-D-galactosamine, and L-fucose [Vorob'ev and Lorie, 1979].

We tested the agglutinating properties of lectins from *L. edodes* strains F-249 and 2T with various purification degrees were tested with intact and trypsin-treated erythrocytes from the rabbit, ram, horse, cattle and four blood types of man [Vetchinkina *et al.*, 2008].

Our experiments revealed hemagglutinating activity towards various erythrocyte types in mycelial extracts obtained at all morphogenetic stages from cultures of both shiitake strains grown on synthetic and wort agar media. The data indicate that the most sensitive test objects for L. edodes lectins were rabbit and human erythrocytes. Treatment of erythrocytes with trypsin increased the reaction sensitivity significantly. This phenomenon can be explained by liberation of lectin receptors on the erythrocyte surface and a four to tenfold increase in their binding by lectins in comparison with intact erythrocytes. Trypsin-treated bovine erythrocytes proved to be less sensitive. The lectins under study did not interact with intact bovine erythrocytes or intact or protease-treated equine or ram erythrocytes.

High hemagglutination titer was a common feature of interaction of the lectins with rabbit and human erythrocytes, but the patterns of this interaction at various shiitake morphogenetic stages were different. The highest titer of human erythrocyte hemagglutination was observed at the white mycelium stage, but it was half as high at the brown mycelial film stage. With rabbit erythrocytes, the behavior of agglutinins was the opposite: white mycelium showed the lowest titer, and the lectins of brown mycelial film had the highest hemagglutinating activity. The patterns of interaction of lectins with trypsin-treated bovine and human erythrocytes were identical: the titer decreased from the white mycelium stage to brown mycelial film. With human erythrocytes of blood type I(O) and in most cases of IV(AB), hemagglutination titers were twice as high as with II(A) or III(B).

The manifestation of lectin activity depended on nutrient media. For both basidiomycete strains grown on the synthetic medium, the hemagglutination titers were higher in comparison with the wort agar medium at various morphogenetic stages. This fact is in agreement with our earlier observations that media unfavorable for culture growth stimulate elevated lectin activity in *L. edodes* [Nikitina *et al.*, 2004].

The sensitivity of intracellular shiitake lectins towards rabbit and human erythrocytes demonstrated strain-specific differences. In case of strain 2T, the hemagglutinating activity of extracts was higher than with F-249 at all morphogenetic stages for both nutrient media. These differences were most clearly pronounced in experiments with trypsin-treated rabbit erythrocytes. The same regularities were observed in experiments with intact erythrocytes, but hemagglutination titers were four to tenfold lower.

We studied the hemagglutinating potential of *L. edodes* lectins at various steps of their gel chromatographic purification on Sephadex G-25 and Sephadex G-75. Their sensitivity towards human erythrocytes decreased seventyfold in comparison with mycelial extracts. In some cases, the specific activity of purified lectins reduced by factors of 155 and even 380 in comparison with crude extracts: in experiments with the white mycelium of strain 2T grown on wort agar in the reaction with trypsin-treated human erythrocytes of types I(O) and IV(AB), respectively.

In the course of purification, the specific lectin activity reduced first about twofold after chromatography on G-25 and even more drastically, after purification on G-75. Interaction with human erythrocytes at the lower boundary of hemagglutination reaction sensitivity was observed only with lectins of white or, in some cases, pigmented mycelium. The highest sensitivity was observed towards trypsin-treated erythrocytes of human blood types I(O) and IV(AB) and the lowest sensitivity, towards intact erythrocytes of human blood types II(A) and III(B). The described higher levels of specific lectin activities of the cultures on synthetic medium in comparison with wort agar were observed at all purification steps of the proteins under study. Differences between strains were subtle, but, as in experiments with crude extracts, higher hemagglutination titers were recorded with strain 2T. Interaction of lectins with trypsin-treated bovine erythrocytes followed the same regularities.

The opposite dependence of specific lectin activity on lectin purification degree was observed in the hemagglutination reaction with rabbit erythrocytes. In the course of purification, the sensitivity of intracellular lectins of both strains towards intact and trypsin-treated rabbit erythrocytes increased significantly at both the vegetative and generative stages. The phenomenon of higher lectin activity towards trypsin-treated erythrocytes observed for crude extracts was noted in these experiments as well. Purified intracellular lectins of strain F-249 were more sensitive towards trypsin-treated rabbit erythrocytes than those of strain 2T. Under certain experimental conditions (hemagglutination with trypsin-treated rabbit erythrocytes and synthetic nutrient medium), the specific activity of lectins from *L. edodes* strain F-249 increased with purification by factors of 11, 23, and 71 in cases of white, weakly pigmented, and brown mycelium, respectively.

In this connection, the following remarks are pertinent. Specific lectin activity and the direction of change of the titer : total protein ratio during purification of intracellular hemagglutinins from crude mycelial extracts to pure protein preparations are discussed in many studies concerning other higher fungi just to characterize the efficiency of agglutinin isolation methods, e.g., [Kawagishi *et al.*, 1990]. In these studies, use is made of the erythrocyte types most prone to agglutination by the purified protein preparations.

In the case of *L. edodes* lectins, such erythrocyte type is trypsin-treated rabbit erythrocytes. Therefore, it is natural that the agglutinating ability increases with regard to just this erythrocyte type but not with, say, human erythrocytes, to which more or less pure lectins are low sensitive. In our opinion, the agglutination of other (nonrabbit) erythrocyte types by crude mycelium extracts, which is still observable in the study, may result from an appropriate combination of physicochemical factors, such as complexation and aggregation of target proteins with admixtures and nonproteinaceous components of the crude extracts.

Therefore, the trends in the change of specific lectin activity during purification are opposite to optimal receptor molecules (on the surface of rabbit erythrocytes) and are observed with other erythrocyte types as well.

The decrease in the sensitivity towards human erythrocytes by tens of times can be explained by the above reasoning. Simultaneously, it was found that the hemagglutination reaction with rabbit erythrocytes was characterized by the opposite dependence of specific lectin activity on the degree of lectin purification.

Our results indicate that the manifestation of lectin activity in *L. edodes* depends mainly on the morphogenetic stage of the culture (In some experiments, the specific activity at the brown mycelial film stage was 3–4 times as high as in nonpigmented mycelium) and the type of erythrocytes used in the hemagglutination reaction.

The activity is less dependent on the composition of the nutrient medium. The same regularities of specific activity changes were observed in experiments with fungi grown on different media.

It should be also emphasized that trypsin treatment of all erythrocyte types increased their sensitivity towards the lectins under study. Purified intracellular *L. edodes* lectins were highly selective in recognition of certain structures on the surface of trypsin-treated rabbit erythrocytes. They did not react with erythrocytes of other animals or man.

The constant presence of lectin activity in shiitake and its change in the succession of morphogenetic stages is an interesting feature of this fungus, deserving close investigation. The lectin activity of mycelium together with other traits can be an additional parameter in the biochemical characterization of mycelium in the course of fruit formation. Further substantiation of the role of lectins as potential morphogenetic proteins can add to the development of an efficient method of obtaining shiitake mycelium for inoculation.

3. Trypsin-treated Erythrocytes as a Perfect Test-system for Extracellular Lectin Activity of *L. Edodes*

Our latest research has been directed to isolation, purification, and characterization of preparations of *L. edodes* F-249 extracellular lectins. The culture of *L. edodes* F-249 occured to synthesize two extracellular lectins. We have isolated those from fungal culture liquid and purified to electrophoretic homogeneity [Tsivileva *et al.*, 2008**a**]. The lectins differ in physicochemical properties, composition, carbohydrate specificity, and ability for agglutination of erythrocytes of various types. Extracellular lectin *L*1 from *L. edodes* is a glycoprotein of mono-subunit structure with molecular weight of 43 kDa. *L*1 is comprised of 10.5 ± 1.0% (w/w) carbohydrates represented by glucose. Extracellular lectin *L*2 is a proteoglycan of mono-subunit structure with molecular weight of 37 kDa. *L*2 is comprised of 90.3 ± 1.0% (w/w) carbohydrates represented by glucose (73% of the total mass of the carbohydrate moiety of the lectin molecule) and galactose (27% of the total mass of the carbohydrate part of the lectin molecule). The content of Asn in *L*2 is high, i.e. 42% (w/w) of total amino acids. This fact along with the composition of the carbohydrate part of the molecule (glucose + galactose) allows one to assign *L*2 to *N*-asparagine-bound proteins. The high content of aspartic acid amide in *L*2 is in agreement with our data on the selective positive effect of Asn on formation of the brown mycelial film of *L. edodes* in submerged culture [Tsivileva *et al.*, 2004].

Both lectins are specific to *D*-galactose and lactose at an equal for *L*1 and *L*2 minimal inhibiting concentration of these carbohydrates (2.08 mM Gal and 8.33 mM Lac). Other carbohydrates to which the lectins show affinity are different for the two lectins: *L*-rhamnose (4.16 mM) for *L*1 and *L*-arabinose (4.16 mM) and mannitol (8.33 mM) for *L*2. The purified extracellular lectins of *L. edodes* are highly selective at recognition of definite structures on the surface of trypsinized rabbit erythrocytes and do not react with the erythrocytes of other animals and humans.

An arabinose-binding fungal lectin was reported solely in one work by H.-X. Wang and T.B. Ng [Wang and Ng, 2005]. This lectin was isolated from a wild discomycete mushroom, *Peziza sylvestris* [Wang and Ng, 2005]. In the course of our research, the arabinose-specific lectin of mono-subunit structure with molecular mass of 37 kD (proteoglycan *L*2) has been isolated and purified from the culture liquid of the xylotrophic basidiomycete *Lentinus edodes* F-249 [Tsivileva *et al.*, 2008*a*]. Along with an unusual carbohydrate specificity, the lectin is unique as to be the extracellular lectin from basidiomycete. Submerged mycelium produces an extracellular glycolipid, *S*3, associated with the lectin *L*2. Galactose glycan residue, as well as the lipid pool composition, which includes nonhydroxylated short-chain fatty acids, is uncommon for basidiomycetes. The glycolipid consisits of *D*-galactopyranose (15 % of *S*3 contains galactose sulphate) acylated by octanoic and nonanoic fatty acids residues (28 and 72 %, respectively). The glycolipid is assumed to be a regulator of lectin activity [Tsivileva *et al.*, 2008*b*].

The distinctive features of some fungal lectins comprise a unique sugar specificity. Carbohydrate specificities of mushroom lectins involve mainly galactose (Gal), lactose (Lac) and *N*-acetylgalactosamine; a small number of mushroom lectins are specific for fucose, raffinose, *N*-glycolylneuraminic acid and *N*-acetyl-D-lactosamine [Wang *et al.*, 1998; Han *et al.*, 2005; Konska, 2006], D-galactosamine [Ngai and Ng , 2004], melibiose and xylose [Liu *et al.*, 2006; Zheng *et al.*, 2007]. For the first time, an arabinose (Ara)-binding fungal lectin with a high specific hemagglutinating (HA) activity was isolated in the study [Wang and Ng, 2005] from a wild discomycete mushroom, *Peziza sylvestris*. Since that, only few mushroom crude isolates, but not the purified lectin preparations, have been shown to exhibit the Ara-binding specificity, i.e. liquid culture mycelia extracts from *Omphalotus olearius* and biomass extracts from *Ganoderma lucidum* grown on agar plate [Mikiashvili *et al.*, 2006].

On discovery of *L. edodes* exolectins, the endogenous regulators of its biological activity were to be revealed. The research was not aimed at glycolipids initially, since there is no literature data on glycolipid regulatory activity towards lectins. Success was achieved upon finding that lectin activity changed in the course of purification. The foremost role of various glycolipids secreted by yeastlike fungi is generally believed to be that of biosurfactants, which promote solubilization of organic hydrophobic substances and their uptake from the media by microbial cells [Kulakovskaya *et al.*, 2007]. In recent years these glycolipids have been found to display biological activity as well. According to the data of chemical and elemental analysis, the principal components of *S*3 are galactose (1-sulfogalactose) acylated by octanoic and nonanoic acids. The methods were complemented by IR spectrometry data. Principal points are that in the IR spectrum of *S*3 there are bands that probably correspond to sulfate group, and that other frequency assignments are in agreement with the presence of carbohydrate units and fatty acid residues in the structure of *S*3 [Tsivileva *et al.*, 2008*b*].

It should be mentioned that *L. edodes* galactolipid *S*3 is not only homologous to the glycolipids of lower fungi in major structural components, but also resembles widely known glycolipids of non-fungal origin. Secreted glycolipids were found in yeast species [Golubev *et al.*, 2001; Cheng *et al.*, 2003; Puchkov *et al.*, 2002]. The extracellular cellobiosolipids containing the derivatives of hydroxyhexadecanoic acid were reported [Golubev *et al.*, 2004; Kulakovskaya *et al.*, 2007]. Lipid A, the major cytoplasmic membrane component in gram-negative bacteria, is known to be phosphorylated 2-amino-2-desoxy-*D*-glucopyranose disaccharide acylated with 3-hydroxyalkane acids at the 2, 3, 2', and 3' positions [quoted from Vorob'eva *et al.*, 2006]. Lipid X (LX) is a monosaccharide (glucosamine) precursor of lipid A acylated by (3-OH-14:0) acid residues at carbons 2 and 3. In the work [Vorob'eva *et al.*, 2006], the isolation of lipid A of an unusual monosaccharide structure from marine gram-negative *Chryseobacterium scophtalmum* was described. The only difference between *Chr. scophtalmum* LA and lipid X structures consists in the *iso*-structures, (3-OH-*iso*-15:0) and (3-OH-*iso*-17:0), of acyl substituents with a hydrocarbon chain longer than in LX.

Another glycolipid of a similar structure, LXLS, is not of microbial origin [Pluzhnikov *et al.*, 2006]. It was isolated from the poison of the South American ant *Paraponera clavata*, and represents 3-myristoyl-2-acetamido-2-desoxy-α-*D*-dlucopyranosylphosphate. Structural homology between the ant glycolipid and LX is not complete, as LXLS contains only one nonxydroxylated fatty acid residue per molecule of N-acetylglucosamine (albeit of the same acyl chain length), while LX contains two β-hydroxylated residues. Therefore, *L. edodes* extracellular galactolipid *S*3 contains one nonhydroxylated fatty acid residue, similarly to LXLS; on the other hand, *S*3 is not a glucosamine derivative, as yeast cellobiosolipids; its glycan part is represented by galactose. Glycolipids producers are diverse in their biological origin. Glycolipids possess similar features, and, as revealed by modern investigations, functionally significant differences in their molecular structure [Vorob'eva *et al.*, 2006; Pluzhnikov *et al.*, 2006; Kulakovskaya *et al.*, 2007; Cheng *et al.*, 2003; Golubev *et al.*, 2004].

It is no wonder, therefore, that *L. edodes* and, probably, other basidiomycetes, are able to synthesize similar compounds. However, no information of the kind concerning this systematical group is available.

Why *S*3 Could Play a Regulatory Role?

Accumulation of short-chain fatty acids in the galactolipid of shiitake mycelium takes place only during the brown mycelium film formation stage and correlates with a sharp increase in extracellular lectin activity in mycelium washouts. Neither $C_{8:0}$ or $C_{9:0}$ fatty acids accumulation nor increase in lectin activity were observed during nondifferentiated fruiting bodies formation on white mycelium. A more detailed description of the changes in fatty acids content in mycelium in relation with cultural lectin activity in the course of morphogenesis is given in our earlier publication [Tsivileva *et al.*, 2007]. In addition to the correlation between *S*3 component accumulation and the increase in lectin activity, other observations contribute to the idea of the glycolipid possible participation in the regulation of this activity. In the mixtures of preparation *S*3 + *L*1 and *S*3 + *L*2 with equal mass concentration of the components, HA titer increases 8 and 16 times, respectively (no HA activity was registered for *S*3 alone). Furthermore, in the course of purification of *L*2 preparation, its specific activity reached a peak at the stage when *L*2 is bound to *S*3 and then decreases significantly with further purification. Earlier we enabled to suggest that lectins could be involved in culture adaptation to unfavourable environmental factors. Under unfavorable mycelium growth conditions (temperature, starvation), we have observed significant increase in lectin activity, which is probably due to stabilizing and adaptogenic activity of *L. edodes* lectins [Nikitina *et al.*, 2004]. Nonspecific reactions of microbial cells towards various external stimuli have been discussed in the literature for a long time [Andreev *et al.*, 1988]. The general mechanism of adaptation to unfavorable conditions or stress includes excretion of regulatory compounds (stress factors) into the extracellular medium. Uracyl, phosphates, fatty acids ($C_{9:0}$ and $C_{10:0}$) and oligosaccharides were identified among the stress factor components. Stress factor is one of the first to be synthesized at a time when normal metabolic processes fade [Feofilova, 1994]. We assume that an unfavorable change in environmental conditions (starvation, or transferring to cell differentiation because of nutrients exhaustion), induces, in addition to secondary metabolites extreted by *L. edodes*, secretion of lectin activity regulators, including *S*3.

4. Human Trypsinized Erythrocytes for Exploring a Blood-group Specificity of Mushroom Lectins

The studies on natural occurrence of lectins was aimed, to a considerable extent, at elucidating and obtaining the blood-group specific preparations capable of agglutinating selectively the erythrocytes of definite human blood group. Blood-group specific lectins have played an important role for establishing the determinants' chemical structure of the erythrocytes antigens [Lutsik *et al.*, 1981]. However, the overwhelming majority of all the known blood-group specific lectins are the toxic ones of plant origin, and almost all the rest are the lectins of animal origin. Those lectins are severely hard to obtain due to considerable technological difficulties. At present, only very limited fungal lectins are known to possess the anti-*O(H)*, anti-*A*, anti-*B*, anti-*(A+B)*, anti-*(B+H)* specificity, among which the data on blood-group specific lectins of xylotrophic basidiomycetes *Armillariella mellea, Flammulina velutipes, Ganoderma applanatum, Ganoderma lucidum, Grifola frondosa, Grifola umbellata* were absent. We examined the listed fungal cultures for blood-groop specificity of their lectins [Nikitina *et al.*, 2005].

A preferable agglutination of human trypsinized erythrocytes compared to untreated ones was not observed under any experimental conditions when exploring the blood-group specificity of the lectins of basidial xylotrophs from different systematic groups. The extent of manifestation of the hemagglutinating activity in respect to human erythrocytes had the peculiarities general for all the cultures along with somewhat differences caused obviously by the individual characteristics of each basidiomycete. The maximal values of hemagglutination titers for all the fungi were on the agar media. Judging from the results of solid-phase cultivation, the agglutinins of *Armillariella mellea* 1346 should be considered to be *H(O)* blood-group specific.

5. Trypsin-assisted Revision of the Erythrocytes Surface Opposes *Grifola Frondosa* Lectin

The protein fractions of the biomass of *Grifola frondosa* contain substances with a high functional activity towards human cells and tissues. It has been established that the hydrophilic proteins of *G. frondosa* fruit bodies include a lectin with the specificity to N-acetyl-D-galactosamine [Kawagishi *et al.*, 1990].

Our works have shown that the mycelium of this fungus also has a lectin activity [Stepanova *et al.*, 2007]. From the surface of the dikaryotic mycelium of the xylotrophic basidiomycete *G. frondosa* 0917, a hemagglutinating protein was isolated with a molecular mass of 68 ± 1 kDa, consisting of two subunits of 33–34 kDa each.. The hemagglutinin was a hydrophilic glycoprotein with the protein : glycan ratio of 3 : 1. It exhibited high affinity to native rabbit erythrocytes and to human erythrocytes of the *O* blood group, but not to trypsin-treated ones. The hemagglutination caused by lectin was not blocked by any of the 25 tested mono-, di-, and amino sugars; it was also not blocked by some of glyco derivatives. Only 13.9 μg/ml of the homogeneous preparation of a polysaccharide, a linear D-rhamnan with the structure of the repeated component →2)-β-*D*-Rha*p*-(1→3)-α-*D*-Rha*p*-(1→3)-α-*D*-Rha*p*-(1→2)-α-*D*-Rha*p*-(1→2)-α-s*D*-Rhap-(1→ blocked hemagglutination completely. The analysis of the amino acid composition of the lectin showed the greatest percentage of amino acids with positively charged R groups, arginine, lysine, and histidine, as well as the complete absence of sulfur-containing amino acids, cysteine, and methionine. *D*-glucose and *D*-glucosamine were detected in the carbohydrate part.

In accordance with the classification proposed by J. T. Gallagher [Gallagher, 1984], the affinity to specific carbohydrate sequences allows us to define the *G. frondosa* mycelial agglutinin as endolectin. The above *D*-rhamnan containing a monosaccharide rhamnose in naturally uncommon *D*-configuration, is one of two O-specific polysaccharides (O-PS) entering a composition of lipopolysaccharide (LPS, or O antigen) of gram-negative soil bacteria *Azospirillum brasilense* Sp245 [Fedonenko *et al.*, 2002]. It should be noted that according to the chemical analysis data, two O-PS from *A. brasilense* Sp245 strain do not differ in their structure presenting *D*-rhamnan homopolymer [Fedonenko *et al.*, 2002], whereas the immunochemical assay reveals differences in the antigen determinants' structure for the given O-PS [Matora *et al.*, 2008], being in agreement with their distinct capability of interacting with the mycelial lectin from *G. frondosa* mushroom. All the aforesaid enables one to conclude on a rather precise carbohydrate-recognizing specificity of the fungal lectin. In the course of comparing (that is quite acceptable) the above lectin selectivity with the antibodies' selectivity in respect to the said O-PS from azospirilla, of special interest appeared the elucidation of immunochemical peculiarities of the lectin.

The complex of immunochemical methods was applied to study the ability of the lectin from *G. frondosa* to interact with homologous and non-homologous rabbit and human polyclonal antibodies.

The results of immunodot assay with the fragments of proteolytically cleaved antibodies demonstrated the binding of the lectin only with the *Fab* fragments (antigen-binding center) of homologous antibodies, which is evidence of specific "antigen–antibody" interaction. The revealed interaction of the lectin with non-homologous antibodies (rabbit antibodies to bacterial O-antigens and the commercial preparation of human γ-globulin) is most likely accomplished due to the contact of the carbohydrate-binding region of the lectin with the carbohydrate moiety of the antibodies ("lectin–carbohydrate"). Immunofluorescence microscopy with homologous antibodies revealed that lectin was diffusely and unevenly distributed over the surface of the hyphae, forming agglomerates in the region of buckles and young shoots [Stepanova *et al.*, 2009].

6. Trypsin-treated Erythrocytes in Visualization of Fungal Lectin - antibodies Interactions

Quantitative estimations of the mushroom lectins binding to the specific and non-specific polyclonal rabbit antibodies were attempted. For the two extracellular *L. edodes* lectins, *L*1 and *L*2, the anti-lectin *L*1 antibodies bound crude *L*2 with ten-fold-greater ELISA results compared to crude *L*1, but showed only limited reaction with *L*2 in the course of this lectin purification [unpublished results]. The data obtained could give new insight into the phenomenon of these biospecific interactions. Obviously, the actual specificity in the above processes of bio-recognition should be discussed in the especial case of the lectins and antibodies incorporation into a living system.

6.1. Results

The rabbit polyclonal antibodies against the homogeneous preparations of the mushroom *L. edodes* extracellular lectin *L*1 [Tsivileva *et al.*, 2008**a**] were obtained, and the immunochemical specificity of their interaction with the antigenic preparation examined.

The ELISA results have demonstrated the presence of common antigenic determinants in the composition of two *L. edodes* extracellular lectins (Figure 1).

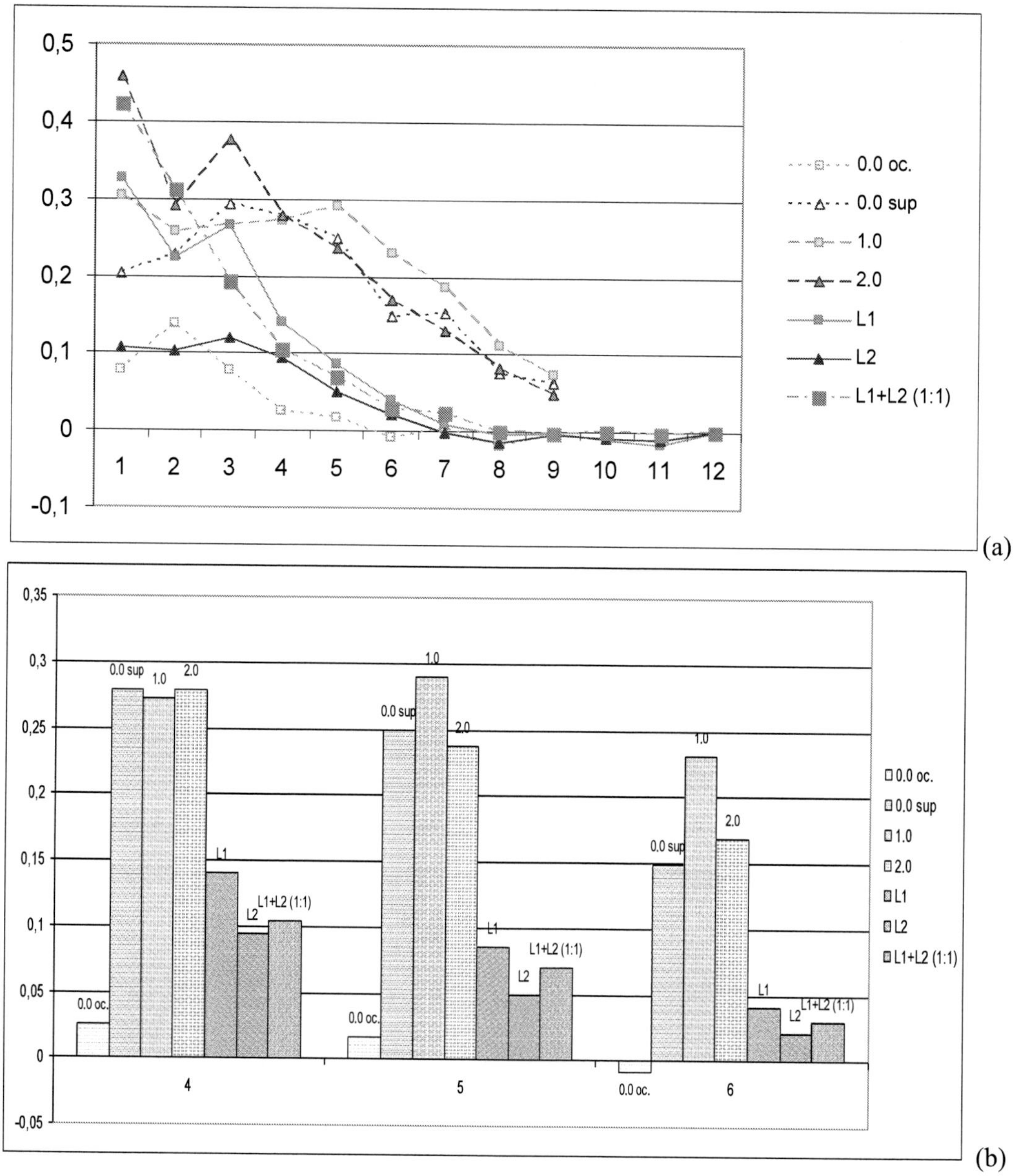

Figure 1. ELISA-detected interactions between *L. edodes* extracellular lectins and antibodies raised against *L*1: a) as introduced into microtiter wells in a series of double dilutions (abscissa); b) as a diagram constructed for linear parts of (a) curves, where 0.0 oc, 1.0 and *L*1 are the successive steps of lectin 1 purification;0.0 sup, 2.0 and *L*2 are the successive steps of lectin 2 purification; Oy axis is for A_{490} values.

At the first step of purification the lectin 2 occurs in supernatant over the solid phase (just crude lectin 1) precipitated using acetone from the culture liquid filtrate [Tsivileva *et al.*, 2008a]. This crude *L*2 capability of interacting with the anti-*L*1 antibodies appears to be about one order of magnitude greater (judging from the A_{490} values, Figure 1) than the corresponding quantity for crude *L*1. Only in the process of further purification, the lectin 1 becomes more superior as compared to lectin 2 in this context (see 1.0 and 2.0 notations, respectively, in Figure 1).

Table 1. Activity of *L. edodes* extracellular lectins at different stages of purification with erythrocytes of various types used in the hemagglutination reaction

Purification stage	Lec-tin	Erythrocytes in the reaction of hemagglutination (HA), HA titer															
		human blood group								animals							
		O		A		B		AB		rabbit		horse		sheep		cow	
		nt	tr	nt	tr	nt	tr	nt	tr	nt	tr	nt	tr	nt	tr	nt	tr
Culture liquid precipitated by acetone	1	128	128	32	8	64	16	128	128	512	512	–	–	**4**	**4**	–	–
	2	1024	256	16	16	128	32	64	512	2048	2048	–	–	–	–	-	-
Sephadex G-25	1	8	-	-	-	4	-	-	-	256	256	–	–	**4**	**4**	–	–
	2	128	-	-	-	**4**	-	-	-	1024	2048	–	–	**4**	**4**	–	–
Sephadex G-75	1	-	-	-	-	-	-	-	-	4096	32800	–	–	**4**	**4**	–	–
	2	-	-	-	-	-	-	-	-	**512**	4096	–	–	**4**	**4**	–	–

Note: "–", absence of hemagglutination reaction; tr, trypsinized erythrocytes; nt, native erythrocytes.

We tested the agglutinating properties of *L. edodes* extracellular lectins of different purification rate using native and trypsin-treated erythrocytes of rabbit, cow, sheep, horse, and humans (of the four blood groups, Table 1). Both lectins gradually become sensitive not at all to the human erythrocytes of four blood groups, in spite of initially high hemagglutination titers in the system "lectin 2+native I (O) blood group erythrocytes" and "lectin 2+trypsinized IV (AB) blood group erythrocytes" (1024 and 512, respectively).

6.2. Discussion

Commonly recognized high specificity of "antigen-antibody" recognition is a kind of biological postulate. However, various lectins are noted to be capable of bonding also non-specific immunoglobulins [Kalinin and Kulyakina, 1998] *via* oligosaccharides incorporated in the latter; with the allowance for the fact just mentioned, a term of antigenicity should be regarded as unclear. In spite of that, the lectin's ability for non-specific binding with antibodies is not a paradox due to the uniform principle of biomolecular surfaces complementarity central for the aforesaid intermolecular contacts. Since those substances are involved in biosystems of actual interest, in our opinion, establishing the parameters of their interaction seems to be important and aimed at deeper insight into the phenomenon of bilateral biospecificity of the lectin.

The experiments conducted to see whether antibodies raised against *L*1 protein from *L. edodes* F-249 would react with *L*2 used as purified preparation, in crude culture liquid and in artificial mixture *L*1+*L*2, have led us to the following indications. There are few antigenic determinants in common between the two extracellular lectins of shiitake, therewith crude *L*2 is much more effective in binding the anti-*L*1 antibodies compared with not only purified *L*2, but also the crude *L*1 as itself (Figure 1). It seems reasonable to suppose that crude *L*2 being admixed with *L*1 *in vivo*, i.e. in culture liquid, presumably displays the more profound reaction with antibodies raised against one of them, *L*1. The more so that our earlier observations [Nikitina *et al.*, 2007] revealed the considerable mutual influence of *L*1 and *L*2 in respect to the change in their lectin activity: hemagglutination titer increased from 16 (for either of two proteins in diluted buffer solutions) up to 1024 (*i.e.* by 128 times) when the lectins' solutions mixing (1:1, v/v) and incubating at 26°C for 30 min.

Obviously, the spatial arrangement of *L*1 + *L*2 complex assists greater accessibility of carbohydrate-binding sites, in the given case of the glycoconjugates binding on the test erythrocytes surface. Nevertheless, the Figure 1 shows that mixing the lectins preparations to form *L*1+*L*2 could not result in the high-selectivity (crude *L*2 toward non-specific antibodies) phenomenon mentioned just above.

And what occurs with the shiitake lectins' selectivity in respect to carbohydrate structure binding during the process of proteins purification? The reaction of hemagglutination is based on specific binding of lectins with carbohydrates present on the surface of erythrocytes; therefore, it is possible to judge their carbohydrate-binding properties by the character of agglutination of erythrocytes by lectins. Erythrocytes from various organisms differ from each other in carbohydrate dominants.

Apparently, the loosely-bound low-molecular admixtures (released *via* the Sephadex G-25 treatment [Tsivileva *et al.*, 2008*a*]) facilitated the crude lectins interaction with human erythrocytes. Purified preparations did not cause the agglutination of human erythrocytes (Table 1). The same is for the trypsin-treated rabbit erythrocytes, the extent of complementarity to which increased by 64 and 2 times in the course of purification of *L*1 and *L*2, respectively.

Thus, the purified extracellular lectins of *L. edodes* displayed high selectivity on recognition of definite structures on the surface of trypsinized rabbit erythrocytes. Table 1 shows also the absence of agglutination reaction when using the erythrocytes other than rabbit and human. Hemagglutination titer 4 with sheep blood cells seems to be neglected compared with the values of 256 to 32800 with rabbit erythrocytes. The treatment of erythrocytes with trypsin significantly increased the sensitivity of the reaction (by 8 times for both purified lectins), that is commonly explained by the higher accessibility of lectin receptors on the trypsinized erythrocytes' surface compared to native cells.

One can suggest therefore that the binding properties of lectins *in vivo* complicated by appropriate admixtures exert the system "lectin - non-specific antibody" characteristics to be opposite to those with isolated and purified lectin preparations. That is obviously due to the common hapten, carbohydrate specific to the given lectin, is a component of fungal culture medium and of antibodies raised against the lectin.

The availability of antibodies to the lectin *L*1 of *L. edodes* F-249 made it possible to test the degree of antigenic similarity among the lectins *in vivo* and *in vitro*. The results presented here indicate that while antibodies raised against *L*1 lectin will strongly react with culture liquid (first of all the *L*2 lectin component of that), it will react only slightly with the *L*2 preparations purified from culture liquid. The non-specificity of antibodies against the fungal lectin appears to be manifested *in vitro* only.

The discussion presented is concerned with the isolated substance-level assays. Probably we couldn't transform exactly the results obtained at a molecular level toward the knowledge on biological specificity of macromolecules at the level of living tissue. The lectins are potentially capable of revealing the unambiguous carbohydrate specificity, therefore the results of *in vitro* assays using lectins should be interpreted carefully when concluding on their behaviour in living systems.

References

Aleksandrova, E. A., Zav'yalova, L. A, Tereshina, V. M., Garibova, L. V., and Feofilova, E. P. (1998). Obtaining of fruiting bodies and submerged mycelium of *Lentinus edodes* (Berk.) Sing [*Lentinula edodes* (Berk.) Pegler]. *Microbiology, 67*, 535-539.

Andreev, V. S., Popov, V. G., and Dronova, N. V. (1988). Electrobiochemical regulation mechanism of microbial physiological activity on the population level. *Biotekhnologiya, 4,* 32-36.

Banerjee, P. C., Ghosh, A. K., and Sengupta, S. (1982). Hemagglutinating activity in extracts of mycelia from submerged mushroom cultures. *Appl. Environ. Microbiol., 44*, 1009-1011.

Barondes, S. H. (1988). Bifunctional Properties of Lectins: Lectins Redefined. *Trends in Biochemical Sciences, 13*, 480-482.

Batterbury, M., Tebbs, C. A., Rhodes, J. M., and Grierson, I. (2002). *Agaricus bisporus* (edible mushroom) lectin inhibits ocular fibroblast proliferation and collagen lattice contraction. *Exp. Eye Res., 74*, 361-370.

Bernardi, A., Arosio, D., Manzoni, L., Monti, D., Posteri, H., Potenza, D., Mari, S., and Jiménez-Barbero, J. (2003). Mimics of Ganglioside GM1 As Cholera Toxin Ligands: Replacement of the GalNAc Residue. *Organic and Biomolecular Chemistry*, *1*, 785-792.

Bernardi, A., Arosio, D., Potenza, D., Sánchez-Medina, I., Mari, S., Cañada, F. J., and Jiménez-Barbero, J. (2004). Intramolecular Carbohydrate-Aromatic Interactions and Intermolecular van der Waals Interactions Enhance the Molecular Recognition Ability of GM1 Glycomimetics for Cholera Toxin. *Chemistry - A European Journal*, *10*, 4395-4406.

Bobrovnik, S. A. (2003). Ligand-receptor interactions: a new method for determining the binding parameters. *J. Biochem. Biophys. Methods, 55*, 71-86.

Bobrovnik, S. A. (2004). Effect of ligand concentration on the precision of determining the parameters of ligand-receptor interaction by serial dilution methods. *Ukr. Biochim. Zh., 76*, 142-148.

Cheng, Y., McNally, D. J., Labbe, C., Voyer, N., Belzile, F., and Belanger, R. R. (2003). Insertional mutagenesis of a fungal biocontrol agent led to discovery of a rare cellobiose lipid with antifungal activity. *Appl. Environ. Microbiol., 69,* 2595-2602.

Fedonenko, Yu. P., Zatonsky, G. V., Konnova, S. A., Zdorovenko, E. L., and Ignatov, V. V. (2002). Structure of the O-specific polysaccharide of the lipopolysaccharide of *Azospirillum brasilense* Sp245. *Carbohydr. Res., 337*, 869-872.

Feofilova, E. P. (1994). Biochemical adaptation of fungi to thermal stress: Review. *Mikrobiologiya, 63*, 757-776.

Feofilova, E. P., Tereshina, V. M., and Gornova, I. B. (1994). Changes in the Carbohydrate Composition of Fungal Cells during Their Adaptation to Temperature Stress. *Mikrobiologiya*, *63*, 792-798.

Feofilova, E. P., Tereshina, V. M., Khokhlova, N. S., and Memorskaya, A. S. (2000). Different Mechanisms of the Biochemical Adaptation of Mycelial Fungi to Temperature Stress: Changes in the Cytosol Carbohydrate Composition. *Mikrobiologiya*, *69*, 606-611.

Feofilova, E. P., Tereshina, V. M., Memorskaya, A. S., Zav'yalova, L. A., and Maryshova, N. S. (1999). Changes in the Cytosol Carbohydrate Composition during the

Cytodifferentiation Process in Fungi of the Order *Agaricales*. *Mikrobiologiya*, *68*, 360-365.

Gabius, H.-J. (1994). Non-Carbohydrate Binding Partners/Domains of Animal Lectins. *International Journal of Biochemistry*, *26*, 469-477.

Gallagher, J. T. (1984). Carbohydrate-binding properties of lectins: a possible approach to lectin nomenclature and classification. *Biosci. Rep.*, *4*, 621-632.

Gendreau, S. (2004). *Modulation of Protein Functions by Homo- and Heterophilic Protein Interactions As Studied with P2X Receptors and Glutamate Transporters*, Dissertation zur Erlangung des Doktorgrades der Naturwissenschaften. Frankfurt am Main: Johann Wolfgang Goethe-Universität in Frankfurt am Main, 162 S.

Giollant, M. (1991). *Les lectines des lactaires du groupe Dapetes: (L. deliciosus, L. deterrimus, L. salmonicolor). Purification, etude biochimique et specificite. Intervention des lectines dans les phenomenes de reconnaissance moleculaire au cours des evenements precoces de la mycorhization avec les coniferes associes*. Clemont-Ferrand: These de Doctorat en Pharmacie.

Golubev, V. I., Kulakovskaya, T. V., and Golubeva, E. V. (2001). The yeast *Pseudozyma fusiformata* VKM Y-2821 producing an antifungal glycolipid. *Microbiology, 70*, 553-556.

Golubev, V. I., Kulakovskaya, T. V., Kulakovskaya, E. V., and Golubev, N. V. (2004). The fungicidal activity of an extracellular glycolipid from *Sympodiomycopsis paphiopedili* Sugiyama *et al. Microbiology, 73*, 724-728.

Han, C. H., Liu, Q. H., Ng, T. B., and Wang, H.-X. (2005). A novel homodimeric lactose-binding lectin from the edible split gill medicinal mushroom *Schizophyllum commune*. *Biochem. Biophys. Res. Commun.*, *336*, 252-257.

Ignatov, P. E. (2002). *Immunity and Infection* (in Russian, 352 p.), Moscow: Vremya.

Ikekawa, T., Uehara, N., Maeda, J., Nakanishi, M., and Fukuoka, F. (1969). Antitumor Acvtivity of Aqueous Extracts of Edible Mushrooms. *Cancer Res.*, *29*, 734-735.

Jeune, K. H., Moon, I. J., Kim, M. K., and Chung, S. R. (1990). Studies on lectins from Korean higher fungi; IV. A mitogenic lectin from the mushroom *Lentinus edodes*. *Planta Med., 56,* 592.

Kalinin, N. L., and Kulyakina M.N. (1998). Method of evaluation of carbohydrate specific interactions between immunoglobulins and biotin-conjugated lectins. *Appl. Biochem. Microbiol.*, *34*, 61-64.

Kawagishi, H., Mitsunaga, S. I., Yamawaki, M., Ido, M., Shimada, A., Kinoshita, T., Murata, T., Usui, T., Kimura, A., and Chiba, S. (1997). A lectin from mycelia of the fungus *Ganoderma lucidum*. *Phytochemistry, 44,* 7-10.

Kawagishi, H., Nomura, A., Mizuno, T., Kimura, A., and Chiba, S. (1990). Isolation and Characterization of Lectin from *Grifola frondosa* Fruiting Bodies. *Biochim. Biophys. Acta, 1034*, 247-252.

Kent, D., Sheridan, C., Tomkinson, H. A., White, S., Hiscott, P., and Grierson, I. (2003). Edible mushroom (*Agaricus bisporus*) lectin modulated human retinal pigment epithelial cell behaviour *in vitro*. *Exp. Eye Res., 76,* 213-219.

Kirichuk, V. F. (2002). *Fiziologiya krovi (Blood Physiology)*. Saratov: Izd. SGMU.

Klotz, I. M. (1946). The application of the law of mass action to binding by proteins. Interaction with calcium. *Arch. Biochem.*, *9*, 109-116.

Kocourek, J., and Horejsi, V. (1981). Defining a Lectin. *Nature*, *290*, 188.

Konska, G. (2006). Lectins of Higher Fungi (Macromycetes) - Their Occurrence, Physiological Role, and Biological Activity. *Int. J. Med. Mush., 8*, 19-30.

Korolev, N. P. (1984). Lectin functions in cells. In *Reviews of sciense and engineering. Ser. General Problems of Physicochemical Biology. Vol. 1.* Moscow: VINITI.

Kulakovskaya, E. V., Kulakovskaya, T. V., Golubev, V. I., Shashkov, A. C., Grachev, A. A., and Nifant'ev, N. E. (2007). Fungicidal activity of cellobiose lipids from culture broth of yeast *Cryptococcus humicola* and *Pseudozyma fusiformata. Russ. J. Bioorg. Chem., 33,* 156-160.

Kulkarni, R. K. (1990). Mannitol metabolism in *Lentinus edodes*, the Shiitake Mushroom. *Appl. Environ. Microbiol., 56*, 250-253.

Laine, R. A. (1997). The information-storing potential of the sugar code. In H.-J. Gabius, and S. Gabius (Eds.), *Glycosciences: Status and Perspectives* (pp. 1-14). London, Weinheim: Chapman and Hall.

Li, Y. R., Liu, Q. H., Wang, H.-X., and Ng, T. B. (2008). A novel lectin with potent antitumor, mitogenic and HIV-1 reverse transcriptase inhibitory activities from the edible mushroom *Pleurotus citrinopileatus. Biochim. Biophys. Acta (BBA) - General Subjects, 1780*, 51-57.

Liener, I. E., Sharon, N., and Goldstein, I. J. (Eds.) (1986). *The Lectins: Properties, Functions, and Applications in Biology and Medicine*. Orlando: Academic Press.

Lin, Yu., and Su, A. (2004). Isolation, characterization and haemagglutination of the lectin from *Fistulina hepatica. Natur. Prod. Res. Develop., 16*, 420.

Lis, H., and Sharon, N. (1986). Biological Properties of Lectins. In I. E. Liener, N. Sharon, and I. J. Goldstein (Eds.), *The Lectins: Properties, Functions, and Applications in Biology and Medicine* (pp. 266-269). Orlando, Florida: Academic Press Inc.

Lis, H., and Sharon, N. (1998). Lectins: carbohydrate-specific proteins that mediate cellular recognition. *Chem. Rev., 98*, 637-674.

Liu, Q., Wang, H.-X., and Ng, T. B. (2006). First report of a xylose-specific lectin with potent hemagglutinating, antiproliferative and anti-mitogenic activities from a wild ascomycete mushroom. *Biochim. Biophys. Acta (BBA) - General Subjects, 1760,* 1914-1919.

Lutsik, M. D., Panasyuk, E. N., and Lutsik, A. D. (1981). *Lektiny (Lectins).* Lvov: Vyssh. Shkola, Izd. L'vov. Univ.

Mahajan, R. G., Patil, S.,I., Mohan, D. R., and Shastry, P. (2002). *Pleurotus eous* mushroom lectin (PEL) with mixed carbohydrate inhibition and antiproliferative activity on tumor cell lines. *J. Biochem. Mol. Biol. Biophys., 6,* 341-345.

Mari, S., Serrano-Gómez, D., Cañada, F. J., Corbí, A. L., and Jiménez-Barbero, J. (2005). 1D Saturation Transfer Difference NMR Experiments on Living Cells: The DC-SIGN/Oligomannose Interaction. *Angewandte Chemie International Edition, 44*, 296-298.

Matora, L. Yu., Burygin, G. L., and Shchegolev, S. Yu. (2008). Study of immunochemical heterogeneity of *Azospirillum brasilense* lipopolysaccharides. *Microbiology,* 77, 166-170.

Metzler, D. (1980). *Biochemistry* (Volume 1). Moskow: Mir.

Mikiashvili, N., Elisashvili, V., Wasser, S. P., and Nevo, E. (2006). Comparative study of lectin activity of higher basidiomycetes. *Int. J. Med. Mush., 8,* 31-38.

Miyazaki, Y., Kaneko, S., Sunagawa, M., Shishido, K., Yamazaki, T., Nakamura, M., and Babasaki, K. (2007). The fruiting-specific Le.flp1 gene, encoding a novel fungal fasciclin-like protein, of the basidiomycetous mushroom *Lentinula edodes*. *Curr. Genet., 51,* 367-375.

Mizuno, T., and Zhuang, C. (1995). Maitake, *Grifola frondosa*: Pharmacological Effects. *Food Rev. Int., 11*, 135-149.

Morton, N., Hammond, J. B. W., and Dickerson, A. G. (1985). The *Agaricus bisporus* mannitol pathway during sporophore growth. *Trans. Br. Mycol. Soc., 85*, 671-675.

Musilek, M., Ticha, M., Volc, J., and Kocourek, J. (1990). Studies on lectins. LXXI. Lectins in mycelial cultures of *Kuehneromyces mutabilis, Pholiota squarrosa*, and *Flammulina velutipes*. In J. Kocourek, and D. L. J. Freed (Eds.), *Lectins - Biology, Biochemistry, Clinical Biochemistry* (Vol. 7, pp. 53-56). St. Louis: Sigma Chemical Company.

Ngai, P. H., and Ng, T. B. (2004). A mushroom (*Ganoderma capense*) lectin with spectacular thermostability, protein mitogenic activity on splenocytes, and antiproliferative activity toward tumor cells. *Biochem. Biophys. Res. Commun., 314*, 988-993.

Nikitina, V. E., Tsivileva, O. M., and Garibova, L.V. (2004). Stimulants of Lectin Activity of *Lentinus edodes* on Synthetic Agar Media. *Biotechnology in Russia, 3,* 53-58.

Nikitina, V. E., Tsivileva, O. M., Pankratov, A. N., and Bychkov, N. A. (2007). *Lentinula edodes* Biotechnology - From Lentinan to Lectins. *Food Technol. Biotechnol., 45,* 228-235.

Nikitina, V. E., Tsivileva, O. M., Stepanova, L. V., and Loshchinina, E. A. (2005). Searching for the blood-group specific lectins of mushroom origin. In Yu. V. Sergeev (Ed.), *Advances in Medicinal Mycology* (Vol. V, pp. 201-205). Moscow: National Academy of Mycology.

Paul, W. E. (Ed.) (1987). *Fundamental Immunology*. New York: Raven Press Books, Ltd.

Pluzhnikov, K. A., Bocharov, D. N., Kononova, N. V., Sukhanov, S. V., Balashova, T. A., Arsen'ev, A. S., and Grishin, E. V. (2006). Identification and structural analysis of a glycophospholipid component from the venom of ant *Paraponera clavata*. *Russ. J. Bioorg. Chem., 32*, 478-484.

Przybylowicz, P., and Donoghue, J. (1991). *Shiitake Growers Handbook: the Art and Science of Mushroom Cultivation*. Dubuque: Kendall / Hunt Publ. Co.

Puchkov, E. O., Zahringer, U., Lindner, B., Kulakovskaya, T. V., Seydel, U., and Wiese, A. (2002). Mycocidal, membrane-active complex of *Cryptococcus humicola*, a new type of cellobiose lipid with detergent features. *Biochem. Biophys. Acta (Biomembranes), 1558,* 161-170.

Quiocho, F. A., Vyas, N. K., and Spurlino, J. C. (1991). Atomic interactions between proteins and carbohydrates. *Trans. Am. Crystallogr. Asoc., 25,* 23-35.

Raju, T. S., Briggs, J. B., Borge, S. M., and Jones, A. J. (2000). Species-specific variation in glycosylation of IgG: evidence for the species-specific sialylation and branch-specific galactosylation and importance for engineering recombinant glycoprotein therapeutics. *Glycobiology, 10,* 477-486.

Richard, T. (1995). *Contribution a l'etude de la lectine du champignon basidiomycete Rigoporus lignosus. Purification, proprietes physicochimiques et localisation de la lectine et de ses sites d'affinite*. Nancy: These de Doctorat en Sciences.

Roitt, I. M. (1988). *Essential Immunology*. Oxford, London, Edinburgh, Boston, Palo Alto, Melbourne: Blackwell Scientific Publications.

Sacchettini, J. C., Baum, L. G., and Brewer, C. F. (2001). Multivalent protein–carbohydrate interactions. A new paradigm for supermolecular assembly and signal transduction. *Biochemistry, 40*, 3009-3015.

Solis, D., Jimenez-Barbero, J., Kaltner, H., Romero, A., Siebert, H. C., von der Lieth, C. W., and Gabius, H. J. (2001). Towards defining the role of glycans as hardware in information storage and transfer: basic principles, experimental approaches and recent progress. *Cells Tissues Organs, 168,* 5-23.

Stamets, P. (1993). *Growing Gourmet and Medicinal Mushrooms* (pp. 259-260). Berkeley: Ten Speed.

Stepanova, L. V., Burygin, G. L., Matora, L. Yu., Bogatyrev, V. A., Sokolova, M. K., and Nikitina, V. E. (2009). Immunochemical Properties and Localization of Lectin from the Basidiomycete *Grifola frondosa* (Fr.) S.F. Gray. *Microbiology*, *78*, 202-207.

Stepanova, L. V., Burygin, G. L., Nikitina, V. E., and Tsivileva, O. M. (2011). On the role of carbohydrate-protein highly-selective interactions in the biological activity of glycoconjugates: *Grifola frondosa* (Fr.) S.F. Gray lectin binding to specific and non-specific antibodies. *World Journal of Microbiology and Biotechnology, 27,* DOI: 10.1007/s11274-010-0610-5.

Stepanova, L. V., Nikitina, V. E., and Boyko, A. S. (2007). Isolation and characterization of lectin from the surface of the mycelium of *Grifola frondosa* (Fr.) S.F. Gray. *Microbiology, 76*, 429-434.

Ticha, M., Dudova, V., Kocourek, J., and Volc, J. (1985). Studies on lectins. LXII. A nonspecific erythroagglutinating lectin and a blood-group A specific lectin in the mushroom *Agrocybe aegerita* (Brig.) Sing. In T. C. Bog-Hansen, and J. Breborowicz (Eds.), *Lectins - Biology, Biochemistry, Clinical Biochemistry* (Vol. 4, pp. 505-514). Berlin: Walter de Gruyter.

Tsivileva, O. M., Makarov, O. E., Nikitina, V. E., and Garibova, L. V. (2007). Changes in fatty acid composition of total lipids and lectin activity during morphogenesis of *Lentinus edodes*. *Mycol.andPhytopathol., 41*, 450-455.

Tsivileva, O. M., Nikitina, V. E., and Garibova, L. V. (2005**a**). Effect of culture medium composition on the activity of extracellular lectins of *Lentinus edodes*. *Appl. Biochem. Microbiol., 41*, 174-176.

Tsivileva, O. M., Nikitina, V. E., Garibova, L. V., and Ignatov, V. V. (2001). Lectin activity of *Lentinus edodes*. *Int. Microbiol., 4*, 41-45.

Tsivileva, O. M., Nikitina, V. E., Garibova, L. V., Zav'yalova, L. A., and Ignatov, V. V. (2000). Hemagglutinating activity of the fungus *Lentinus edodes* (Berk.) Sing [*Lentinula edodes* (Berk.) Pegler]. *Microbiology, 69*, 30-35.

Tsivileva, O. M., Nikitina, V. E., and Loshchinina, E. A. (2008**a**). Isolation and Characterization of *Lentinus edodes* (Berk.) Singer Extracellular Lectins. *Biochemistry (Moscow), 73*, 1154-1161.

Tsivileva, O. M., Nikitina, V. E., and Makarov, O.E. (2008b) Characterization of an Extracellular Glycolipid from *Lentinus edodes* (Berk.) Sing [*Lentinula edodes* (Berk.) Pegler]. *Microbiology, 77*, 436-440.

Tsivileva, O. M., Nikitina, V. E., Makarov, O. E., and Garibova, L. V. (2005b). Relationship between the Carbohydrate Specificity of Lectins and the Carbohydrate Composition of the *Lentinus edodes* (Berk.) Sing [*Lentinula edodes* (Berk.) Pegler] Mycelium at Different Stages of Its Morphogenesis. *Microbiology, 74*, 621-623.

Tsivileva, O. M., Pankratov, A. N., Nikitina, V. E., and Garibova, L. V. (2004). Relationship between the molecular structure of nitrogen source and the activity of the extracellular lectins of *Lentinus edodes* (Berk.) Sing [*Lentinula edodes* (Berk.) Pegler] upon submerged cultivation. *Microbiology, 73*, 410-413.

Tsivileva, O. M., Pankratov, A. N., Nikitina, V. E., and Garibova, L. V. (2005**c**). Effect of media components on the mycelial film formation in submerged culture of *Lentinus edodes* (Shiitake). *Food Technol. Biotechnol., 43*, 227-234.

Tsivileva, O. M., Stepanova, L. V., Burygin, G. L., and Nikitina, V. E. (2011). How much would the fungal lectin - antibodies interactions be selective? *Current Topics in Biotechnology*. In press.

Ukawa, I., Ito, H., and Hisamatsu, M. (2000). Antitumor effects of (1→3) β-D-glucan and (1→6)β-D-glucan purified from newly cultivated mushroom Hatakeshimeju (Lyophyllum decastes Sing.). *J. Biosci. Bioeng., 90*, 98-104.

Vetchinkina, E. P., Nikitina, V. E:, Tsivileva, O. M., and Garibova, L. V. (2008). Activity of *Lentinus edodes* intracellular lectins at various developmental stages of the fungus. *Applied Biochemistry and Microbiology, 44*, 66-72.

Vorob'ev, A. I., and Lorie, Yu. I. (Eds.) (1979). *Rukovodstvo po gematologii (A Handbook on Hematology)*. Moscow: Meditsina.

Vorob'eva, E. V., Krasikova, I. N., Dmitrenok, A. S., Dmitrenok, P. S., Isakov, V. V., Nedashkovskaya, O. I., and Solov'eva, T. F. (2006). An unusual lipid A from a marine bacterium *Chryseobacterium scophtalmum* CIP 104199^{T}. *Russ. J. Bioorg. Chem., 32*, 485-491.

Wang, P. H., Hsu, C. I., Tang, S. C., Huang, Y. L., Lin, J. Y., and Ko, J. L. (2004). Fungal immunomodulatory protein from *Flammulina velutipes* induces interferon-gamma production through p38 mitogen-activated protein kinase signaling pathway. *J. Agric. Food. Chem., 52*, 2721-2725.

Wang, H.-X., and Ng, T.-B. (2005). First report of an arabinose-specific fungal lectin. *Biochem. Biophys. Res. Commun., 337*, 621-625.

Wang, H.-X., Ng, T.B., and Ooi, V. E. C. (1998). Lectins from mushrooms. *Mycol. Res., 102*, 897-906.

Wang, H. X., Ng. T. B., and Ooi, V. E. C. (1999). Studies on purification of a lectin from fruiting bodies of the edible shiitake mushroom *Lentinus edodes. Int. J. Biochem. Cell Biol., 31*, 595-599.

Wasser, S. P. (2002). Medicinal Mushrooms as a Source of Antitumor and Immunomodulating Polysaccharides. *Appl. Microbiol. Biotechnol., 60*, 258-274.

Zheng, S., Li, C., Ng, T. B., and Wang, H.-X. (2007). A lectin with mitogenic activity from the edible wild mushroom *Boletus edulis. Process Biochemistry, 42*, 1620-1624.

Zhou, H., Hou, W., Denis, N. J., Zhou, H., Vasilescu, J., Zou, H., and Figeys, D. (2009). Glycoproteomic Reactor for Human Plasma. *J. Proteome Res., 8*, 556–566.

In: Trypsin: Structure, Biosynthesis and Functions
Editors: Kirk Weaver and Clayton Kelley
ISBN 978-1-61942-319-0

Chapter V

Protease-Activated Receptor 2 in the Enteric Nervous System

Danielle M. Fritze, Michael W. Mulholland and Weizhen Zhang**
Department of Surgery, University of Michigan,
Ann Arbor, US

Abstract

The enteric nervous system (ENS) integrates local neuroendocrine signaling with central autonomic input to regulate the motor and secretory function of the gastrointestinal (GI) tract. Exposure to inflammatory mediators such as trypsin or mast cell tryptase is postulated to affect ENS signaling, contributing to both protective and pathologic changes in GI function.

Protease-activated receptor 2 (PAR-2) is a receptor specifically activated by the serine-proteases trypsin and tryptase. Within the mammalian ENS, PAR-2 expression has been identified in neurons of both the submucosal and myenteric plexus. Myenteric neurons respond to trypsin with prolonged depolarization, suppression of fast excitatory post-synaptic potentials, and phospholipase C (PLC) - dependent cytosolic calcium transients. Trypsin also activates PAR-2 in enteroglial cells, causing activation of PLC and sphingosine kinase.

This signaling cascade results in cytosolic calcium transients, subsequent capacitative calcium entry, and c-fos expression. Activation of PAR-2 by trypsin within the ENS may ultimately alter intestinal ion channel permeability and secretory function. PAR-2 may therefore contribute to the physiological function and pathophysiological response in the ENS.

* Corresponding author: Weizhen Zhang. Department of Surgery, University of Michigan Medical Center, Ann Arbor, MI . Tel: 734-615-0360; Fax: 734-763-4135; E-mail: weizhenz@umich.edu

Introduction

The human gastrointestinal tract serves a myriad of functions ranging from nutrient absorption to hormone secretion to protection against ingested pathogens. These processes are subject to several levels of regulation; input from the central nervous system (CNS), endocrine and paracrine signals, and information from receptors within the gut are integrated within the enteric nervous system (ENS). The ENS provides coordination of gastrointestinal motility, secretory function, and local blood flow.

Protease-activated receptor 2 (PAR2) is a receptor expressed by both neurons and glial cells within the ENS. Activation of either neuronal or glial PAR2 by trypsin or tryptase results in physiologic responses involving changes in intracellular calcium concentration. Ultimately, the activity of PAR2 may modulate gastrointestinal motility, ion flux, intestinal barrier function, and sensitivity to noxious stimuli.

Gastrointestinal (GI) conditions such as inflammatory bowel disease (IBD), Irritable Bowel Syndrome (IBS), post-operative ileus, and various gastrointestinal infections may affect and be affected by the enteric nervous system via trypsin/tryptase-induced activation of PAR2. An understanding of the role of these pathways in disease pathophysiology may yield new therapeutic approaches. Indeed, mast cell stabilization, tryptase inhibition, and PAR2 blockade have each shown promise as treatment options for different gastrointestinal diseases.

Enteric Nervous System Structure and Function

The enteric nervous system is located within the intestinal wall, spanning the entire length of the GI tract. Nicknamed the "second brain," the ENS is capable of regulating gastrointestinal function independent of central nervous system input[1]. Neuronal cell bodies are housed in ganglia in two distinct locations. The myenteric ganglia are located between the longitudinal muscle of the muscularis externa and the circular muscle of the muscularis interna, while submucous ganglia are located within the submucosa. Processes from these neurons then form the myenteric and submucous plexuses. While neurons of the myenteric ganglia primarily affect gastrointestinal motility and those located in the submucous plexus regulate GI secretory and endocrine function, there are also numerous connections between the two networks.

Neurons of the ENS form reflex pathways entirely contained within the gut. Sensory information is transmitted from gastrointestinal mucosa, muscle fibers, vasculature, and endocrine cells via afferent nerve processes. Afferent neurons then synapse on interneurons within the two enteric plexuses. Interneurons travel longitudinally along the gastrointestinal tract to synapse with other interneurons and eventually with efferent motor neurons. These motor neurons may project locally or travel longitudinally along the bowel to transmit functional signals back to the effector organs. Efferent enteric nerves innervate gastrointestinal smooth muscle, secretory glands, endocrine cells, and intestinal blood vessels. Those motor neurons with proximal projections are primarily excitatory whereas those projecting distally are inhibitory, allowing for coordinated peristalsis.

While the enteric nervous system can function independent of central input, there are nonetheless important connections between the central and enteric nervous systems. These may be characterized by their involvement with either the sympathetic or parasympathetic pathway. Afferent parasympathetic fibers carry sensory information from GI mechanoreceptors and chemoreceptors to the brainstem via the vagus nerve. Efferent fibers in the vagus nerve then transmit motor signals from the brainstem back to the GI tract, with greatest synaptic density in the foregut. Parasympathetic activation causes increased gastrointestinal motor and secretory function, as well as vasodilation and sphincter relaxation.

Afferent sympathetic fibers serve a nociceptive function, transmitting information from gastrointestinal mechanical, chemical, and thermal stimuli to the brain. Efferent sympathetic fibers from the brain innervate the various GI sphincters and submucosal blood vessels. Sympathetic fibers also terminate on ENS vasoactive intestinal polypeptide (VIP) neurons and pre-synaptic cholinergic nerve endings to modulate their activity. In addition to the sympathetic pathways involving the brain, the sympathetic nervous system has a unique reflex pathway. In certain sympathetic neurons, excitation of one limb of an axon is propagated into the other limb, projecting back to the GI tract. This pathway results in an "axon reflex" arc which translates sensory information into a sympathetic response without central involvement. Sympathetic activation typically causes splanchnic vasoconstriction, sphincter contraction, and inhibition of gastrointestinal motor and secretory function.

Enteric neurons may be characterized by their primary function and by the neurotransmitters that they produce. Excitatory motor neurons innervating gastrointestinal muscle, for example, produce primarily acetylcholine and substance P [2,3]. In contrast, the main neurotransmitter released by inhibitory motor neurons is nitric oxide, with lesser production of ATP, VIP, and other neuropeptides[4-7]. Ascending interneurons are largely excitatory and almost exclusively cholinergic[8]. There are several distinct subtypes of descending interneurons, each producing a combination of neurotransmitters including acetylcholine, serotonin, nitric oxide, VIP, γ-amino butyric acid (GABA), neuropeptide Y, bombesin, and somatostatin[9]. Secretomotor neurons fall into three subtypes: those producing acetylcholine and NPY which innervate the intestinal mucosal glands, those producing acetylcholine and calretinin which innervate mucosal glands and arterioles, and those producing only VIP which also innervate intestinal arterioles[9]. Primary afferent neurons are primarily cholinergic, with additional production of other neurotransmitters such as tachykinins and calbindin[10]. The presence of neuronal subtypes characterized by different neurotransmitter expression profiles allows for precise tailoring of gastrointestinal function to local and systemic conditions.

Neurons of the ENS may be further characterized by their morphological and corresponding electrophysical properties. Dogiel I (DI) neurons are uniaxonal, and function as motor neurons or interneurons. They display S-type electrophysiology with prominent fast excitatory post-synaptic potentials (EPSPs), narrow action potentials, and an absence of prolonged afterhyperpolarization (AHP) [11]. Dogiel II (DII) neurons have multiple axons, and function as interneurons or intrinsic primary afferent neurons. In contrast to DI neurons, DII neurons have AH electrophysiology characterized by broad action potentials, prolonged AHP, and only rare fast EPSPs [11]. Alterations in enteric neuronal electrophysiology may contribute to ENS dysfunction in various gastrointestinal disease states.

In addition to its neurons, the enteric nervous system contains a large population of enteroglial cells. These cells envelop the nerve bodies of enteric neurons throughout the ENS. While enteroglia were once believed to provide only structural support to enteric neurons, further study has suggested additional roles in maintenance of intestinal homeostasis.

Enteroglial cells have antigen-presenting capabilities, and can be activated by exposure to inflammatory mediators. Specifically, they are responsive to acetylcholine, serotonin, histamine, proteases including trypsin, and other neuropeptides [12,13]. They secrete neuronal growth factors, cytokines, ATP, and nitric oxide [12]. The exact functions of enteroglial cells have not been fully characterized, but are presumed to include modulation of the gastrointestinal immune milieu, intestinal barrier function, and GI motility[14,15].

The Enteric Nervous System and Gastrointestinal Disease

The enteric nervous system is involved in many different gastrointestinal and systemic diseases. Congenital or acquired absence of enteric ganglia results in disordered motility within the aganglionic segment. Hirschprung's disease is a classic congenital condition in which failure of neural crest migration during embryogenesis results in aganglionosis of the distal GI tract, usually the distal colon.

The aganglionic colon lacks inhibitory innervation, resulting in tonic contraction of colonic smooth muscle and functional obstruction. Chagas disease, caused by *Trypanosoma cruzi* infection, is variably characterized by acquired enteric hypoganglionosis.

This manifests as achalasia and chronic intestinal pseudo-obstruction in affected patients. Hyperganglionic states such as neurofibromatosis are also characterized by dysmotility, either from hyper or hypotonic intestinal smooth muscle. Enteric neurons which are dysfunctional despite normal population can be equally problematic. In congenital infantile hypertrophic pyloric stenosis, the myenteric plexus around the gastric pylorus is populated by neurons lacking nitric oxide synthase. This results in tonic contraction of the circular smooth muscle of the pylorus and gastric outlet obstruction.

States of gastrointestinal inflammation, including inflammatory bowel disease (IBD), may also affect the enteric nervous system. Conversely, enteric nervous system dysfunction may play a role in the pathophysiology of such inflammatory conditions and influence their manifestations. It remains unclear whether neuro-inflammation is part of the inciting event in the development of IBD; more probably, alterations in enteric nervous system function result from the local and systemic inflammation associated with IBD. Patients with IBD often exhibit abnormal colonic motility which is hypothesized to result from enteric nervous system dysfunction.

Alterations in levels of substance P, VIP, and other neuropeptides, as well as increased expression of their receptors have been observed in enteric nerves and surrounding tissues of patients with IBD. Furthermore, there are fewer nerve terminals and synapses, and evidence of degenerating axons within the intestine of patients with Crohn's disease as compared to healthy controls.

Despite these observations, there are many aspects of enteric nervous system function and dysfunction in inflammatory bowel disease that remain unclear. One area of recent interest involves the potential role of trypsin, tryptase, and other agonists of protease-activated receptor 2 (PAR2) in the ENS in the pathophysiology of inflammatory bowel disease and other GI conditions.

Par2 in the Enteric Nervous System

Protease-activated receptors represent a unique receptor class in which cleavage by a serine protease reveals a tethered ligand which can then bind the receptor's active site, resulting in activation and physiologic response. There are several different types of protease-activated receptors, with different ligands and expression patterns. Each class functions through the activation of G-proteins, Raf/Ras, and calcium signaling. PAR2 is known to be activated by trypsin and tryptase, but not by thrombin. Trypsin and tryptase are also capable of activating PAR4, but research involving the enteric nervous system has focused primarily on PAR1 (activated by thrombin but not trypsin) and PAR2.

PAR2 expression has been identified within different cells of the gastrointestinal tract, including enteric neurons and glial cells. In porcine ileum, PAR2-like immunoreactivity was detected in neurons of the submucosal and myenteric plexuses as well as in fibers innervating smooth muscle, mucosa, and entero-endocrine cells [16]. PAR2 cloning by RT-PCR confirmed the presence of PAR2 transcripts in primary myenteric neuron cultures [17].

In primary culture of guinea pig myenteric plexus, PAR2 immunoreactivity was also noted on myenteric glial cells [13]. The proportion of cultured guinea pig myenteric neurons expressing PAR2 has been estimated at approximately 65% by co-localization of PAR2 and various neuronal markers [17]. PAR2 has also been co-localized with VIP, calbindin, calcitonin gene-related peptide, and substance P [18,19].

Trypsin and Tryptase in the Enteric Nervous System

The primary agonists of protease-activated receptor 2 are trypsin and tryptase, although active coagulation factors such as Factor VIIa and Xa are also capable of receptor cleavage and activation [20]. In specific circumstances such as periodontal inflammatory disease, bacteria may produce serine proteases with the capacity for protease-activated receptor 2 activation [21,22]. Within the enteric nervous system, however, trypsin and tryptase are likely the most significant stimuli for protease-activated receptor 2.

Trypsin is a serine protease produced by proteolytic cleavage of the zymogen trypsinogen. There are several isoforms of trypsinogen, expressed in different tissues, each of which is a precursor to active trypsin. The pancreas is the largest producer of trypsinogens, primarily secreting trypsinogen I and II. Within the duodenum, these zymogens are cleaved by enterokinase to yield the active enzyme. While the primary target of pancreatic trypsin is intra-luminal proteins within the proximal GI tract, trypsinogens are also produced in the more distal bowel and other tissues. Trypsinogen and enteropeptidase mRNA transcripts have been detected in human epithelial cell lines from the colon, prostate, and airway[23]. Using in situ hybridization and immunohistochemistry, trypsinogen mRNA and trypsin protein have also been detected in human and mouse skin, brain, lung, kidney, splenic leukocytes, liver, the extra-hepatic biliary tree, and the luminal GI tract from the esophagus through the colon[24]. While trypsin expression has been documented in gastrointestinal mucosa and neurons of the central nervous system, production of trypsin in neurons and glia of the enteric nervous system has not been investigated.

Tryptase is a serine protease with action similar to trypsin. It is produced and secreted by mast cells, derived from hematopoietic progenitors. Mast cells play a role in immunity and inflammation, and are particularly important factors in allergic reactions and parasitic infections. Located primarily in the skin, lung, and gastrointestinal tract where exposure to pathogens is particularly high, mast cells participate in host-defense mechanisms. While the concentration is lower than in the epithelial tissues, mast cells also reside within the brain. In each of these organs, including the intestine, mast cells are often found clustered around blood vessels and nerve endings[25,26]. Mast cells are activated primarily by IgE, however other substances including cytokines, neuropeptides, and some medications can also result in stimulation of mast cells. Upon activation, mast cells are induced to release pre-formed substances stored in granules. These compounds include histamine, TNF-alpha, and proteases such as tryptase. Prostaglandins, interleukins, and other such mediators may also be produced and secreted by activated mast cells.

In the gastrointestinal tract, mast cells may maintain a baseline level of activation, presumably due to the ubiquity of intra-luminal pathogens[27]. Activation of gastrointestinal mast cells above this basal level has a myriad of potential effects related to the compounds that they secrete. Cytokines and chemokines contribute to the recruitment of other inflammatory cells and increase capillary permeability. Histamine changes intestinal ion transport and may contribute to diarrhea. Tryptase may cleave and activate PAR2 on enteric neurons, glia, and smooth muscle cells. Eventually, these mediators can lead to changes in tissue composition, such as angiogenesis or fibrosis, and organ function.

Myenteric Neuron Response to Trypsin and Tryptase

The interaction between the serine proteases and enteric neurons is complex and at least partially mediated by protease-activated receptor 2. Anatomic proximity of mast cells and enteric nerve endings in vivo suggests a functional relationship between these two elements within the intestinal wall[25]. While the location of mast cells relative to protease-activated receptor 2 has not been specifically evaluated, PAR expression has been demonstrated in neurons located within both the myenteric and submucous plexuses[16]. This provides indirect evidence that protease-activated receptors expressed by enteric neurons may be exposed to the products of mast cell degranulation, including tryptase. Trypsin mRNA has been co-localized with that of enteropeptidase and protease-activated receptor 2 in colon epithelial cell lines, also suggesting that activated trypsin may exist in close proximity to mucosal and enteric neuronal PAR2[20,23].

In vitro, cultured neurons of the myenteric plexus respond to both trypsin and mast cell tryptase with a dose-dependent rise in intracellular calcium. Analogous calcium transients were observed in these neurons following exposure to PAR2 agonist peptide, but not the inactive reverse-sequence peptide [17]. Calcium transients persist in the absence of extra-cellular calcium, indicating mobilization of an intra-cellular calcium source. Neuronal response to both trypsin and tryptase decreased with repeated exposure demonstrating desensitization concordant with a receptor activated by proteolytic cleavage. Treating cultured myenteric nerves with the mixed products of mast cell degranulation also resulted in mobilization of intra-cellular calcium. Neuronal response to the degranulated mast cell filtrate was nearly abolished by pre-treatment with a tryptase inhibitor [17,18]. Furthermore, exposure to PAR2 agonist peptide prior to trypsin or mast cell lysate exposure resulted in a desensitized trypsin response similar to that observed after repeated trypsin stimulation [18] . Taken together, these results indicate that myenteric neurons may be stimulated to mobilize intra-cellular calcium in response to mast cell degranulation, specifically tryptase exposure. While this response is likely due to tryptase-induced activation of PAR2, the lack of specific PAR2 blocking agents has prevented explicit evidence of PAR2 involvement in the mast-cell response. Ex-vivo electrophysiologic studies of myenteric neurons in segments of guinea pig ileum further characterize the basic enteric neuron response to trypsin. Approximately 60% of AH and S type neurons respond to trypsin with membrane depolarization. A portion of the trypsin-responsive AH neurons also exhibit decreased input resistance. Mast cell tryptase isolated from human lung elicits a comparable response [28]. A separate study using similar methods confirms these results: myenteric neurons respond to trypsin with prolonged but reversible membrane depolarization analogous to that induced by application of the PAR2 agonist peptide [29]. Approximately three-fourths of the trypsin-responsive AH neurons and one half of the S neurons examined in this study exhibited increased input resistance while the remainder exhibited decreased input resistance. Trypsin exposure also increased neuronal excitability in both studies, with increased action potential firing in response to a depolarizing current. Moreover, spontaneous action potentials followed application of trypsin in approximately 1 in 5 myenteric neurons [29]. Application of trypsin (or a peptide consisting of the active sequence of the PAR2 tethered ligand) to sheets of porcine mucosa and submucosa results in elevated short-circuit currents. Currents are attenuated by the addition of soybean trypsin inhibitor, the neurotoxin saxitoxin, and the Na+/K+/Cl- co-transport inhibitor furosemide[16]. These findings suggest that trypsin activates protease-activated receptor 2 in ileal mucosa/submucosa leading to excitation of enteric neurons and changes in ileal ion transport. Opioid antagonism and cyclooxegenase inhibition also attenuated the effects of PAR2 activation by trypsin, suggesting that the effects on ion transport in this model can be mediated by opioids and prostaglandins. As atropine had no effect on the currents elicited in response to trypsin, muscarinic cholinergic receptors are likely not involved.

Enteroglial Cell Response to Trypsin and Tryptase

In addition to affecting enteric neurons, evidence suggests that trypsin and tryptase may cleave protease-activated receptor 2 present on enteroglia cells to elicit a functional response. In primary culture of enteroglial cells derived from the myenteric plexus of neonatal guinea pigs, glia respond to trypsin with a rise in cytoplasmic calcium concentration [13]. Calcium transients were found to be independent of neurally-mediated effects, dose-dependent, and analogous to activation with PAR2 agonist peptide. Enteroglial response to repeated trypsin or protease-activated receptor 2 agonist peptide exposure results in significantly diminished calcium rise. This receptor desensitization is similar to that observed in enteric neurons, and is consistent with the mechanism of receptor activation by proteolytic cleavage. As in enteric neurons, the trypsin-induced cytoplasmic calcium transient results from the release of calcium from intracellular stores. Capacitative calcium entry across the plasma membrane follows depletion of intracellular stores. The pathway from receptor activation to calcium transient is dependent upon activation of both phospholipase C and sphinosine kinase, however, the exact cascade of signaling events has yet to be elucidated. While PAR2 agonist peptide exposure does lead to c-fos positivity, the downstream effects of calcium signaling following activation of protease-activated receptor 2 in enteroglial cells also remain undefined.

Trypsin, Tryptase and Par2 in Gastrointestinal Disease

Inflammatory Bowel Disease

As the enteric nervous system plays a central role in the regulation of gastrointestinal function, it also is affected by and contributes to various forms of gastrointestinal disease. The enteric nervous system has been most extensively studied in inflammatory bowel sisease, including Crohn's disease and ulcerative colitis. Evidence from both human IBD patients and animal models of experimental colitis indicates changes in enteric nervous system structure and function in the affected gut. The exact character of the structural changes remains controversial due to conflicting data from different studies. In left colon biopsy specimens from patient with ulcerative colitis, myenteric Hu C/D positive neuron density was decreased by over 61%. There was a 38% reduction in density of S100β enteroglial cells, corresponding to an increased glial-neural cell ratio as compared to controls [30]. In another study of human colonic biopsy specimens, however, glial-fibrillary acidic protein (GFAP) positive enteroglial cell density was significantly *increased* in the inflamed colon of patients with ulcerative colitis and, to a lesser extent, Crohn's disease as compared to specimens from patients without inflammatory bowel disease[31]. Biopsy specimens from the non-inflamed colon of the same IBD patients revealed increased GFAP and glia-derived neurotrophic factor (GDNF) expression in ulcerative colitis patients, but decreased GFAP and GDNF expression in Crohn's disease patients as compared to controls. With some conflicting results as described, the bulk of the evidence suggests enteric nervous system hypertrophy in IBD. A study using transgenic mice with either greater or less than normal enteric neuron density supports this observation. Mice with greater than normal, normal, and less than normal ENS neuron density were treated with 2,4,6-trinitrobenzene sulfonic acid (TNBS) to establish a hapten-based model of inflammatory bowel disease. Transgenic mice with a hyperplastic enteric nervous system developed more severe inflammation than those with a hypoplastic enteric nervous system [32]. These results suggest that the enteric nervous system may contribute to the pathogenesis of experimental colitis.

Further investigation of the functional changes associated with and potentially contributing to inflammatory bowel disease revealed increased enteric neuron excitability in experimental colitis. Myenteric AH neurons demonstrated more spontaneous activity and more action potentials in response to depolarizing current in guinea pigs with chronic colon inflammation than in controls[33]. A similar observation was made regarding the increased excitability of AH neurons from the submucous plexus. S-type neurons also demonstrated larger stimulus-evoked fast and slow excitatory post-synaptic potentials (EPSPs), and more frequent spontaneous EPSPs in the colitis as compared to control group [34,35]. The enteric neurons of inflamed guinea pig ileum demonstrated similar electrophysical changes [36].

Enteroglial cells are also affected by inflammation. In primary culture of human small bowel enteroglia, exposure to lipopolysaccharide (LPS) and interferon-gamma results in enteroglial cell activation. Enteroglia exposed to inflammatory mediators exhibit increased c-fos positivity, proliferation rate, and expression of major histocompatibility complex (MHC) II, S100B, and GFAP. Human enteroglia also demonstrate increased production of nitric oxide in response to inducible nitric oxide synthase activation [37].

As enteroglial gene expression is altered by inflammation, so too is gene expression in enteric neurons. The changes in mediators released by these two cell types within the enteric nervous system may explain some of the symptoms associated with inflammatory bowel disease. For example, vasoactive intestinal peptide (VIP) serves to inhibit circular smooth muscle contraction and peristalsis and modulate intestinal vascular tone. Several studies suggest increased VIP content in enteric nerves of patients with Crohn's disease and in animal models of colitis [38-40]. Exogenous administration of VIP has been associated with reduced severity of intestinal inflammation [41].

Finally, inflammatory bowel disease has been associated with enteric nervous system infiltration by immune cells. Among these, mast cells have demonstrated increased numbers in the intestinal and colonic wall of patients with Crohn's disease and ulcerative colitis. Accompanying the increase in cell number is an increase in the products of mast cell degranulation, including mast cell tryptase [42]. Another study confirmed elevated levels of mast cell tryptase release from both inflamed and non-inflamed tissue of patients with ulcerative colitis, but failed to demonstrate increased mast cell tryptase release in patients with Crohn's disease as compared to controls [43].

The interaction between mast cell tryptase and protease-activated receptor 2 in the enteric nervous system may play a significant role in the pathogenesis of inflammatory bowel disease. Protease-activated receptor 2 expression is higher in the intestinal wall of patients with ulcerative colitis as compared to controls. Methylation of the protease-activated receptor 2 promotor region in patients with ulcerative colitis is associated with pancolitis, steroid-dependence, and refractory disease [44]. Moreover, PAR2 agonist application has actually been used as a model of inflammatory colitis [45]. Animals treated with trypsin, tryptase, or the PAR2 agonist peptide develop intestinal inflammation with inflammatory cell infiltrate, increased wall thickness, and paracellular permeability leading to increased bacterial translocation through the colonic mucosa [45]. In animals with a congenital paucity of capsaicin-sensitive sensory nerves, the severity of inflammation is significantly less than that observed in control animals, indicating neural mediation of the PAR2 effect[46]. Studies examining gastrointestinal inflammation in mast-cell deficient animals support the hypothesis that mast cells affect enteric nervous system function. In the TNBS colitis model, rats with colitis display visceral hypersensitivity manifested as a decreased pain threshold following colonic distension. In mast cell deficient rats, this visceral hypersensitivity is abolished, suggesting that enteric nervous system nociceptive pathways are not triggered or are not transmitted effectively in mast-cell deficient animals [47].

Although the exact pathway has not been determined, indirect evidence suggests that intestinal inflammation leads to influx of mast cells, which then produce tryptase. Tryptase and trypsin cleave and activate PAR2 expressed by enteric neurons and glial cells, leading to physiologic responses such as altered gastrointestinal motility, ion channel permeability, and blood flow. Each facet of the pathway – mast cell activation, tryptase release, PAR2 activation, and neurologic response - may be potentially be manipulated to attenuate signs and symptoms of inflammation in IBD. Mast cell stabilizers or modulating agents have not been fully studied as pharmacotherapy for Inflammatory Bowel Disease, but may merit examination given the attenuated visceral hypersensitivity in mast cell deficient rats [47]. The tryptase-specific serine protease inhibitor nafamostat mesilate is another potential pharmacologic therapy for IBD. In a TNBS model of colitis, nafamostat mesilate-treated animals demonstrated significantly less mucosal damage than controls [48]. A different tryptase inhibitor, APC 2059 was evaluated in a phase 2 clinical trial involving 56 patients with mild to moderate ulcerative colitis. Twenty-nine percent of these patients demonstrated a significant clinical response, with 9% experiencing complete remission [49]. PAR2 blockade is as yet unstudied, but may represent another novel target in the treatment of inflammatory bowel disease.

Irritable Bowel Syndrome

Irritable bowel syndrome (IBS) is characterized by alterations in gastrointestinal function, with individual patients experiencing either primarily constipation, primarily diarrhea, or alternating diarrhea and constipation. These motility changes are accompanied by abdominal pain, bloating, and urgency. The root etiology and pathophysiology underlying these symptoms remain undefined, however interactions between trypsin or tryptase, PAR2, and the enteric nervous system are believed to play a role.

The evidence for the involvement of the enteric nervous system in IBS is based on both anatomic and functional studies. In patients with IBS as compared to healthy controls, more than 3 times as many mast cells were located within 5 microns of intestinal nerve fibers. Biopsy specimens also demonstrated more mast cells, more degranulating mast cells, and higher mucosal tryptase content in colonic biopsy specimens from patients with IBS. The proximity of mast cells and enteric nerve fibers was significantly correlated with abdominal pain severity and frequency [50]. This observation was further studied in cultured neurons from rat dorsal root ganglia. Mast cell degranulation products from IBS patients but not controls led to excitation of nociceptive nerves. This neuronal activation was sensitive to serine-protease inhibitors, suggesting a mechanism for the pain symptoms which accompany IBS [51]. A similar study used colonic biopsy specimens containing intact submucosal plexus from healthy humans. These neurons were treated with the supernatant from colon biopsy specimens from either IBS patients or healthy controls. The IBS biopsies had higher mast cell density than controls, as well as increased supernatant concentrations of histamine and tryptase. IBS patient biopsy supernatants elicited a significantly increased spike frequency in submucosal neurons as compared to controls; specimens from diarrhea and constipation predominant IBS patients caused equal neuronal stimulation. Activation of submucosal neurons was diminished by inhibition of serine proteases as well as antagonism of the serotonin and histamine receptors [52].

More direct evidence for PAR2 involvement in the abdominal pain associated with IBS was obtained using PAR2 deficient mice. Fecal supernatants from patients with IBS were evaluated in comparison to specimens from healthy controls. IBS patients had a threefold higher level of fecal serine protease activity than controls. Supernatants were then applied to the colonic mucosa of wild-type and transgenic PAR2 deficient mice. Allodynia and paracellular permeability were then evaluated in the mice. Normal mice treated with IBS specimens demonstrated significantly increased allodynea and paracellular permeability, whereas PAR2 deficient mice did not experience these changes as compared to control animals treated with fecal supernatant from healthy patients [53]. This study strongly supports PAR2 involvement in the abdominal pain and altered intestinal permeability associated with IBS.

Based on these and other data, several potential therapeutic targets have been identified for IBS, including mast cell activation, serine protease activity, and PAR2 receptor activation. Mast cell stabilizers have been evaluated in animal studies as well as a clinical trial. Decreased mast cell activation was hypothesized to lead to decreased release of tryptase, diminished PAR2 cleavage, less activation of nociceptive enteric neurons, and ultimately less abdominal discomfort for patients affected by IBS. In one clinical trial, patients with IBS were randomized to receive the mast cell stabilizer ketotifen or placebo for eight weeks. Patients with baseline visceral hypersensitivity in the ketotifen group experienced significantly decreased hypersensitivity at eight weeks compared to the placebo group. Abdominal pain was also diminished and quality of life improved in the ketotifen group, however, tryptase levels were not changed by therapy [54]. While mast cell stabilization shows some degree of promise as evaluated in this study, the absence of an effect on tryptase levels suggests the influence of other mast cell products. Serine protease inhibition and PAR2 blockade have not been specifically studied in the treatment of IBS.

Conclusions

While the basic mechanism of PAR2 proteolytic cleavage and activation by trypsin and tryptase is well characterized, the physiologic triggers of this reaction and its downstream effects are subjects of ongoing study. Within the enteric nervous system, PAR2 has been identified in both submucosal and myenteric neurons as well as enteric glia. Enteric neuron and glial PAR2 activation by trypsin causes a cascade of signaling involving PLC and cytoplasmic calcium gradients, and ultimately results in alterations in gastrointestinal motility and ion transport. In certain gastrointestinal diseases including Inflammatory Bowel Disease and Irritable Bowel Syndrome, mast cells release results in increased intestinal tryptase content. Tryptase-induced activation of PAR2 on enteric neurons and glial cells may contribute to the manifestations of these diseases including abnormal gastrointestinal motility and abdominal pain.

Improved understanding of this pathophysiologic mechanism may lead to the use of novel therapeutics including mast cell stabilizers, serine protease inhibitors, and PAR2 blocking agents.

Acknowledgments

This work is supported by National Institutes of Health Grant 4R37DK043225.

References

[1] Gershon MD. The enteric nervous system: a second brain. *Hosp Pract (Minneap).* Jul 15 1999;34(7):31-32, 35-38, 41-32 passim.

[2] Borody TJ, Quigley EM, Phillips SF, et al. Effects of morphine and atropine on motility and transit in the human ileum. *Gastroenterology,* Sep 1985;89(3):562-570.

[3] Galligan JJ, Furness JB, Costa M. Effects of cholinergic blockade, adrenergic blockade and sympathetic denervation on gastrointestinal myoelectric activity in guinea pig. *The Journal of pharmacology and experimental therapeutics,* Sep 1986;238(3):1114-1125.

[4] Burnstock G. Purinergic nerves. *Pharmacological reviews,* Sep 1972;24(3):509-581.

[5] Crist JR, He XD, Goyal RK. Both ATP and the peptide VIP are inhibitory neurotransmitters in guinea-pig ileum circular muscle. *The Journal of physiology,* Feb 1992;447:119-131.

[6] Fahrenkrug J. Vasoactive intestinal polypeptide: measurement, distribution and putative neurotransmitter function. *Digestion,* 1979;19(3):149-169.

[7] Furness JB, Costa M. Projections of intestinal neurons showing immunoreactivity for vasoactive intestinal polypeptide are consistent with these neurons being the enteric inhibitory neurons. *Neuroscience letters,* Dec 1979;15(2-3):199-204.

[8] Kunze WA, Furness JB. The enteric nervous system and regulation of intestinal motility. *Annual review of physiology,* 1999;61:117-142.

[9] Furness JB. Types of neurons in the enteric nervous system. *Journal of the autonomic nervous system,* Jul 3 2000;81(1-3):87-96.

[10] Furness JB, Kunze WA, Bertrand PP, Clerc N, Bornstein JC. Intrinsic primary afferent neurons of the intestine. *Progress in neurobiology,* Jan 1998;54(1):1-18.

[11] Nurgali K. Plasticity and ambiguity of the electrophysiological phenotypes of enteric neurons. *Neurogastroenterology and motility: the official journal of the European Gastrointestinal Motility Society,* Sep 2009;21(9):903-913.

[12] Ruhl A. Glial cells in the gut. *Neurogastroenterology and motility : the official journal of the European Gastrointestinal Motility Society,* Dec 2005;17(6):777-790.

[13] Garrido R, Segura B, Zhang W, Mulholland M. Presence of functionally active protease-activated receptors 1 and 2 in myenteric glia. *Journal of neurochemistry,* Nov 2002;83(3):556-564.

[14] Burnstock G, Lavin S. Interstitial cells of Cajal and purinergic signalling. *Autonomic neuroscience : basic and clinical.* Apr 18 2002;97(1):68-72.

[15] Flamant M, Aubert P, Rolli-Derkinderen M, et al. Enteric glia protect against Shigella flexneri invasion in intestinal epithelial cells: a role for S-nitrosoglutathione. *Gut.* Apr 2011;60(4):473-484.

[16] Green BT, Bunnett NW, Kulkarni-Narla A, Steinhoff M, Brown DR. Intestinal type 2 proteinase-activated receptors: expression in opioid-sensitive secretomotor neural circuits that mediate epithelial ion transport. *The Journal of pharmacology and experimental therapeutics,* Oct 2000;295(1):410-416.

[17] Corvera CU, Dery O, McConalogue K, et al. Thrombin and mast cell tryptase regulate guinea-pig myenteric neurons through proteinase-activated receptors-1 and -2. *The Journal of physiology,* Jun 15 1999;517 (Pt 3):741-756.

[18] Reed DE, Barajas-Lopez C, Cottrell G, et al. Mast cell tryptase and proteinase-activated receptor 2 induce hyperexcitability of guinea-pig submucosal neurons. *The Journal of physiology,* Mar 1 2003;547(Pt 2):531-542.

[19] Steinhoff M, Vergnolle N, Young SH, et al. Agonists of proteinase-activated receptor 2 induce inflammation by a neurogenic mechanism. *Nature medicine,* Feb 2000;6(2): 151-158.

[20] Cottrell GS, Amadesi S, Schmidlin F, Bunnett N. Protease-activated receptor 2: activation, signalling and function. *Biochemical Society transactions,* Dec 2003;31 (Pt 6):1191-1197.

[21] Holzhausen M, Spolidorio LC, Vergnolle N. Proteinase-activated receptor-2 (PAR2) agonist causes periodontitis in rats. *Journal of dental research,* Feb 2005;84(2): 154-159.

[22] Holzhausen M, Spolidorio LC, Vergnolle N. Role of protease-activated receptor-2 in inflammation, and its possible implications as a putative mediator of periodontitis. *Memorias do Instituto Oswaldo Cruz,* Mar 2005;100 Suppl 1:177-180.

[23] Cottrell GS, Amadesi S, Grady EF, Bunnett NW. Trypsin IV, a novel agonist of protease-activated receptors 2 and 4. *The Journal of biological chemistry,* Apr 2 2004;279(14):13532-13539.

[24] Koshikawa N, Hasegawa S, Nagashima Y, et al. Expression of trypsin by epithelial cells of various tissues, leukocytes, and neurons in human and mouse. *The American journal of pathology,* Sep 1998;153(3):937-944.

[25] Bienenstock J, Tomioka M, Matsuda H, et al. The role of mast cells in inflammatory processes: evidence for nerve/mast cell interactions. *International archives of allergy and applied immunology,* 1987;82(3-4):238-243.

[26] Dimitriadou V, Rouleau A, Trung Tuong MD, et al. Functional relationships between sensory nerve fibers and mast cells of dura mater in normal and inflammatory conditions. *Neuroscience,* Apr 1997;77(3):829-839.

[27] Argenzio RA. Neuro-immune pathobiology of infectious enteric disease. *Advances in experimental medicine and biology,* 1997;412:21-29.

[28] Gao C, Liu S, Hu HZ, et al. Serine proteases excite myenteric neurons through protease-activated receptors in guinea pig small intestine. *Gastroenterology,* Nov 2002;123(5):1554-1564.

[29] Linden DR, Manning BP, Bunnett NW, Mawe GM. Agonists of proteinase-activated receptor 2 excite guinea pig ileal myenteric neurons. *European journal of pharmacology,* Nov 23 2001;431(3):311-314.

[30] Bernardini N, Segnani C, Ippolito C, ct al. Immunohistochemical Analysis of Myenteric Ganglia and Interstitial Cells of Cajal in Ulcerative Colitis. *Journal of cellular and molecular medicine,* Mar 22 2011.

[31] von Boyen GB, Schulte N, Pfluger C, Spaniol U, Hartmann C, Steinkamp M. Distribution of enteric glia and GDNF during gut inflammation. *BMC gastroenterology,* 2011;11:3.

[32] Margolis KG, Stevanovic K, Karamooz N, et al. Enteric neuronal density contributes to the severity of intestinal inflammation. *Gastroenterology,* Aug 2011;141(2):588-598 e582.

[33] Linden DR, Sharkey KA, Mawe GM. Enhanced excitability of myenteric AH neurones in the inflamed guinea-pig distal colon. *The Journal of physiology,* Mar 1 2003;547(Pt 2):589-601.

[34] Lomax AE, Fernandez E, Sharkey KA. Plasticity of the enteric nervous system during intestinal inflammation. *Neurogastroenterology and motility : the official journal of the European Gastrointestinal Motility Society,* Feb 2005;17(1):4-15.

[35] Lomax AE, Mawe GM, Sharkey KA. Synaptic facilitation and enhanced neuronal excitability in the submucosal plexus during experimental colitis in guinea-pig. *The Journal of physiology,* May 1 2005;564(Pt 3):863-875.

[36] Nurgali K, Nguyen TV, Matsuyama H, Thacker M, Robbins HL, Furness JB. Phenotypic changes of morphologically identified guinea-pig myenteric neurons following intestinal inflammation. *The Journal of physiology,* Sep 1 2007;583(Pt 2):593-609.

[37] Cirillo C, Sarnelli G, Turco F, et al. Proinflammatory stimuli activates human-derived enteroglial cells and induces autocrine nitric oxide production. *Neurogastroenterology and motility : the official journal of the European Gastrointestinal Motility Society,* Sep 2011;23(9):e372-382.

[38] Linden DR, Couvrette JM, Ciolino A, et al. Indiscriminate loss of myenteric neurones in the TNBS-inflamed guinea-pig distal colon. *Neurogastroenterology and motility : the official journal of the European Gastrointestinal Motility Society,* Oct 2005;17(5): 751-760.

[39] Belai A, Boulos PB, Robson T, Burnstock G. Neurochemical coding in the small intestine of patients with Crohn's disease. *Gut,* Jun 1997;40(6):767-774.

[40] Kishimoto S, Kobayashi H, Shimizu S, et al. Changes of colonic vasoactive intestinal peptide and cholinergic activity in rats with chemical colitis. *Digestive diseases and sciences,* Nov 1992;37(11):1729-1737.

[41] Arranz A, Abad C, Juarranz Y, Leceta J, Martinez C, Gomariz RP. Vasoactive intestinal peptide as a healing mediator in Crohn's disease. *Neuroimmunomodulation,* 2008;15(1):46-53.

[42] He SH. Key role of mast cells and their major secretory products in inflammatory bowel disease. *World journal of gastroenterology, WJG.* Feb 1 2004;10(3):309-318.

[43] Raithel M, Winterkamp S, Pacurar A, Ulrich P, Hochberger J, Hahn EG. Release of mast cell tryptase from human colorectal mucosa in inflammatory bowel disease. *Scandinavian journal of gastroenterology,* Feb 2001;36(2):174-179.

[44] Tahara T, Shibata T, Nakamura M, et al. Promoter methylation of protease-activated receptor (PAR2) is associated with severe clinical phenotypes of ulcerative colitis (UC). *Clinical and experimental medicine,* Jun 2009;9(2):125-130.

[45] Cenac N, Coelho AM, Nguyen C, et al. Induction of intestinal inflammation in mouse by activation of proteinase-activated receptor-2. *The American journal of pathology,* Nov 2002;161(5):1903-1915.

[46] Nguyen C, Coelho AM, Grady E, et al. Colitis induced by proteinase-activated receptor-2 agonists is mediated by a neurogenic mechanism. *Canadian journal of physiology and pharmacology,* Sep 2003;81(9):920-927.

[47] Ohashi K, Sato Y, Kawai M, Kurebayashi Y. Abolishment of TNBS-induced visceral hypersensitivity in mast cell deficient rats. *Life sciences,* Feb 13 2008;82(7-8):419-423.

[48] Isozaki Y, Yoshida N, Kuroda M, et al. Anti-tryptase treatment using nafamostat mesilate has a therapeutic effect on experimental colitis. *Scandinavian journal of gastroenterology,* Aug 2006;41(8):944-953.

[49] Tremaine WJ, Brzezinski A, Katz JA, et al. Treatment of mildly to moderately active ulcerative colitis with a tryptase inhibitor (APC 2059): an open-label pilot study. *Alimentary pharmacology and therapeutics,* Mar 2002;16(3):407-413.

[50] Barbara G, Stanghellini V, De Giorgio R, et al. Activated mast cells in proximity to colonic nerves correlate with abdominal pain in irritable bowel syndrome. *Gastroenterology.* Mar 2004;126(3):693-702.

[51] Barbara G, Wang B, Stanghellini V, et al. Mast cell-dependent excitation of visceral-nociceptive sensory neurons in irritable bowel syndrome. *Gastroenterology,* Jan 2007;132(1):26-37.

[52] Buhner S, Li Q, Vignali S, et al. Activation of human enteric neurons by supernatants of colonic biopsy specimens from patients with irritable bowel syndrome. *Gastroenterology,* Oct 2009;137(4):1425-1434.

[53] Gecse K, Roka R, Ferrier L, et al. Increased faecal serine protease activity in diarrhoeic IBS patients: a colonic lumenal factor impairing colonic permeability and sensitivity. *Gut,* May 2008;57(5):591-599.

[54] Klooker TK, Braak B, Koopman KE, et al. The mast cell stabiliser ketotifen decreases visceral hypersensitivity and improves intestinal symptoms in patients with irritable bowel syndrome. *Gut,* Sep 2010;59(9):1213-1221.

In: Trypsin: Structure, Biosynthesis and Functions
Editors: Kirk Weaver and Clayton Kelley
ISBN 978-1-61942-319-0

Chapter VI

Trypsin Acts as an Activating Enzyme in Gut Innate Immunity

Hiroki Tanabe, Mikihiro Fujiya and Yutaka Kohgo*
Division of Gastroenterology and Hematology/Oncology,
Department of Medicine, Asahikawa Medical University, Japan

Abstract

Digestive enzymes in the human gut play major roles in digesting food so that nutrients can be absorbed through epithelial sheets in the intestinal lumen. Trypsin, one of the digestive enzymes, is mainly produced in the pancreas and secreted in the duodenum. Recent finding have shown that small intestinal epithelial cells produce trypsin peptide, which plays an important role in the human innate immune system. The digestive organs, contributing to the absorption of nutrients on one side and protecting the host from the numerous bacteria residing in the gut microbiota, also protects against external infectious microbes on the other side. Paneth cells, one of the secretory epithelial cells in the small intestine, express and secrete antimicrobial peptide, human alpha-defensin (HD). HD is an innate immune molecule that directly eliminates bacteria to maintain homeostasis in the gut's ecosystem. A specific pattern of trypsin isozymes is also expressed in Paneth cells, and trypsin co-localizes with HD to cleave propeptides to mature forms identical to those isolated *in vivo*. HD is stored in secretory vesicles as a propeptide, but the mature peptides isolated from the intestinal lumen are proteolytically processed forms. HD is produced and stored as a propeptide in Paneth cell granules, secreted in response to stimulation by cholinergic reagents or bacterial antigens, and finally activated by trypsin in the intestinal lumen in order to produce mature functional HD. Therefore, trypsin is involved in the regulation of innate immunity in the small intestine by acting as a prodefensin convertase in human Paneth cells. The activating process is critical for its antibacterial role and it is also a bridge to acquired immunity.

---

* Corresponding author: Hiroki Tanabe. Address: Division of Gastroenterology and Hematology/Oncology, Department of Medicine, Asahikawa Medical university, Midorigaoka-Higashi 2-1-1-1, Asahikawa Hokkaido 078-8510, Japan. Tel: +81-166-68-2462. Fax: +81-166-68-2469. E-mail: tant@asahikawa-med.ac.jp

This chapter reviews the novel functional role of trypsin which is produced in the small intestine.

Pancreatic Enzymes are Produced in Small Intestinal Paneth Cells

Pancreatic trypsin, a member of the serine protease family, is produced in the pancreas, and hydrolyses proteins in the digestive tract. The peptides are secreted as propeptide trypsinogens from pancreatic acinar cells into the small intestine, where they are cleaved by enterokinase, which is produced by duodenal epithelial cells. Three different isoforms of trypsinogen are secreted, namely cationic trypsinogen, anionic trypsinogen and mesotrypsinogen, classified based on their pI value [1-3]. Their active forms are also termed trypsin-1, -2 and -3, respectively. Trypsin-1 and -2 account for most of the pancreatic secretory trypsin, and trypsin-3 (mesotrypsin) is secreted in only a trace amounts from the pancreas [2].

Immunohistochemical determination and biochemical purification performed in the 1980's and 1990's demonstrated that some pancreatic enzymes are also produced heterotopically in the gastrointestinal tract [4-6].

Paneth cells, one of the intestinal cell lineages in the small intestine, were found to express trypsin-like immunoreactivities. Paneth cells are pyramid-shaped columnar epithelial cells located at the bottom of the small intestine and were thought to act as extrapancreatic endocrine cells in the intestine because of the similarity in their dense granules observed by electron microscopy [7, 8].

Transgenic mice with altered the cells and oral infection models in various animals have been used to study the function of these cells in living animals [9, 10], but their full activities were not identified [11]. In a detailed immunohistochemical study using specific antiserum absorbed with the antigens, both cationic and anionic trypsins were detected [12]. Recent progress in the analytical technology using reverse transcription-PCR and hybridization demonstrated that human ileal tissues express anionic and mesotrypsin with no cationic trypsin, which differs from the pancreatic distribution mentioned above [13, 14].

Paneth cells were found to express trypsins, lysozyme, and pancreatic secretory trypsin inhibitor (PSTI) [11, 12]. Since the shape of Paneth cells and acinar cells in the pancreas with dense granules are similar, the physiological roles of Paneth cells were thought to be the production of digestive enzyme until recently [11, 15].

The cells were eventually demonstrated to be negative for the expression of other endocrine digestive enzymes, such as lipase, amylase, chymotrypsin, elastase and pancreatic phospholipase A2 [11, 14, 16-17].

The Functional Role of Paneth Cells

The physiological roles of Paneth cells were estimated based on the histochemical changes of the granules released from the cells. The explosion of the granules from the cells was stimulated by cholinergic reagents through calcium influx into the cells [18-20].

An excellent study using crypts isolated from mouse small intestinal tissue clarified the roles of Paneth cells, and demonstrated that they release their granules, including antibacterial peptides, in response to Gram-negative and Gram-positive bacteria, lipopolysaccharide, lipoteichoic acid, lipid A and muramyl dipeptide [19-22].

Paneth cell granules consist of some antimicrobial peptides and the pancreatic enzymes mentioned above, and possess antibacterial activity, of which up to 70% are alpha-defensins [19].

The physiological roles of the defensins *in vivo* were demonstrated by gene targeting mice which are deficient matrilysin, the mouse defensin (cryptdin, named for "crypt defensin") activating enzyme [9, 23, 24]. The mice which lacked the active cryptdins are highly sensitive to oral challenge with bacteria, such as *Salmonella typhymurium*.

The studies in these mice demonstrated that the defensin peptides contribute to protection from bacterial exposure in the intestine, and are important molecules involved in innate immunity.

Paneth Cell Trypsin Mediates the Activation of Antimicrobial Peptides Involved in Human Innate Immunity

Paneth cells in the human small intestine produce two isoforms of α-defensin, human defensin (HD)-5 and HD-6, as precursor forms termed proHD-5 and proHD-6 [25-27]. The proHD-5 peptide is cleaved at the Arg^{62}-Ala^{63} position by trypsin to produce the mature form of HD-5. The trypsinogen is expressed in Paneth cell granules and HD-5 is positive in the granules as well (Figure 1). The immunoreactivity of the anti-trypsin monoclonal antibody is more apparent in the basal portion of the cells, as determined using the reactivity of the anti-sera against recombinant HD-5. The role of the complexity in granule distribution still needs to be elucidated. Upon degranulation from Paneth cells, trypsinogen is cleaved to trypsin, and then proHD-5 is cleaved by trypsin (Figure 2).

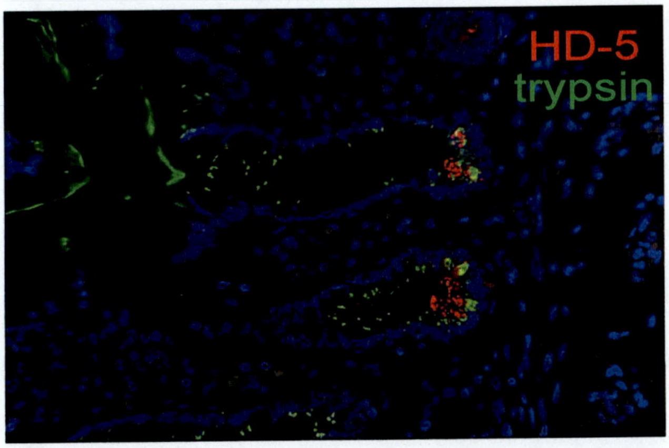

Figure 1. Trypsin co-localizes with HD-5 in human small intestinal Paneth cells. Sections were incubated with anti-HD-5 rabbit serum (red) and anti-trypsin monoclonal IgG (green). DAPI was used for nuclear counterstaining (blue).

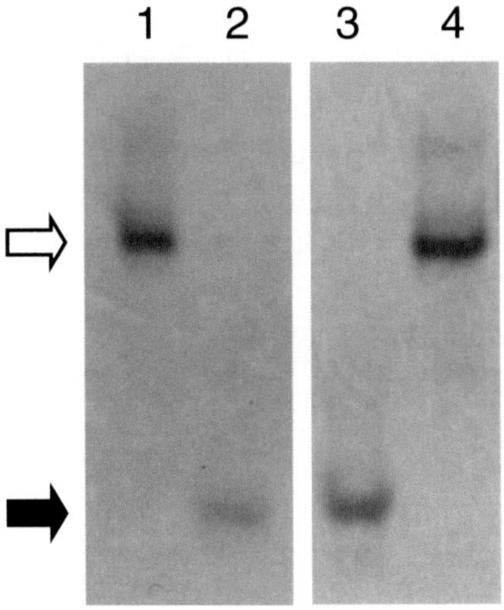

Figure 2. Trypsin cleavage to produce mature HD-5. Recombinant peptides were loaded in acid-urea PAGE and stained with coomassie blue. Pro HD-5 (lane 1) was treated with a 1:10 molar ratio of trypsin in order to produce mature HD-5 (lane 2). Recombinant HD-5 and proHD-5 were loaded as standards in lanes 3 and 4, respectively. The closed arrow denotes HD-5, and the open arrow indicates proHD-5.

HD-5 is a multifunctional peptide showing not only antibacterial activity but also immunomodulatory activity. Since the HD-5 peptide is preserved as a propeptide, the proHD-5 can be purified from the small intestinal tissue [28, 29]. The cleavage by the trypsin (HD-5 convertase) occurs after the release from Paneth cells into the intestinal lumen, and processed HD-5 is detected in the luminal flow. Interestingly the propeptide itself is already bactericidal against Gram-positive and Gram-negative bacteria, but lacks the immunomodulatory activity of the mature peptide [30, 31]. The active antimicrobial peptides bind and insert into the lipid bilayer of bacterial membranes to eventually kill the bacteria [32]. However, a high concentration of the defensin peptide in the granules can lead to disruption of the human cell membrane, potentially causing adverse effects. It has been speculated that the enzymatic cleavage by trypsin in Paneth cell granules is impeded by the co-expressed enzymatic inhibitor, e.g. serpin or PSTI. After secretion from storage granules to the luminal surface, trypsin takes part in the activation process. The differences between activities of proHD-5 and those of the mature form have been demonstrated *in vivo* as well as *in vitro*. The mature HD-5 is useful against mouse DSS colitis models arising from external peritoneal injection, and demonstrates potential for application to treat human disorders, such as inflammatory bowel disease [31, 33]. Taken together, Paneth cell trypsin contributes to the gut innate immunity, activating antimicrobial peptides to protect against harmful intestinal bacteria.

Future Studies with Paneth Cell Trypsin

To elucidate the physiological role of tissue-specific molecules, gene-targeting mice have proven invaluable during the last decade. Tissue-specific expression of Cre-mediated recombination can control the expression of the gene of interest, and the villin-Cre transgenic mouse has become useful tools to examine the loss of many molecules.

It should be mentioned that the key enzymes activating defensins are different between mice and humans [34-36]. Mouse Paneth cell defensins are cleaved by matrilysin, while HD-5 is cleaved by trypsin. Whether the results of the former study with the matrilysin knockout mouse can be applied to humans is controversial. A detailed pathological observation will need to be performed to obtain a better understanding of the physiological roles of Paneth cell trypsin in humans. There was an interesting observation that described a luminal complex formed by proHD-5, trypsin, and chymotrypsinogen/chymotrypsin in the small intestine [35].

ProHD-5 and trypsin are secreted from Paneth cells and form a complex with chymotrypsin, and then mature HD-5 and chymotrypsin are processed by trypsin and released to the lumen of the intestine. The details of the process are still unclear, but impairment of the process may be associated with human intestinal disorders [37-40].

Therefore, although it is an enzyme identified many decades ago, trypsin is still at the forefront of the newest research fields. Future studies will need to be performed to elucidate the role(s) of Paneth cell trypsin in innate immunity.

Reference

[1] Rinderknecht, H., Renner, I. G., Abramson, S. B. and Carmack, C. (1984). Mesotrypsin: a new inhibitor-resistant protease from a zymogen in human pancreatic tissue and fluid. *Gastroenterology*, 86 (4), 681-692.

[2] Nyaruhucha, C. N., Kito, M. and Fukuoka, S. I. (1997). Identification and expression of the cDNA-encoding human mesotrypsin(ogen), an isoform of trypsin with inhibitor resistance. *J. Biol. Chem.,* 272 (16), 10573-10578.

[3] Szmola, R., Kukor, Z. and Sahin-Toth, M. (2003). Human mesotrypsin is a unique digestive protease specialized for the degradation of trypsin inhibitors. *J. Biol. Chem.,* 278 (49), 48580-48589.

[4] Bohe, M., Borgstrom, A., Lindstrom, C. and Ohlsson, K. (1984). Trypsin-like immunoreactivity in human Paneth cells. *Digestion*, 30 (4), 271-275.

[5] Bohe, M., Lindstrom, C. and Ohlsson, K. (1986). Immunohistochemical demonstration of pancreatic secretory proteins in human paneth cells. *Scand. J. Gastroenterol. Suppl.,* 126 , 65-68.

[6] Bohe, M., Borgstrom, A., Lindstrom, C. and Ohlsson, K. (1986). Pancreatic endoproteases and pancreatic secretory trypsin inhibitor immunoreactivity in human Paneth cells. *J. Clin. Pathol.,* 39 (7), 786-793.

[7] Satoh, Y., Yamano, M., Matsuda, M. and Ono, K. (1990). Ultrastructure of Paneth cells in the intestine of various mammals. *J. Electron. Microsc.* Tech, 16 (1), 69-80.

[8] Selsted, M. E., Miller, S. I., Henschen, A. H. and Ouellette, A. J. (1992). Enteric defensins: antibiotic peptide components of intestinal host defense. *J. Cell Biol.,* 118 (4), 929-936.

[9] Wilson, C. L., Ouellette, A. J., Satchell, D. P., Ayabe, T., Lopez-Boado, Y. S., Stratman, J. L., Hultgren, S. J., Matrisian, L. M. and Parks, W. C. (1999). Regulation of

intestinal alpha-defensin activation by the metalloproteinase matrilysin in innate host defense. *Science*, 286 (5437), 113-117.

[10] Masty, J. and Stradley, R. P. (1991). Paneth cell degranulation and lysozyme secretion during acute equine alimentary laminitis. *Histochemistry*, 95 (5), 529-533.

[11] Senegas-Balas, F. O., Figarella, C. G., Amouric, M. A., Guy-Crotte, O. M., Bertrand, C. A. and Balas, D. C. (1991). Immunocytochemical demonstration of a pancreatic secretory protein of unknown function in human duodenum. *J. Histochem. Cytochem.*, 39 (7), 915-919.

[12] Freeman, T. C., Playford, R. J., Quinn, C., Beardshall, K., Poulter, L., Young, J. and Calam, J. (1990). Pancreatic secretory trypsin inhibitor in gastrointestinal mucosa and gastric juice. *Gut*, 31 (11), 1318-1323.

[13] Bohe, M., Lindstrom, C. G. and Ohlsson, K. (1987). Varying occurrence of gastroduodenal immunoreactive pancreatic secretory trypsin inhibitor. *J. Clin. Pathol.*, 40 (11), 1345-1348.

[14] Ghosh, D., Porter, E., Shen, B., Lee, S. K., Wilk, D., Drazba, J., Yadav, S. P., Crabb, J. W., Ganz, T. and Bevins, C. L. (2002). Paneth cell trypsin is the processing enzyme for human defensin-5. *Nat. Immunol.,* 3 (6), 583-590.

[15] Satoh, Y., Ishikawa, K., Oomori, Y., Yamano, M. and Ono, K. (1989). Effects of cholecystokinin and carbamylcholine on Paneth cell secretion in mice: a comparison with pancreatic acinar cells. *Anat. Rec.,* 225 (2), 124-132.

[16] Porter, E. M., Bevins, C. L., Ghosh, D. and Ganz, T. (2002). The multifaceted Paneth cell. *Cell Mol. Life Sci.,* 59 (1), 156-170.

[17] Bohe, M., Lindstrom, C. and Ohlsson, K. (1988). Immunoreactive pancreatic secretory trypsin inhibitor in gastrointestinal mucosa. *Adv. Exp. Med. Biol.,* 240 , 101-105.

[18] Satoh, Y. (1988). Atropine inhibits the degranulation of Paneth cells in ex-germ-free mice.. *Cell Tissue Res.,* 253 (2), 397-402.

[19] Ayabe, T., Satchell, D. P., Wilson, C. L., Parks, W. C., Selsted, M. E. and Ouellette, A. J. (2000). Secretion of microbicidal alpha-defensins by intestinal Paneth cells in response to bacteria. *Nat. Immunol*., 1 (2), 113-118.

[20] Ayabe, T., Wulff, H., Darmoul, D., Cahalan, M. D., Chandy, K. G. and Ouellette, A. J. (2002). Modulation of mouse Paneth cell alpha-defensin secretion by mIKCa1, a Ca2+-activated, intermediate conductance potassium channel. *J. Biol. Chem.,* 277 (5), 3793-3800.

[21] Ayabe, T., Ashida, T., Kohgo, Y. and Kono, T. (2004). The role of Paneth cells and their antimicrobial peptides in innate host defense. *Trends Microbiol.,* 12 (8), 394-398.

[22] Tanabe, H., Ayabe, T., Bainbridge, B., Guina, T., Ernst, R. K., Darveau, R. P., Miller, S. I. and Ouellette, A. J. (2005). Mouse paneth cell secretory responses to cell surface glycolipids of virulent and attenuated pathogenic bacteria. *Infect. Immun.,* 73 (4), 2312-2320.

[23] Ouellette, A. J. (2005). Paneth cell alpha-defensins: peptide mediators of innate immunity in the small intestine. *Springer Semin. Immunopathol.,* 27 (2), 133-146.

[24] Shirafuji, Y., Tanabe, H., Satchell, D. P., Henschen-Edman, A., Wilson, C. L. and Ouellette, A. J. (2003). Structural determinants of procryptdin recognition and cleavage by matrix metalloproteinase-7. *J. Biol. Chem.,* 278 (10), 7910-7919.

[25] Porter, E. M., Liu, L., Oren, A., Anton, P. A. and Ganz, T. (1997). Localization of human intestinal defensin 5 in Paneth cell granules. *Infect. Immun.,* 65 (6), 2389-2395.

[26] Mallow, E. B., Harris, A., Salzman, N., Russell, J. P., DeBerardinis, R. J., Ruchelli, E. and Bevins, C. L. (1996). Human enteric defensins. Gene structure and developmental expression. *J. Biol. Chem.*, 271 (8), 4038-4045.

[27] Cunliffe, R. N. and Mahida, Y. R. (2000). Antimicrobial peptides in innate intestinal host defence. *Gut*, 47 (1), 16-17.

[28] Cunliffe, R. N., Rose, F. R., Keyte, J., Abberley, L., Chan, W. C. and Mahida, Y. R. (2001). Human defensin 5 is stored in precursor form in normal Paneth cells and is expressed by some villous epithelial cells and by metaplastic Paneth cells in the colon in inflammatory *bowel disease. Gut,* 48 (2), 176-185.

[29] Tanabe, H., Ayabe, T., Maemoto, A., Ishikawa, C., Inaba, Y., Sato, R., Moriichi, K., Okamoto, K., Watari, J., Kono, T., Ashida, T. and Kohgo, Y. (2007). Denatured human alpha-defensin attenuates the bactericidal activity and the stability against enzymatic digestion. *Biochem. Biophys. Res. Commun.*, 358 (1), 349-355.

[30] Rajabi, M., de Leeuw, E., Pazgier, M., Li, J., Lubkowski, J. and Lu, W. (2008). The conserved salt bridge in human alpha-defensin 5 is required for its precursor processing and proteolytic stability. *J. Biol. Chem.*, 283 (31), 21509-21518.

[31] Ishikawa, C., Tanabe, H., Maemoto, A., Ito, T., Watari, J., Kono, T., Fujiya, M., Ashida, T., Ayabe, T. and Kohgo, Y. (2009). Precursor processing of human defensin-5 is essential to the multiple functions in vitro and in vivo. *J. Innate. Immun.*, 2 (1), 66-76.

[32] Ouellette, A. J. (2006). Paneth cell alpha-defensin synthesis and function. *Curr. Top. Microbiol. Immunol.*, 306 , 1-25.

[33] Motzkus, D., Schulz-Maronde, S., Heitland, A., Schulz, A., Forssmann, W. G., Jubner, M. and Maronde, E. (2006). The novel beta-defensin DEFB123 prevents lipopolysaccharide-mediated effects in vitro and in vivo. *FASEB J.*, 20 (10), 1701-1702.

[34] Salzman, N. H., Ghosh, D., Huttner, K. M., Paterson, Y. and Bevins, C. L. (2003). Protection against enteric salmonellosis in transgenic mice expressing a human intestinal defensin. *Nature*, 422 (6931), 522-526.

[35] Elphick, D., Liddell, S. and Mahida, Y. R. (2008). Impaired luminal processing of human defensin-5 in Crohn's disease: persistence in a complex with chymotrypsinogen and trypsin. *Am. J. Pathol.*, 172 (3), 702-713.

[36] Ayabe, T., Satchell, D. P., Pesendorfer, P., Tanabe, H., Wilson, C. L., Hagen, S. J. and Ouellette, A. J. (2002). Activation of Paneth cell alpha-defensins in mouse small intestine. *J. Biol. Chem.*, 277 (7), 5219-5228.

[37] Tanabe, H., Sato, T., Watari, J., Maemoto, A., Fijiya, M., Kono, T., Ashida, T., Ayabe, T. and Kohgo, Y. (2008). Functional Role of Metaplastic Paneth Cell Defensins in Helicobacter pylori-Infected Stomach. *Helicobacter.*, 13 , 370-379.

[38] Nuding, S., Fellermann, K., Wehkamp, J. and Stange, E. F. (2007). Reduced mucosal antimicrobial activity in Crohn's disease of the colon. *Gut*, 56 (9), 1240-1247.

[39] Salzman, N. H., Underwood, M. A. and Bevins, C. L. (2007). Paneth cells, defensins, and the commensal microbiota: a hypothesis on intimate interplay at the intestinal mucosa. *Semin Immunol.*, 19 (2), 70-83.

[40] Wehkamp, J. and Stange, E. F. (2006). A new look at Crohn's disease: breakdown of the mucosal antibacterial defense. *Ann. NY Acad. Sci.*, 1072, 321-331.

In: Trypsin: Structure, Biosynthesis and Functions
Editors: Kirk Weaver and Clayton Kelley
ISBN 978-1-61942-319-0

Chapter VII

Two Independent Reactive Sites in the Bifunctional Inhibitor of Alfa-Amylase and Trypsin*

A. Rinat Islamov
Aitkhozhin Institute of Molecular Biology and Biochemistry,
Ministry of Education and Science, Republic of Kazakhstan,
Almaty, Kazakhstan

Abstract

Using cytraconic anhydride and 1,4-cyclohexadione, lysine and arginine of bifunctional inhibitor α-amylase/trypsin from wheat (Triticum aestivum L.) has been modified. These results found that two independent reactive sites are present in the bifunctional wheat inhibitor. The experimental data obtained that the lactoperoxidase-catalyzed reaction is accompanied by oxidation aromatic and sulfur-containing amino acids of the inhibitor. This can point out one of the mechanisms inactivating proteins in sprouting seeds.

Introduction

Serine proteases and α-amylase inhibitors are widespread in the biosphere and are found in prokaryotic as well as eukaryotic organisms [1]. In plants their role is consist in inhibited exogenous enzymes of pathogenic organisms such as fungi, bacteria and insects [2]. The Republic of Kazakhstan is a country producing and exporting of wheat. In this connection the research of the wheat is actual and paramount.

---

* A version of this chapter also appears in *Food Supplies and Food Safety: Production, Conservation and Population Impact*, edited by Marion B. Walsch, published by Nova Science Publishers, Inc. It was submitted for appropriate modifications in an effort to encourage wider dissemination of research.

Inhibitors have been grouped into families and subfamilies and into different clans on the basis of sequent relationship and the relationship of protein fold of the inhibitory domains or units. The members of family bifunctional inhibitors (BI) have an activity against serine protease and α-amylase of exogenous and endogenous natures [3]. These proteins are characterized by a high content of cysteines that form four or five intramolecular disulfide bridges [4, 5]. The BI-s has a monomeric structure, basic protein (pI > 10) and consists of two independent active centers. However, one of the fault properties of bifunctional inhibitors is an ability to cause the allergy known as baker's asthma [6]. Specific chemical modifications of proteins can be used to study the involvement of particular residues in both the biological and the antigenic sites of these proteins [7]. The acylate of lysine, iodinated of aromatic and sulfur-containing amino acid were used often methods [8, 9, 10, 11]. In this connection the bifunctional inhibitors of α-amylase/trypsin type were of most interest for our research. In our work were modified of amino acid residues of the inhibitor.

Materials and Methods

BI of mammalian α-amylase and trypsin (BIAT) was extracted from flours wheat (*Triticum aestivum* L.) of Saratovskay-29 and inhibition assays as described previously [12].

Homogeneity of inhibitor preparation was investigated by electrophoreses in denaturation conditions and natives conditions, and also under use of the bioanalyzer Agilent Technologies 2100. Kinetic properties, specific and physic and chemical characterization was made as described previously [12]. Chemical modification of arginine and lysine residues was realized by 1,4-cyclohexandione, citraconic anhydride accordingly [8]. Bifunctional inhibitor has been processed by lactoperoxidase and H_2O_2 at presence of iodide ion for oxidized tyrosine, tryptophan and methionine [10, 11, 13].

Results and Discussion

BI was obtained by affinity chromatography and ultrafiltration (Amicon UM 10). Homogeneity was checked by electrophoresis (not shown) and bioanalyzer (Figure 1).

The homogenous is every important parameter of BIAT, as the contamination with another protein can be critical for characterization of inhibitor [14]. The results presented in figure 1 confirm the high degree of the purity substance of BIAT. The peak 14.0 according to BIAT is molecular weigh 14 kDa. The following steps were investigated: physical and chemical characterization of BIAT. The detailed results are presented in previous researches [12]. We shall only enumerate the most important ones. Protein BIAT was termostabile (80°C, 15 min), pI > 9 and had five disulfide bridges. The competitive inhibition of trypsin and the substrate character of the inhibitor are in full agreement with the so called standard mechanism of serine proteinases inhibitor interaction. The measured K_i value of inhibitor was 10^{-9} M. The trypsin inhibitors are subdivided on lysine and arginine contained. For checking what residues are found in active centre chemical modification of lysine and arginine was organized. The specific reagents for lysine (ε-NH_2) are citraconic anhydride, for arginine is

1,4-cyclohexandione. There were modified amino acid residues of lysine and arginine. The results of the studies were presented in figure 2.

As a result of chemical modification it has been established, that arginine is a part of the active center of inhibitor responsible for interaction with trypsin. Lysine participates in interaction of the inhibitor with α-amylase.

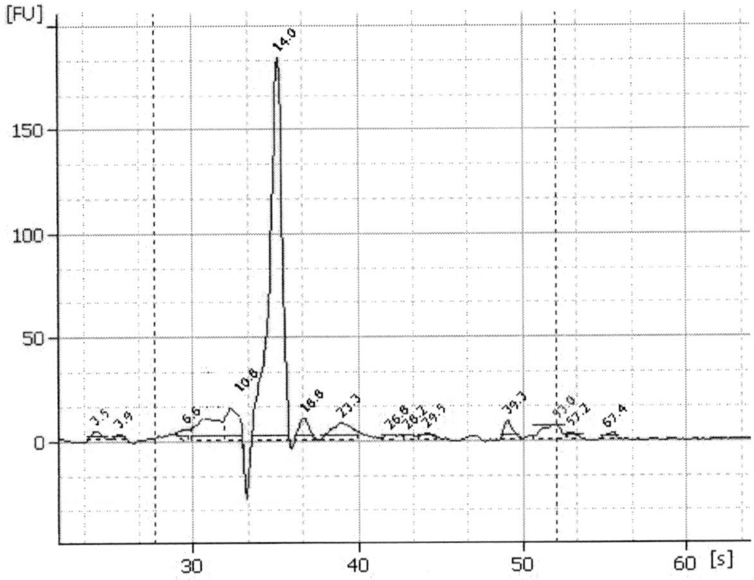

Figure 1. Densitogramm of fraction BIAT after affinity chromatography and ultrafiltration.

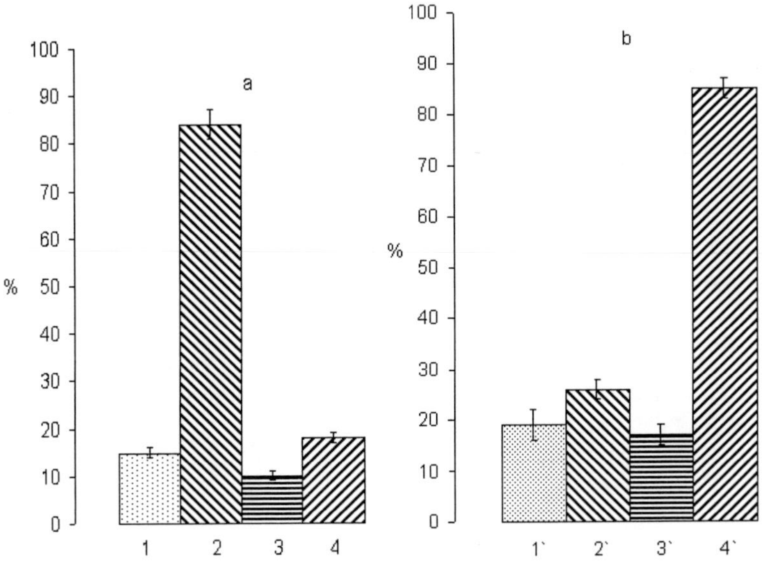

Figure 2. Results of acylated arginine (a) and lysine (b) of inhibitor. 1(1`), 3(3`) – non modif. BIAT; 2(2`), 4(4`) – modif. BIAT. Axis (y) - activity of the enzymes in %; 1(1`), 2(2`) – trypsin, 3(3`), 4(4`) – α-amylase.

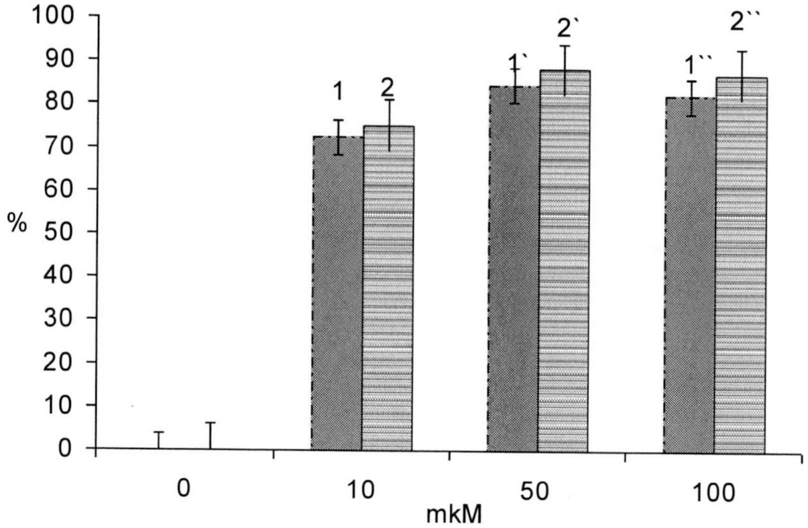

Figure 3. Results of enzymatic method of modification of tyrosine of BIAT. 1-1``- trypsin, 2-2``- α-amylase. Axis (y) - activity of the enzymes. Axis (y) mkM - I- ions.

Really, the residues of arginine can fall into reactive centre of inhibitor responsible for binding with trypsin. The lysine is localized in the area of polypeptide chain responsible for amylase binding site. Chemical modification experiments indicated that (Lys 96) in bifunctional inhibitor from ragi (*Eleusine coracana* Gaertneri) RBI may be involved in binding with mammalian amylases [4]. The researchers [4] showed residues tyrosine and tryptophan RBI is involved in the stabilization of the trypsin binding loop. The proposal that tyrosine (tryptophan and methionine) residues of inhibitor are involved in amylase binding is not supported by the inhibitor structure, as these residues are mainly involved in the stabilization of the trypsin binding loop [4]. For study of the participation of aromatic and sulfur-containing amino acids in stabilization of the structure BIAT the oxidation residues tyrosine (tryptophan and methionine) by hydrogen peroxide - lactoperoxidase and iodide ion was organized. Results presented in figure 3.

As a result of experiment the following data have been received. The inactivation of inhibitor occurred at presence of lactoperoxidase - H_2O_2 - I^-. It showed that there is an oxidation of aromatic and sulfur-containing amino acids, which can play the main role in the active center, but also they can support native conformation of molecule. This way of oxidation also can specify a probable inhibitor inactivation during germination of the grains when an activation of oxidation-reduction processes take part. Thereby full inactivated of bifunctional inhibitor amylase/trypsin occurred. Considering that at germination seed occurs increase the contents of the active forms of the oxygen and activity of the peroxidase, possible expect the oxidation of the inhibitor by such way.

Conclusion

Plants have evolved proteinaceous inhibitors against endogenous and exogenous carbohydrate-active enzymes as well as against enzymes of animals, insect or microbial pathogens. The understanding of the structural bases of active enzyme, involved into amino acid residues, may enable the rational design of more efficient inhibitors with more desirable functional properties. Moreover, it may be possible to reinforce plant protection against pathogens and to improve agronomic traits by possible transgenic technology. The high thermostability, specificity of BIAT and a strong complex with enzymes is perspective in the use for protection of plants against pathogens.

References

[1] Zhaoa, Y; Jin, Y; Weia, Sh.-Sh; Lee, W.-H; Zhang, Y. Purification and characterization of an irreversible serine protease inhibitor from skin secretions of *Bufo andrewsi. Toxicon*, 2005 volume 46, p. 635-640.

[2] Valueva, T. A. and Mosolov, V. V. (2004) Role of inhibitors of proteolytic enzymes in plant defense against phytopathogenic microorganisms. *Biochemistry (Moscow)*, volume 69, p. 1305-1309.

[3] Franco, OL; Rigden, DJ; Melo, FR; Grossi-de-Sa, MF; Plant α-amylase inhibitors and their interaction with insect α-amylases. *European Journal Biochemistry*, 2002 volume 269, p. 397-412.

[4] Strobl, S; Muhlhahn, P; Bernstein, R; Wiltscheck, R; Maskos, K; Wunderlich, M; Huber, R; Glockshuber, R; Holak, TA; Determination of the three-dimensional structure of the bifunctional α-amylase/trypsin inhibitor from Ragi seeds by NMR spectroscopy. *Biochemistry*, 1995 volume 34, p. 8281-8293.

[5] Zemke, KJ; Muller-Fahrnow, A; Jany, K; The three-dimensional structure of the bifunctional proteinase K/ α-amylase inhibitor from wheat (PKI3) at 2.5 A resolution. *FEBS letters*, 1991 volume 397, p. 240-242.

[6] Constantin, C; Quirce, S; Grote, M; Touraev, A; Swoboda, I; Stoecklinger, A; Mari, A; Thalhamer, J; Heberle-Bors, E; Valenta, R; Molecular and immunological characterization of a wheat serine proteinase inhibitor as a novel allergen in baker's asthma. *The Journal of Immunology*, 2008 volume 180, p. 7451-7460.

[7] Elayeb, M; Darbon, H; Bahraoui, M; Vargas, O; Rochat, H; Differential effects of defined chemical modifications on antigenic and pharmacological activities of scorpion α and β toxins. *European Journal of Biochemistry*, 2005 volume 155, p. 289 – 294.

[8] Lundblad, RL. *Chemical reagents for protein modification*. Third Edition. Boca Raton: CRC Press; 2004.

[9] Moyse, E., and Krantic, S. M. (2001). Visualization of receptors in situ: Application of radioligand binding. *Methods in visualization.* Boca Raton, CRC Press.

[10] Yamakura, F. and Ikeda, K. (2006). Modification of tryptophan and tryptophan residues in proteins by reactive nitrogen species. *Nitric Oxide*, volume 14, p. 152-161.

[11] Morrison, M. and Schonbaum, G. R. (1976). Peroxidase-catalyzed halogenation. *Annual Review of Biochemistry*, volume 45, p. 861-888.

[12] Islamov, R. A. and Fursov, O. V. (2007). Bifunctional inhibitor of α-amylase/trypsin from wheat grain. *Applied Biochemistry and Microbiology*, volume 43, p. 379-382.

[13] Gvozdeva, EL; Valueva, TK; Mosolov, VV; Enzymatic oxidation of the bifunctional wheat inhibitor of subtilisin and endogenous α-amylase. *FEBS Letters*, 1993 volume 334, p. 72-74.

[14] Gomez-Leyva J. F. and Blanco-Labra A. (2001). Bifunctional α-amylase/trypsin inhibitor activity previously ascribed to the 22 KDa TL protein, resided in a contaminant protein of 14 KDa. *Journal of Plant Physiology*, volume 158, p. 177-183.

In: Trypsin: Structure, Biosynthesis and Functions
Editors: Kirk Weaver and Clayton Kelley

ISBN 978-1-61942-319-0

Chapter VIII

Quantitative LC-MS Analysis of Proteins Using Trypsin and CNBr Generated Marker-Peptides: Proof-of-Concept Study on Cystatin C*

Michael L. Storme and Jan F. Van Bocxlaer
Laboratory of Medical Biochemistry and Clinical Analysis,
Faculty of Pharmaceutical Sciences, Ghent University, Ghent, Belgium

Abstract

Proteins, either therapeutic or diagnostic, will become increasingly important in the bio-medical and pharmaceutical field. The major efforts invested in e.g. proteomics, in the recent past, will provide us with many new and promising protein type of target molecules in the coming years. Irrespective whether these proteins are intended therapeutics or endogenous, medically diagnostic molecules, their absolute quantitative measurement will become more and more of an issue. In that respect, immunoassays are of paramount importance. Nevertheless, as in the field of small molecules, alternatives based on chromatography and, inevitably, mass spectrometric detection, are attracting the attention of many investigators. Although more complicated and allowing less sample throughput, (ESI)-LC/MS provides much higher selectivity and thus analytical confidence with respect to the particular measurement.

In terms of quantitative target compound analysis, mass spectrometry of intact proteins has the major disadvantage of producing an envelope of multiply charged ions, thus spreading the amount of protein compound over many different species. This results in a major loss of sensitivity as only one of a few species are measured in the (tandem) LC-MS process. In this chapter we report on an alternative approach to analyzing intact proteins based on the proteomic "bottom-up" principle of generating peptides from the protein by proteolysis. These peptides are the stoichiometric representation of the protein

* A version of this chapter also appears in *Handbook on Mass Spectrometry: Instrumentation, Data and Analysis, and Applications*, edited by J. K. Lang, published by Nova Science Publishers, Inc. It was submitted for appropriate modifications in an effort to encourage wider dissemination of research.

and some of them can be selected for LC-MS measurement using the techniques commonly used for small molecules and with comparable analytical complexity.

This chapter will focus on the reproducible generation of a number of so called marker-peptides based on enzymatic (trypsin) and especially chemical protein digestion using cyanogen bromide. Reaction conditions for reproducible protein digestion, internal standardization, liquid chromatographic separation, mass spectrometric detection and quantitative evaluation of the approach are discussed using the endogenous human cystatin C protein, a clinically relevant biochemical marker often used in diagnostic settings, as a proof-of-concept protein.

Absolute Quantitative Analysis of Proteins

Nowadays, the use of liquid chromatography-(tandem) mass spectrometry (LC-MS(/MS)) for the absolute quantitation of target compounds is widespread and probably one of the most applied methodologies in modern bio-analytical work. Especially for small molecular mass compounds, there are many well described approaches, "good-practices", and quality assurance guidclines with regard to their development, routine application and validation. However, the real challenge of future work lies in the extension of such LC-MS (/MS) based procedures to a new application field, being the absolute quantitation of larger bio-molecules such as proteins. Proteins, either therapeutic or diagnostic, will become increasingly important in the bio-medical and pharmaceutical field. The major efforts invested in e.g. proteomics in the recent past will provide us with many new and promising protein type of target molecules in the coming years. Irrespective whether these proteins are intended therapeutics or endogenous, medically diagnostic molecules, their absolute quantitative measurement will become more and more of an issue [1]. In that respect, it is necessary to exactly define quantitative analysis of proteins. In the field of proteomics, the term quantitative protein analysis is frequently used nowadays, often in conjunction with commercialized quantitative techniques such as ICAT®, iTRAQ® and the likes. However, in line with the "omics" philosophy, this remains a relative quantitation, i.e. a relative quantitative comparison of two or more set conditions (between for instance healthy and diseased state). What we in this chapter will refer to as absolute quantitative measurement aims to really quantify a protein in terms of absolute concentration expressed e.g. in μg/mL or nmol/mL.

In the field of protein analysis as a whole, the use of mass spectrometry is already widely accepted but mainly, if not only, for qualitative or semi-quantitative purposes. Historically, in contrast to mass spectrometric based approaches for protein quantitation, almost all protein quantitation methods are based upon immunoassays. These allow high-throughput but can essentially only be applied for the protein they have been developed for. Moreover, development of an immunoassay for a certain protein is a complicated, long-lasting, and specialized multidisciplinary process, often taking anywhere from 6 to 12 months before an assay is established. As such, there is a certain need for more generic methods and LC-MS bears in it the abilities to provide this kind of methodology, being rather chemical than biological of nature.

Nevertheless, LC-MS based approaches for whole protein quantitation are hampered by awkward LC separation, often incompatible with MS, as well as complicated mass spectrometry e.g. spectra dominated by a multiple charge envelope. The latter results in a major loss of sensitivity as only one of a few species are measured in the (tandem) LC-MS process (see later in this chapter). Due to these inconveniences, quantitative LC-MS of whole proteins, especially the bigger ones, is still rather a goal than a practice. In this perspective, the use of marker-peptides as a measure of the protein of interest as a whole, is a potential alternative [2]. Therefore, the protein is cleaved into peptides by means of chemical or enzymatic proteolysis. The peptides obtained as such are then, in a next step, chromatographically separated and quantitatively analyzed using MS(/MS). Using this so-called “bottom-up” approach for mass spectrometric protein analysis, absolute quantitative protein analysis is demoted to the more straightforward quantitation of a small peptide subset. It is quite evident that the most important and critical step in such an approach is the proteolysis. Reproducibility is vital and special attention on internal standardization to compensate for differential proteolysis efficiencies is mandatory. A large part of this chapter is devoted to this aspect, investigating enzymatic (tryptic) and chemical (cyanogen bromide, CNBr) proteolysis and their performance in a LC-MS(/MS) based, absolute quantitative procedure.

Quantitative measurements of proteins will be of great importance to valorize proteomics discoveries in medical-biological application fields. In essence, this means measurement in a biological matrix such as blood, plasma, etc. Consequently, another critical aspect in absolute quantitative protein analysis is the often high complexity of protein samples. For instance, in the case of plasma samples, the 22 most abundant plasma proteins count for more than 99% of the plasma bulk protein mass. Thus, it is clear that the effective removal of the major part of these proteins will be mandatory since the detection of less abundant proteins will be suppressed by these (much) higher abundant ones. Part of this chapter will indeed be devoted to implementing the absolute quantitative analysis of proteins using marker-peptides into measuring such proteins in plasma, thus extending the proteolysis and LC-MS methodology with a suitable sample preparation phase as front-end. Although the quality of an analytical method is determined by the quality of its weakest element, the mass spectrometric part of an LC-MS(/MS) based quantitative protein analysis remains vital for the overall approach.

Mass Spectrometry of Proteins and Peptides

Mass spectrometry (MS) determines the mass-to charge ratio’s *(m/z)* of gas-phase ions. Hence, the analytes need to be transferred to the gas phase and ionized prior to analysis. Besides molecular mass information, the technique also provides structural information. Mass spectrometry as a technique already originates from the early twentieth century. The breakthrough of mass spectrometric (bio-) analysis of bio-molecules, however, came not until the early 1980’s by the discovery of fast-atom bombardment (FAB) by Barber and co-workers [3]. Nevertheless, it was the revolutionizing introduction of soft-ionization techniques like electrospray ionization (ESI) by Fenn further on in the 1980’s [4], and later matrix assisted laser desorption ionization (MALDI) that made mass spectrometry the most important tool to analyze large bio-molecules. Before, mass spectrometry demanded vaporized samples, ionized by either electron impact or chemical ionization. Unfortunately, larger, polar and/or thermally labile bio-molecules like peptides and proteins could not be analyzed using these ionization techniques. This, in contrast to ESI and MALDI which nowadays allow the analysis of bio-molecules as large as a few mega-Dalton [5]. As such, during the last decades, there has been an explosion in instrumentation and applications of mass spectrometry for the analysis of large bio-molecules.

Once the analytes of interest are brought into the gas phase and ionized, whatever the chronological sequence, a number of mass analyzers are these days available to determine their *m/z*, such as quadrupole mass filters [6], double-focusing magnetic and electric sector instruments, time-of-flight (TOF) [7], quadrupole ion traps [8], the recently added orbitrap, and Fourier-transform ion cyclotron resonance [9] mass analyzers. Two or more mass analysers can be put together to form a tandem mass spectrometer, such as a triple quadrupole mass spectrometer [10] or a hybrid instrument, consisting of two different kinds of mass spectrometers, e.g. a quadrupole-TOF (Q-TOF) mass spectrometer [11]. A collision cell positioned in between the two mass analyzing regions is a common feature for this kind of mass spectrometers. This collision cell contains an inert gas (typically argon) in which precursor ions (e.g. a protonated peptide), selected in the first mass analyser, collide and form so-called product ions whose *m/z* is now mass-measured in the second mass analyzer, in a process named collision-induced dissociation (CID) [12]. In the case of peptides, the nature of these product ions can be used to determine the peptide primary structure, i.e. the amino-acid sequence [13]. This complete process is often described as tandem mass spectrometry or MS/MS and is widely used to identify unknown proteins and peptides [14]. As a logical extension of the former, mass spectrometry is nowadays a widespread technique with key functions in a number of fields, including biochemistry, biotechnology, pharmacology, microbiology and the proteomic/functional genomics field [14].

Electrospray Ionization

The development of ESI by Fenn, almost two decades ago, has paved the way to the analysis of large bio-molecules using mass spectrometry and was awarded the Nobel Prize in 2002 [4, 15, 16]. In fact, ESI is a continuous-flow ionisation device used as an interface in the coupling of separation techniques such as LC to mass spectrometric devices. In conventional electrospray, a flow of liquid, either from a chromatographic system or a syringe pump, is passed through a thin conducting needle at high voltage and a potential difference is created between the needle tip and a counter electrode, being the inlet of the mass spectrometer [14]. Due to the electric field gradient created at the tip, charge separation occurs in the solution as anions migrate towards the capillary walls (positively charged) and cations travel towards the meniscus of the droplet formed at the tip [17, 18].

Owing to the presence of an electric field, liquid emerges from the tip of the capillary in the shape of a cone, also known as the "Taylor cone". When the electrostatic repulsion between charged molecules at the surface of the Taylor cone approaches the surface tension of the solution, known as reaching the Rayleigh limit, charged droplets are expelled from the tip. A process, known as "Coulomb explosion", results in the formation of highly charged micro droplets. Evaporation of the offspring droplets' solvent, assisted by the presence of a (warm) nitrogen gas stream, leads to a fission series and the process repeats itself to produce smaller and smaller droplets until ultimately gas phase ions are formed [17].

The exact mechanism of formation of these gas phase ions, together with the exact mechanism of charging the analytes, remains unclear but is thought to be a combination of two mechanisms known as the "ion evaporation mechanism", originally proposed by Iribarne and Thomson [20], and the "charged residue model", put forward by Dole *et al.* [21].

During ionization, the analytes become protonated or cation-adducted positive ions (+ESI), while in –ESI, a proton is extracted from the analyte. The resulting ions themselves have little excess of internal energy and therefore, little fragmentation is noticed during the ionization process.

Many of the ions formed during +ESI occur as $[M+nH]^{n+}$ (or other cations like Na^+, K^+, NH_4^+), alternatively $[M-nH]^{n-}$ in –ESI. In the case of larger bio-molecules like proteins, the formation of multiple charged ions up to 30^+ is very common and typical for ESI.

Electrospray Ionization of Peptides and Proteins

As mentioned above, ESI of larger molecules produces multiply charged ions. As a result, proteins with molecular masses in the mass range of 10-100 kDa will, in general, produce an envelope of ions (see Figure 1), different from each other in the number of attached protons and hence charge state, with *m/z* values below 2500 Da.

Ion transmission throughout the mass spectrometer is generally very good within this region. As a result, mass measurement statistics are excellent. These features make ESI one the most suitable ionization methods for molecular mass determination of large bio-molecules. For structural information, however, the use of MS/MS is needed (*vide infra*) as the ESI process in itself does not produce a substantial number of fragment ions [14].

Protein/Peptide Fragmentation

For protein characterisation, proteins are typically first enzymatically or chemically digested into peptides and these peptides are then fragmented by CID fragmentation in the mass spectrometer.

This so-called "bottom-up" protein analysis process has for years been the gold standard approach in proteomics for protein/peptide identification and characterisation. However, reducing a protein to a collection of peptides could also be interesting for the absolute quantitation of the protein by means of one or more selected marker-peptides. In such a LC-MS(/MS) experiment, the chromatographic separation is used to separate the peptides from a protein digest and the first mass analyzer (MS1) is then set up so as to sequentially "mass-select" these peptides for further analysis.

The selected peptide-ion is focused toward the collision cell where the peptide collides with an inert gas (mostly argon). During these collisions, the translational energy of the precursor peptide-ion will partly be converted into internal energy and the ions become excited to an unstable state. Consequently, the precursor ions dissociate (fragment) into smaller product ions. The mass of these product ions can then be determined in the second mass analyzer (MS2). Because of the standardized way in which polypeptides fragment (largely due to the repetitive nature of the peptide bond), the amino-acid sequence of the peptide can be deduced [22].

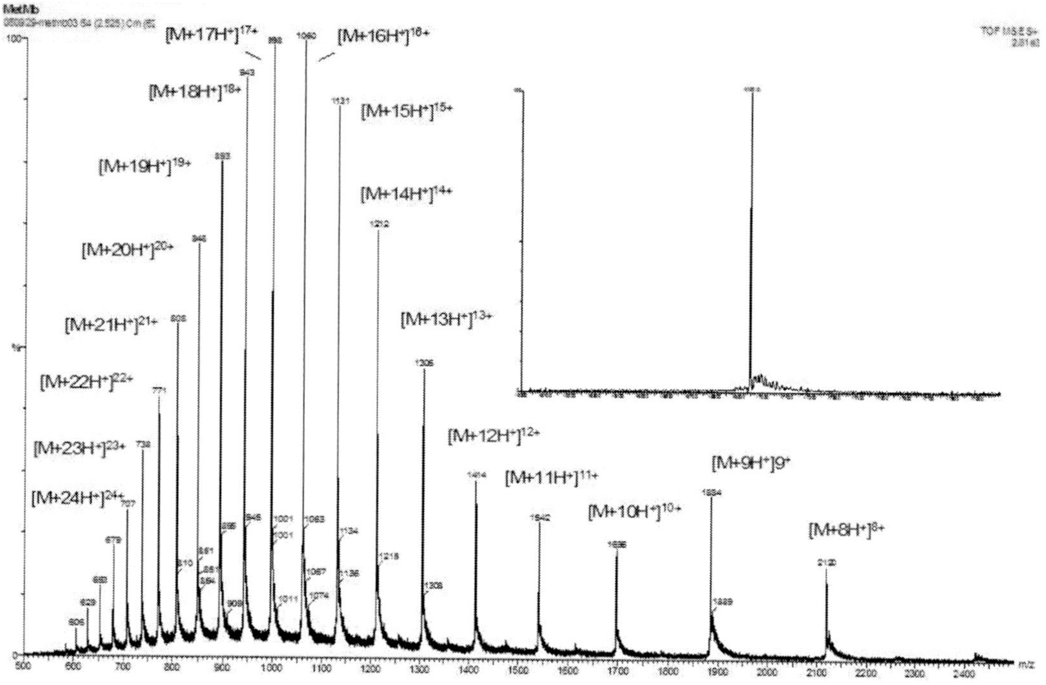

Figure 1. Electrospray mass spectrum (QTof) of metmyoglobin (dissolved in dilute formic acid). The attachment of many protons per protein molecule (from less than 10 to more than 20 here) leads to a series of m/z peaks for this single protein. The inset shows a computer analysis of the data from this series of peaks that generates a single peak at the correct molecular mass (16.950 Da) of the protein.

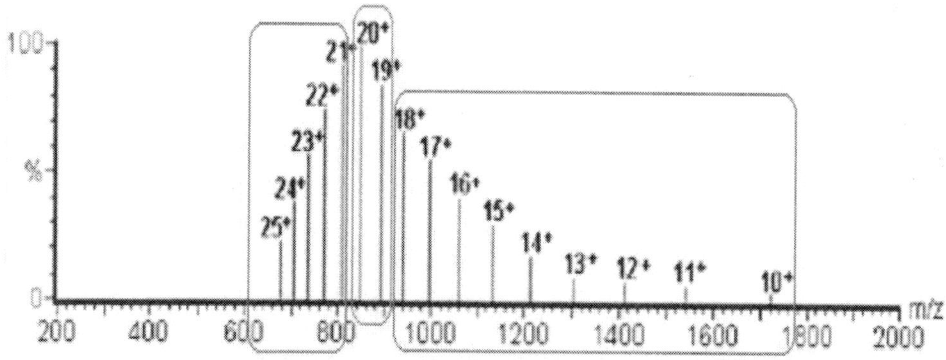

Figure 2. Theoretical example of envelope formation during ESI-MS. In Q3 MRM experiments, only a few of the generated ions can be selected for quantitation of the protein (e.g.. green m/z values). As a result, a loss of sensitivity is inevitable as a major part of the protein is not detected (red m/z values).

Alternatively, in the quantitation approach, one or two product ions could be selected (in MS2) for quantitation. For protein characterization, the use of a Q-TOF tandem mass spectrometer is favoured by virtue of the high full-scan sensitivity of the TOF analyzer; whereas for protein quantitation the use of a triple quadrupole (Q3) tandem mass spectrometer is recommended.

The Marker-Peptide Approach in Absolute Quantitation of Proteins

The mass spectrometric, absolute quantitation of a protein can be performed using 2 different approaches. The "top-down" approach is based on the mass spectrometric analysis of the protein as a whole. However, the use of a Q3 mass spectrometer, as the preferred mass spectrometric device for quantitation purposes, is hampered by the envelope formation during the ESI process. Indeed, with multiple charge states present, multiple *m/z* values are generated. However, only a few of these can be selected as MRM precursor ion and hence, a major sensitivity loss is inevitable (see Figure 2).

Moreover, as mentioned before, whole protein LC separation in a way compatible with MS detection is equally challenging. High-performance size exclusion chromatography has been on-line coupled to mass spectrometry but largely remains a fractionation technique rather than an analytical separation tool.

Reversed phase type of separations with on-line MS detection have been described but in the majority of cases as a second dimension in 2D-separations and in any case for qualitative purposes only [23].

The "bottom-up" approach on the other hand works in the opposite direction and proteins are first digested, enzymatically and/or chemically, into peptides. A subset of the peptides generated from the protein can be used as marker-peptides. Analyzing these peptides instead of the total protein simplifies the quantitation of a protein to the quantitation of a single or a number of chromatographically separated peptides followed by the mass spectrometric detection. Hence, the mass spectrometric quantitative analysis of a protein is demoted to the more straightforward analysis of one or more peptides.

The idea of combining proteolysis with LC-MS for absolute quantitation was first reported by Barr and co-workers [24, 25]. In 2004, Zhang *et al.* [2] described a quantitation tool for human glutathione S-transferase, using trypsin digestion and LC-MS(/MS). Out of the total set of tryptic peptides produced, the four most abundant were used in a quantitative LC-MS(/MS) analysis procedure.

Essential in the "bottom-up" methodology is a reproducible digestion method. A large part of this chapter deals with the evaluation and optimization of two different proteolysis approaches, enzymatically using trypsin and chemically using CNBr, in terms of their quantitative performance, i.e. repeatability. To that end, a proof-of-concept protein, cystatin C, was used. Equally essential in the "bottom-up" methodology is an adequate internal standard (IS).

The main point pertaining to that IS is that it should not only be capable of compensating for analytical variations (e.g.. injection differences, matrix effect, etc.) but especially for differences during sample treatment, including the digestion step(s).

While the performance of quasi all quantitation methods using LC-MS(/MS) is highly dependent on adequate internal standardization, the latter is especially true for proteins. With respect to the analysis of cystatin C, the use of a protein family analogue from a different species, in this case chicken egg white cystatin, is investigated.

The Proof-of-Concept Protein Cystatin C and its Internal Standard Protein Chicken Egg White Cystatin

Why Cystatin C?

Cystatin C is chosen as a model protein for evaluation of the marker-peptide (bottom-up quantitation) methodology for a number of reasons. First of all because of its structure: cystatin C is a non-glycosylated protein of a medium size. Consequently, it represents a model of intermediate difficulty: although being a real protein in terms of its size, it is not too big in size. At the other hand, it is not exactly known in what way glycosylation of a protein might impact on the quantitative nature of the proteolysis step. Finally, there is also the advantage that, even though cystatin C is used merely as a model, this model also has a clinical significance. The latter is based on the fact that cystatin C is expected, in the near future, to act as a measurement alternative of kidney function [26, 27].

Until now, kidney function is expressed by the glomerular filtration rate (GFR) based on the serum creatinine level. Cystatin C could serve this goal better than creatinine because it has, under normal conditions, a constant serum level independent of gender, muscle mass, age and is, for more than 99%, cleared from the circulation by glomerular filtration [28, 29]. Cystatin C levels are, however, not only determined as a measurement of kidney function (serum cystatin C) but also sporadically as a pain-marker in cerebrospinal fluid (CSF) although with limited clinical significance [30]. Also in Alzheimer disease, the cystatin C CSF level can be of some importance [31]. Indeed, cystatin C brain tissue levels are up-regulated with brain tissue damage.

Cystatin C Structure

Cystatin C, previously also named either γ-trace or post-γ-globulin, is part of the cystatin super family, a name proposed by Barett *et al.* in 1981 [32]. The name cystatin refers to the ability to inhibit certain cysteine proteinases. The first cysteine proteinase inhibitors described were obtained from chicken egg white.

Nowadays, the cystatin super family is divided into four main cystatin families [33, 34]. The family of the type 2 cystatins has the largest number of members, including cystatin C and chicken egg white cystatin, considered as the prototypical member. Type 2 cystatins are typically about 120-125 amino-acid residues long, without the signal-peptide, and contain four cysteine residues, which are involved in the formation of two disulphide bonds, characteristic of the family. They are secreted with a secretory peptide leader sequence and hence, are generally known as extracellular. As such, cystatin C is a 120 amino-acids protein, 146 when the signal peptide is included, with an average molecular mass of 13347 Da and with 2 disulphide bridges between amino-acids 99-109 and amino-acids 123-143 [27]. Its complete amino-acid sequence was determined in 1981 by Anders Grubb and Helge Löfberg [35]. The complete cystatin C sequence is shown in Figure 3. In body fluids, cystatin C is present as an active monomer. However, during maturization and before extracellular secretion, cystatin C is present as a transient dimer, probably to prevent interfering with the functioning of cysteine proteases present in the secretion pathway [36].

A Protein Analogue as Internal Standard: Chicken Egg White Cystatin

The ideal IS is an IS chromatographically co-eluting with the analyte. In the case of peptides from a protein digest, this can be achieved by use of isotopically labelled internal standards. Insertion of isotopes changes the mass of the peptide but not its chemical behaviour [1].

Unfortunately, they need to be custom-made and hence, their cost is high, depending on the length of the peptide. More importantly, however, based on the fact that the actual analyte is a protein and the IS is a peptide, severe quantitation errors may result due to the selection of unsuitable reference peptides and/or imperfect protein proteolysis [37]. Taking all of this into consideration, there is a need to implement internal standardization in a different way.

In our view, the best alternative approach, apart from a generally utopical labelled protein, is to use a homologue sequence protein, in this case the commercially available chicken egg white cystatin, as IS.

In doing so, nearly co-eluting internal standard peptides (ISP) can be generated for every selected marker-peptide, obtained by either enzymatic cleavage using trypsin or chemical proteolysis using CNBr. Clearly, the analyte protein and its IS can thus be digested simultaneously and under exactly the same reaction conditions. Such a protein IS can be added to the sample prior to the proteolysis, and even before the eventual sample preparation step, and is thus (theoretically) capable of counterbalancing the majority of the sample treatment induced variability.

Chicken egg white cystatin consists of a chain of 140 amino-acids with 2 disulphide bridges between amino-acids 94-104 and between amino-acids 118-139. As such, the size of the IS is comparable with cystatin C, both proteins share about 44 % of the amino-acid sequence [27]. Moreover, with both proteins belonging to the type 2 cystatins, their higher conformation too is very similar.

Both consist of a five-stranded anti-parallel β-sheet wrapping around a long α_1-helix that is almost perpendicular to the general β-strand direction. In addition, also the number of disulphide bridges and their relative position within the amino-acids sequence provides a good representation of cystatin C. As already stated, the use of a whole protein as internal standard is important to compensate for (minor) differences in cleavage efficiencies. Figure 3 shows the amino-acid sequences of both cystatin C and chicken egg white cystatin. Disulphide bridges and possible cleaving sites are indicated (both enzymatic (trypsin) and chemical cleavage (CNBr) sites).

As can be deduced from the figure, more cleavage sites are present for tryptic cleavage (after, C-terminal side, arginine and lysine residues), compared to CNBr-based chemical cleavage (after methionine residues).

The differences among both techniques will be clearly described in the following sections, as is the selection of the different marker-peptides and their ISP's. In general, for every selected peptide, a co-eluting ISP, or at least an ISP in a close time-window, can be selected out of the peptide subset of proteolyzed chicken egg white cystatin.

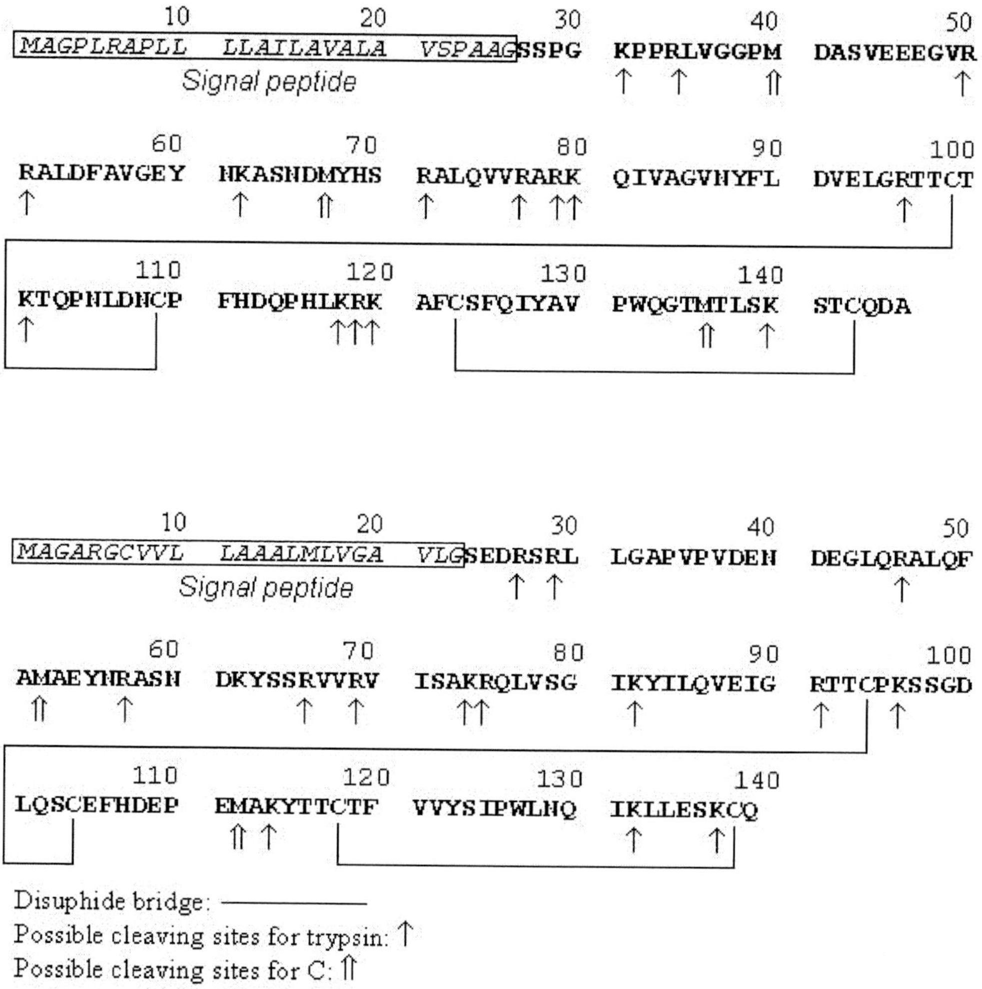

Figure 3. Cystatin C (upper pane) and chicken egg white cystatin (lower pane) amino-acid sequence (www.expasy.org). Possible cleavage sites for both enzymatic cleavage (trypsin) and chemical cleavage (CNBr) are indicated, as well as the disulphide bridges.

Enzymatic Protein Proteolysis: In-Solution Tryptic Digestion

For protein quantitation using marker-peptides, i.e. the bottom-up approach, mass spectrometry is performed on proteolytic peptides. In such a set-up, a given protein is typically proteolyzed with trypsin, followed by LC separation of the proteolytic peptides produced. As already mentioned in this chapter, in a marker-peptide approach, developing a reproducible, in-solution trypsin digest procedure is a vital step. To that end, 4 different denaturing procedures have been evaluated [38]. Denaturing entails reduction of eventual intra-chain disulphide bonds and unfolding of the protein to promote proteolysis. As reducing agents, 5 mM dithiothreitol (DTT) versus 10% betaME in the denaturing buffer of 50 mM Tris-HCl/ 6 M urea (urea is a chaotropic agent which unfolds the protein) have been tested using our proof-of-concept protein cystatin C based on the following procedure. Cystatin C was trypsinized using Promega Sequencing Grade Modified Trypsin. 55 µL of a protein stock-solution (1mg/mL lyophilized powder in 50 mM tris-HCl /1 mM $CaCl_2$) was denatured for one hour at 65°C, alternatively 20 min at 95°C, using 145 µL of a solution of 50 mM Tris-HCl/ 6 M urea/ 10% beta mercapto-ethanol. When denaturing for 1 hour at 65°C the best results have been obtained, and there is another 5 to 8-fold increase of the peptide LC-MS peak areas when using betaME instead of DTT (see Figure 4).

The denatured protein is diluted in 50 mM tris-HCl /1 mM $CaCl_2$ (600 µl, to a total volume of 800 µL), to achieve a urea concentration below 2 M, in essence to prevent self destruction of trypsin. Iodoacetamide (IA) is added to a final concentration of 20 mM. Addition of IA to block free SH-groups is essential for good protein sequence coverage.

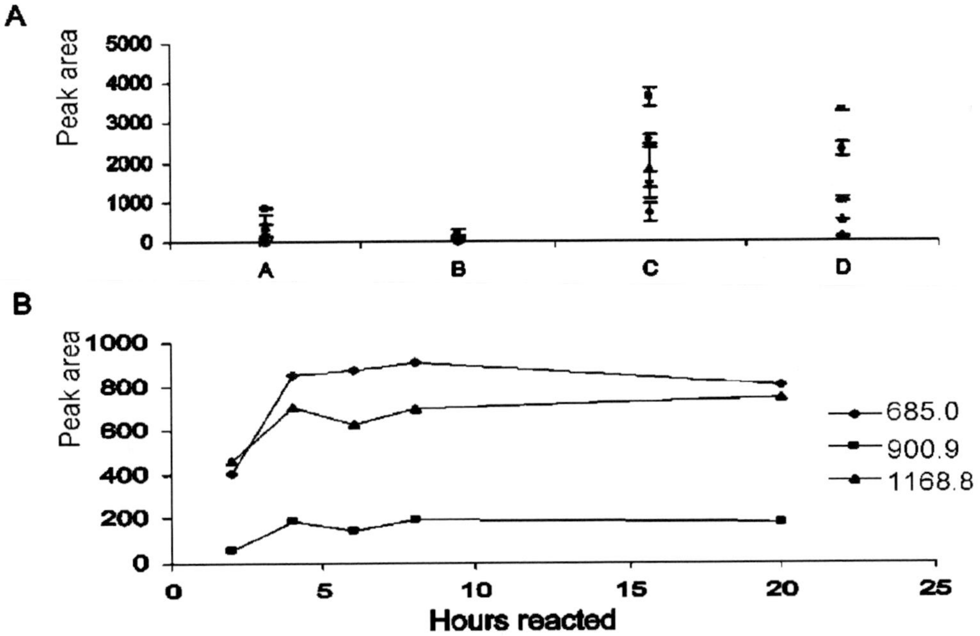

Figure 4. [A] Peptide recovery under different denaturing conditions of three possible marker-peptides in cystatin C. Clearly, for this application betaME is a better reducing agent then DTT: (A) 50 mM Tris.HCl/6 M urea/5 mM DTT, 1h 65° (n=3); (B) 50 mM Tris.HCl/ 6 M urea/ 5 mM DTT, 20min 95° (n=3); (C) 50 mM Tris.HCl/ 6 M urea/ 10%betaME, 1h 65° (n=3); (D) 50 mMTris.HCl/ 6 M urea/ 10% betaME, 20min 95° (n=3) [B] Time course study of trypsin digestion: the peak area of the peptides with m/z 685.0, 900.9 and 1168.8 are plotted against the reaction time [reproduced with permission from [38].

SSPGK(//)**PPR**//**LVGGPMDASVEEEGVR**//R//**ALDFAVGEYNK**//**ASNDMYHSR**//**ALQVVR**//**AR**//K//**QIVAG**

VNYFLDVELGR//TTCTK//**TQPNLDNCPFHDQPHLK**//R//K//**AFCSFQIYAVPWQGTMTLSK**//STCQDA

Figure 5. Cystatin C sequence (without signal peptides sequence). Tryptic peptides are separated by //, peptides in bold are detectable on reversed phase liquid chromatographic separations. Peptides underlined are most suitable as marker peptides. The cysteine residue in peptide 3 is IA cysteinyl carboxyamidomethylated.

In this way, re-uniting of two adjacent SH-groups is prevented. A 20 minutes reaction time at room temperature, under gentle shaking and in total darkness, due to the light-sensitivity of IA, provides good acetylation efficiency. After checking the pH, the trypsinization process is started by adding trypsin (50 µL, as a 1 µg/10 µL solution in 50 mM acetic acid, pH 7.8) to a final protease: protein ratio between 1:10 and 1:50. Different ratios, 1:10; 1:20 and 1:50 have been tested but did not affect the sequence coverage. The optimized trypsin proteolysis procedure yields 100% sequence coverage (only taking peptides of minimum 6 amino-acid residues into account). While a 100% sequence coverage is thus obtained, only a few peptides are necessary as marker-peptides. All potential marker-peptides for cystatin C after tryptic proteolysis are summarized in Table 1.

Also peptides composed of 2 tryptic fragments, thus allowing 1 missed cleavage, have been included. Theoretical masses of the peptide fragments and corresponding m/z values, ranging from $[M+H]^+$ until $[M+3H]^{3+}$, are calculated using Masslynx Biolynx® and PeptideCutter/PeptideMass (ExPASy; Expert Protein Analysis System) proteomics server (www.expasy.org). Cleavage sites with low cleavage probability are not included, thus for trypsin, cleavage sites followed by a proline residue are disregarded.

Logically, the four most abundant peptides, the singly charged peptide with m/z 685.0 and the doubly charged peptides with m/z 897.5, 900.9, and 1168.8, are the most likely marker-peptide candidates (see Figure 5). To allow a selection of marker-peptides to represent the full cystatin C protein as adequately as possible, marker-peptides are chosen from the beginning, the middle and the end part of the protein. Consequently, peptides with m/z 685.0, 900.9 and 1168.8 are most suitable.

These three peptides, selected as marker-peptides, are chromatographically separated using a YMC Pack ODS-AQ™ 2.1 x 150 mm, 5 µm C18 column, eluted at a flow rate of 0.2 mL/min. using 0.1% formic acid (FA) in water as eluent A, and 0.1% FA in methanol or AcN as eluent B.

FA is added to improve electrospray ionization. For quantitation purposes, chromatographic separation of the obtained tryptic peptides with a resolution of at least 1.2 is not absolutely necessary but often desirable. This can be achieved using gradient elution beginning with a 5' equilibration period at 5% eluent B, followed by an increase of B to 40% over 26.5 minutes. The % B is then quickly increased to up to 90% in the next 30 seconds and stays there for 3.5 minutes. After regaining starting conditions within 30 seconds, adequate re-equilibration, essential for reproducible retention times, is mandatory. The chromatographically separated marker-peptides are detected using mass spectrometry (electrospray ionization in the positive ion mode).

Both a Q-TOF hybrid mass spectrometer or triple quadrupole system can advantageously be used. Due to its high "full scan" sensitivity, the Q-TOF is most suitable for the ultimate confirmation in practical conditions of the initial theoretical selection of the marker-peptide subset. Moreover, it is very useful for evaluation of the fragmentation spectra, in order to select the most suitable product ions to be used for quantitation in the MRM mode. The final quantitative MRM analysis is performed on a triple quadrupole system which in this operational mode, provides enhanced sensitivity compared to a Q-TOF.

For the assessment of the trysinization process as part of a quantitative protein assay, evaluation of the reproducibility and linearity of the proteolysis step revealed the following results [38]. Calibration curves were prepared from 3.9 to 1000 µg/mL cystatin C.

Table 1. possible marker-peptides after cleavage using trypsin (T1-T15) of cystatin C. For each peptide, the corresponding theoretical mass and *m/z* values are given. One missed cleavage is allowed (K/R-P cleavage sites are not taken into consideration)

Name	Sequence	Theoretical mass (Da)	$[M+H]^+$	$[M+2H]^{2+}$	$[M+3H]^{3+}$
T1	SSPGKPPR	824.9	825.9	413.5	276.0
T2	LVGGPMDASVEEEGVR	1644.8	1645.8	823.4	549.3
T3	R	174.1	175.1	88.1	59.1
T4	ALDFAVGEYNK	1226.4	1227.4	614.2	409.8
T5	ASNDMYHSR	1080.2	1081.2	541.1	361.1
T6	ALQVVR	684.8	685.9	343.4	229.3
T7	AR	245.2	246.2	123.6	82.7
T8	K	146.1	147.1	74.1	49.7
T9	QIVAGVNYFLDVELGR	1793.1	1794.1	897.5	598.7
T10	TTCTK	552.7	553.7	277.3	185.2
T11	TQPNLDNCPFHDQPHLK	2004.2	2005.2	1003.1	669.1
T12	R	174.1	175.1	88.1	59.1
T13	K	146.1	147.1	74.1	49.7
T14	AFCSFQIYAVPWQGTMTLSK	2278.7	2279.7	1140.4	760.6
T15	STCQDA	623.6	624.7	312.8	208.9
T1-2	SSPGKPPRLVGGPMDASVEE EGVR	2451.7	2452.8	1226.9	818.3
T2-3	LVGGPMDASVEEEGVRR	1799.8	1800.8	900.9	600.9
T3-4	RALDFAVGEYNK	1382.5	1383.6	692.3	461.9
T4-5	ALDFAVGEYNKASNDMYHSR	2288.5	2289.5	1145.3	763.8
T5-6	ASNDMYHSRALQVVR	1747.0	1748.0	874.5	583.3
T6-7	ALQVVRAR	912.1	913.1	457.1	305.0
T7-8	ARK	373.5	374.5	187.7	125.5
T8-9	KQIVAGVNYFLDVELGR	1921.2	1922.2	961.6	641.4
T9-10	QIVAGVNYFLDVELGRTTCT K	2327.7	2328.7	1164.9	776.9
T10-11	TTCTKTQPNLDNCPFHDQPH LK	2538.9	2539.9	1270.4	847.3
T11-12	TQPNLDNCPFHDQPHLKR	2160.4	2161.4	1081.2	721.1
T12-13	RK	302.4	303.4	152.2	101.8
T13-14	KAFCSFQIYAVPWQGTMTLSK	2406.9	2407.9	1204.4	803.3
T14-15	AFCSFQIYAVPWQGTMTLSK STCQDA	2884.3	2885.3	1443.2	962.4

Each standard (1000 (74.92 x 10^3 pmol/mL), 500 (37.46 x 10^3 pmol/mL), 250 (14.98 x 10^3 pmol/mL), 125 (7.499 x 10^3 pmol/mL), 62.5 (3.745 x 10^3 pmol/mL), 31.3 (1.875 x 10^3 pmol/mL), 15.6 (0.9374 x 10^3 pmol/mL, 7.8 (0.4687 x 10^3 pmol/mL, and 3.9 μg/mL (0.2343 x 10^3 pmol/mL)), was trypsinized individually using the same trypsin:cystatin C ratio. [Glu1]-fibrinopeptide B (glufib) was used as a surrogate internal standard. Glufib was chosen as an easily commercially available peptide with an m/z of 785.8 (doubly charged), intermediate between the m/z 685.0 and 1168.8 selected marker-peptides. It can compensate for small variations in the LC-MS measurement part of the analysis. It is, however, not capable of compensating for differences produced during the trypsinization process itself and is therefore less optimal compared to using e.g. chicken egg white cystatin (see later in this chapter). Using a triple quadrupole system in tandem MS, MRM was used as detection technique. To that end, the chromatogram was divided into 3 separate time-dependent MRM functions for the different peptides (min. 12-16: m/z 685.0 to 313.1 and 412.1 (CE 38eV), min. 17.5-20.5: m/z 900.9 to 343.9 and 566.5 (CE 38eV); min. 27.5-31.0: m/z 1168.8 to 1148.5 and 1482.1(CE 38eV)) and a 4th for the internal standard glufib (min. 20.5-24.5: m/z 785.8 to 480.4 and 684.3 (CE 25eV)).

Linear calibration curves were obtained for all three peptides. Peptide m/z 900.9 (amino-terminal end of cystatin C) revealed the best linearity (R^2 0.994, n=3) in calibration (see Figure 6). Unfortunately, such calibration curves could only be constructed from the 7.8 µg/mL cystatin C calibrator upwards. All calibrators were analyzed in triplicate and CV% was below 20%, except for the protein standard of 3.9 µg/mL. This lower calibration point could not be satisfactorily measured. The lower calibrator is, however, roughly 10-fold higher than physiological cystatin C plasma concentration. Clearly, a pre-concentration step (e.g. during sample preparation) will be inevitable to compensate for the dilution effect inherent to the in-solution digestion protocol. Indeed, when starting with 50 µL of cystatin C standard, at the end of this kind of tryptic digestion protocol, the standard solution is almost 20-fold diluted to 930 µL.

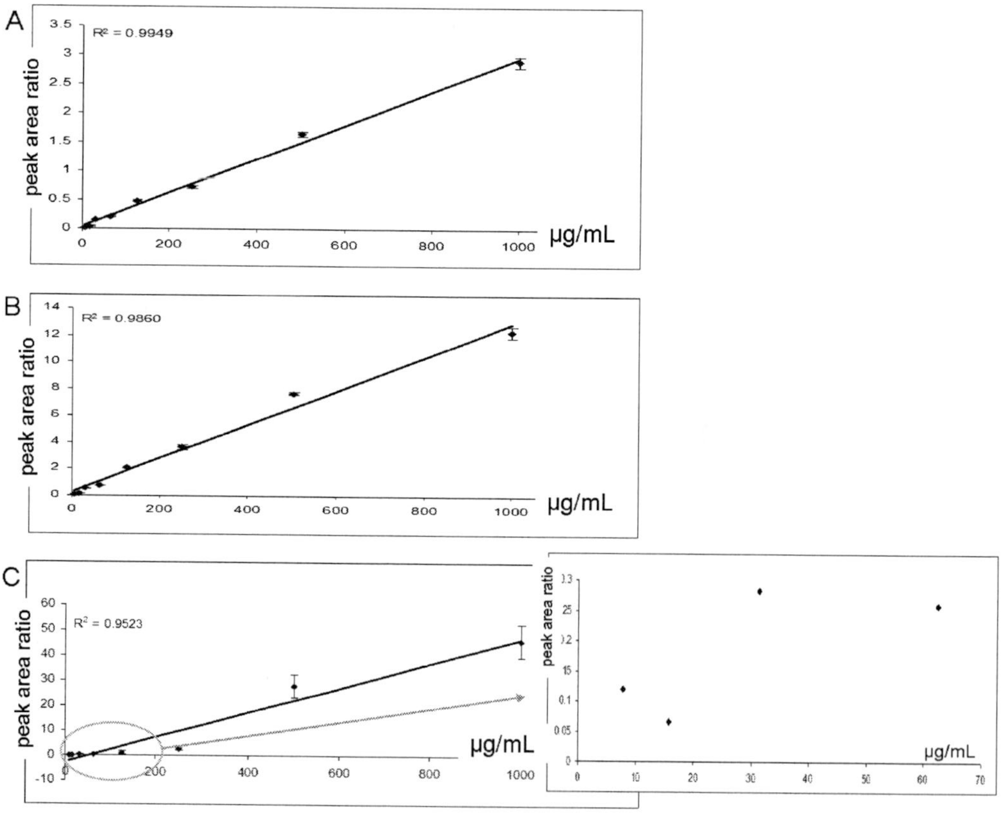

Figure 6. Calibration curves (from 7.8 to 1000 µg/mL) as obtained for the three selected marker-peptides with m/z 900.9 (A), 685.0 (B), and 1168.8 (C). Measurements were performed in the MRM mode using glufib as surrogate internal standard [reproduced with permission from [38].

The experiments essentially show the quantitative potential of the approach of using trypsin in an in-solution enzymatic hydrolysis of a protein into stoichiometrically representative marker-peptides. Nevertheless, it can also be seen that the trypsinization process itself tends to perform better with higher protein concentrations (see inset in Figure 6, C, of the lower calibration concentrations). Moreover, some individual calibration points sometimes had to be excluded from the study due to probably insufficient proteolysis. Better internal standards, e.g. simultaneously hydrolyzed homologue sequence protein, are certainly needed for full quantitation. Transposing basic tools such tryptic digestion, used in semi-quantitative proteomic experiments, to an absolute quantitative level is clearly not that straightforward. Even optimized conditions result in a suboptimal outcome caused by reproducibility and efficiency problems of the enzymatic digestion step. This is especially the case when working with medium to low abundant proteins ($\leq$ 10 µg/mL). Indeed, Strader et al. already confirmed insufficient trypsinization of medium to low abundant proteins because the reaction rate of the enzymatic digestion is proportional to the concentration [39]. Furthermore, most exo-peptidases have a K_m-value in the range from 5 to 50 mM, which means they are operating at 50% of maximum velocity when a protein concentration of 5 to 50 mmol/mL is used [40]. Consequently, with concentrations below 5 to 50 mmol/mL, as is the case with the majority of protein biomarkers, the proteolytic activity toward the substrate will be minimal, while autolysis rates will be relatively high [41]. Additionally, proteolytic enzymes require effective denaturing of the protein in advance. This can only be achieved by the use of heat, chaotropes, or surfactants to render more of the proteins' structure accessible to the proteolytic enzyme [42,43]. In many cases, thermal denaturing results in sample loss due to precipitation because many proteins are susceptible to aggregation when treated with heat. Chaotropes and surfactants on the other hand are very effective but their use is ambiguous. At high concentrations, surfactants and chaotropes also inactivate proteases such as trypsin. Therefore, dilution of the sample to lower their concentration is mandatory. Unfortunately, dilution can result in protein refolding and inevitably lowers, a generally already low, substrate concentration, thus reducing overall proteolytic efficiency. Taking all of this into account, non-enzymatic proteolysis can be an interesting alternative. Chemical reactions are most of the time less influenced by reaction medium and tend to be more robust. That is why cyanogen bromide proteolysis is investigated too in the context of quantitative protein analysis using marker-peptides.

Chemical Protein Proteolysis: The Cyanogen Bromide Alternative

As an alternative to enzymatic methods, various chemically based cleaving methods, in essence independent of protein concentration, have been described in the past. Only a handful of these methods yield relatively predictable cleavage products and have been applied in practice. However, these chemicals may succeed where enzymes fail [44]. During the last decades, only chemical cleavage of proteins based on CNBr hydrolysis has become a common alternative to tryptic digestion [45]. Some of the well known advantages of CNBr protein hydrolysis are the ease of use, the good reproducibility and a high selectivity towards methionine residues. In general, CNBr based proteolysis is performed for 12 to 24 hours with a large excess of CNBr in acidic conditions. CNBr hydrolyses peptide bonds C-terminal to methionine residues through an intermediate cyclic iminolactone. Under acidic conditions, and in the presence of water, this iminolactone undergoes a Schiff base hydrolysis and the actual proteolysis takes place. As such, a homoserine lactone peptide is created at the C-terminal end (the former methionine position) and a N-terminal peptide at the other end [45]. The efficiency of CNBr peptide bond cleavage exceeds 90%, except in situations where in the amino-acid sequence a serine or threonine residue follows methionine. In that particular case, the same iminolactone is formed as in regular cleavage conditions, but, due to the presence of a hydroxyl in the neighbouring amino-acid, the latter can also react with the iminolactone. Homoserine is also formed but without peptide bond cleavage [45].

The peptides formed as such have a homoserine lactone (Δ mass -48 Da), which can undergo further hydrolysis to form homoserine (Δ mass -30 Da) at the C-terminus. Acidic conditions favour the formation of homoserine lactone, whereas under basic conditions the free acid (homoserine) is formed [46-48]. Acidic conditions are obtained by reaction media of 60 to 80% formic acid or trifluoroacetic acid (TFA).

In the past, FA was mostly chosen as reaction medium because of its ability to solubilize most proteins. Itakura *et al.* were first to report CNBr cleavage of peptide bonds using trifluoroacetic acid en found the latter to be superior to FA. They reported a higher yield of cleaved methionine-serine and methionine-threonine bonds [49].

In an effort to explore the possibilities of using CNBr based proteolysis for the absolute quantitation of proteins using marker-peptides and LC-MS(/MS), cystatin C has again been used as a proof-of-concept protein. Moreover, internal standardization using a protein analogue, chicken egg white cystatin, has simultaneously been assessed in terms of improving reproducibility and accuracy. Protein analogues are often relatively easy to obtain as species differences in e.g. endogenous proteins provide a perfect source of an often closely related protein.

The presence of matching cleavage sites within cystatin C and chicken egg white cystatin, producing similar peptides after proteolysis allows this kind of IS to compensate for minor differences in cleavage efficiencies when both the analyte and the internal standard are proteolyzed simultaneously under the same reaction conditions.

The Influence of the Proteolysis Approach to the Selection of the Marker-Peptides

According to the Swiss-Prot database, in general, many more cleaving sites are expected in proteins for trypsin compared to CNBr. Consequently, not only fewer but also larger peptides are generated by CNBr. The latter is advantageous as it is well known that the higher the mass of the peptide, the more distinctive it is. All potential marker-peptides after CNBr based proteolysis are summarized in Table 2 for cystatin C, for chicken egg white cystatin after tryptic- and CNBr based proteolysis in Table 3.

For tryptic cleavage, also peptides composed of 2 tryptic fragments, thus allowing 1 missed cleavage, have been included. Theoretical masses of the peptide fragments and corresponding *m/z* values, ranging from $[M+H]^+$ until $[M+3H]^{3+}$, have again been calculated (Masslynx Biolynx® and PeptideCutter/PeptideMass (ExPASy; Expert Protein Analysis System) proteomics server). Cleavage sites with low cleavage probability have not been not included. As such, for trypsin, cleavage sites followed by a proline residue are disregarded, as are CNBr cleavage sites followed by a serine or threonine residue.

Table 2. Possible marker-peptides after cleavage with CNBr (M1-M4) of cystatin C. For each peptide, the corresponding theoretical mass and *m/z* values are given. (M-S/T cleavage sites are not taken into consideration)

Name	Sequence	Theoretical mass (Da)	$[M+H]^+$	$[M+2H]^{2+}$	$[M+3H]^{3+}$
M1	SSPGKPPRLVGGPM	1379.7	1380.7	690.8	460.9
M2	DASVEEEGVRRALDFAVGEYNKASNDM	2973.2	2974.2	1487.6	992.1
M3	YHSRALQVVRARKQIVAGVNYFLDVELG RTTCTKTQP NLDNCPFHDQPHLKRKAFCSFQIYAVPW QGTM	7995.2	7996.3	3998.6	2666.1
M4	TLSKSTCQDA	1053.2	1054.2	527.6	352.1

When working with chemical instead of enzymatic cleavage, sterical hindrance has almost no influence on the reaction and marker-peptides can often be generated without the necessity to denature the protein in advance. Consequently, the peptide mixtures formed are less complex, also because fewer peptides are generated. Only when a given cleavage site is positioned in between an amino-acid loop formed by a disulphide bridge, denaturing, reduction, and alkylation (to block the free SH-groups, in this way preventing the reformation of the disulphide bridges) is sometimes favoured to disconnect the generated peptides from each other, if these are the only ones suitable as marker-peptide. For cystatin C, e.g., 2 disulphide bridges occur between amino-acids 99-109 and 123-143. As a consequence, CNBr marker-peptides from amino-acid 68 to 136 with $[M+H]^+$ *m/z* 7996 and from amino-acid 137 to 146 with $[M+H]^+$ *m/z* 1053 are linked by the 123-143 disulphide bond and will not be disconnected from each other if samples are not reduced (and alkylated) prior to chemical digestion.

This results in a larger peptide of 79 amino-acid residues. The latter can no longer be taken into consideration as a potential marker-peptide candidate as it is susceptible to the same effects, e.g. envelope formation during the electrospray ionization process, as the cystatin C protein itself. If only this kind of long marker-peptides can be generated, it is better to analyze the whole protein. However, in the case of cystatin C, a representative marker-peptide (from the first part of the protein) can obtained whether or not the protein is reduced and alkylated prior to the chemical digestion. Moreover, for the internal standard, chicken egg white cystatin, no CNBr cleaving sites lie in between a disulphide bridge, thus completely obviating the need for extra treatment before CNBr hydrolysis.

Chemical CNBr Proteolysis Results

As already described, chemical proteolysis using CNBr requires acidic conditions. As such, the reaction medium serves two important functions; (i) it provides an acidic environment propitious for protonation of nucleophilic groups; and (ii) it promotes exposure of methionine residues by acting as a polypeptide unfolding agent, which increases the reaction efficiency [50]. Different reaction media have been investigated, varying in the amount and type of acid used and the presence of water in the reaction mixture. To that end, lyophilized cystatin C powder, reconstituted in 0.1 M sodium acetate buffer pH 4.5 to obtain a stock solution of 1000 µg/mL has been further diluted using milliQ high purity water into the following concentrations: 100 µg/mL (equivalent to 74.9 x 10^2 pmol/mL); 50.0 µg/mL (37.4 x 10^2 pmol/mL); 25.0 µg/mL (18.7 x 10^2 pmol/mL); 10.0 µg/mL (749 pmol/mL); 5.00 µg/mL (374 pmol/mL); 2.50 µg/mL (187 pmol/mL) and 1.00 µg/mL (74.9 pmol/mL).

Physiological plasma concentrations (humans) of cystatin C are expected to lie within this concentration range. Lyophilized chicken egg white cystatin powder, at the other hand was dissolved in the same 0.1 M sodium acetate buffer pH 4.5 to obtain a stock solution of 1000 µg/mL and further diluted to a concentration of 50 µg/mL (average molecular mass 13.148 kDa; 38.0 x 10^2 pmol/mL. Using CNBr, marker-peptides were generated from these standards and the IS, using the following protocol. 50 µL of the cystatin C protein solution was mixed with 500 µL of reaction medium, either H_2O:5 M CNBr in ACN:TFA 20:20:60; H_2O:5 M CNBr in ACN:TFA 15:15:70; or H_2O: 5M CNBr in ACN:FA 15:15:70, overnight at 4°C. The resulting peptide mixture was dried down under a stream of nitrogen gas and re-dissolved in 100 µL of LC mobile phase (eluent A). Considering the limited number of peptides generated in CNBr proteolysis, only one really suitable marker-peptide can be designated. Consequently, only this peptide has been monitored using MRM. For cystatin C, M2 (*m/z* 992.1, triply charged, see Table 2) has been selected as marker-peptide.

Because digestion occurs under acidic conditions, the selected marker-peptide is present as a homoserine lactone (Δ mass of 48, thus *m/z* 992.4 – (48/3) = 976.4). For the chicken egg white cystatin ISP, peptide M3 with *m/z* 1060.0 (triply charged, see Table 3) has been selected. This peptide is, however, not present as a homoserine lactone. The homoserine lactone is formed, during digestion, at the N-terminal side of the cleaved peptide-bond (i.e. from the methionine amino acid). With M3 being the outermost C-terminal peptide of chicken egg white cystatin, the homoserine lactone at the cleaved bond is formed at the M2 peptide and M3 is left unchanged.

The marker-peptides have been analyzed using LC-MS/MS in the MRM mode. Liquid chromatography was performed on an YMC ODS-AQ™ 1 x 150 mm, 3 µm (C18) micro-column with a binary mobile phase consisting of an eluent A, 0.1 % aqueous FA, and an eluent B of 0.1 % FA in ACN. Gradient elution at 40 µl/min in the micro-flow-mode has been used. After an initial 5 min. 5 % B isocratic phase, % B was changed from 5 to 60 % over the next 26.5 min., followed by a sharp increase to 95 % B. The column was then maintained at these conditions for 3.5 min. after which the gradient returns to initial conditions over a 1 min. time period and re-equilibration occurs.

Tandem mass spectrometric detection in the MRM mode was used on a triple quadrupole mass spectrometer. The MRM set-up and collision induced dissociation (collision energy, CE) were all optimized such that both one precursor-to-product ion transition and the precursor-to-precursor (unfragmented, by lack of an additional suitably intense fragment) could be registered. The following conditions have been utilized: for cystatin C, peptide M2, *m/z* 976.4 to 976.4 (CE 25 eV; dwell time 0.8 sec.) and *m/z* 976.4 to 765.0 (CE 30 eV; dwell time 0.5 sec.). For chicken egg white cystatin, peptide M3 (triply charged), *m/z* 1060.0 to 1060.0 (CE 30 eV; dwell time 0.8 sec.) and *m/z* 1060.0 to 1408.5 (CE 30 eV; dwell time 0.5 sec.).

Figure 7 shows the peak areas (means, n=3) obtained after LC-MS/MS MRM analysis of the selected, CNBr generated, cystatin C marker-peptide, depending on the chemical cleavage conditions. The presence of water in the reaction mixture (data not shown) clearly proved to be essential for digestion. The reaction requires water to attack the iminolactone.

Table 3. Possible marker-peptides after cleavage with CNBr (M1-M3) and trypsin (T1-T16) of chicken egg white cystatin. For each peptide, the corresponding theoretical mass and *m/z* values are given. For the tryptic fragments, one missed cleavage is allowed (K/R-P and M-S/T cleavage sites are not taken into consideration)

Name	Sequence	Theoretical mass (Da)	$[M+H]^{+}$	$[M+2H]^{2+}$	$[M+3H]^{3+}$
M1	SEDRSRLLGAPVPVDENDEGLQRALQFAM	3214.5	3215.5	1608.2	1072.5
M2	AEYNRASNDKYSSRVVRVISAKRQLVSGIK YILQVEIGRTTCPKSSGDLQSCEFHDEPEM	6791.7	6792.7	3396.8	2264.9
M3	AKYTTCTFVVYSIPWLNQIKLLESKCQ	3177.8	3178.8	1589.9	1060.3
T1	SEDR	505.5	506.5	253.8	169.5
T2	SR	261.3	262.3	131.7	88.1
T3	LLGAPVPVDENDEGLQR	1822.0	1823.0	912.0	608.3
T4	ALQFAMAEYNR	1313.5	1314.5	657.8	438.8
T5	ASNDK	533.5	534.6	267.8	178.9
T6	YSSR	511.5	512.5	256.8	171.5
T7	VVR	372.5	373.5	187.2	125.2
T8	VISAK	516.6	517.7	259.3	173.2
T9	R	174.1	175.1	88.1	59.1
T10	QLVSGIK	743.9	744.9	373.0	249.0
T11	YILQVEIGR	1090.3	1091.3	546.2	364.4
T12	TTCPK	548.7	549.7	275.3	183.9
T13	SSGDLQSCEFHDEPEMAK	2010.2	2011.2	1006.1	671.1
T14	YTTCTFVVYSIPWLNQIK	2176.6	2177.6	1089.3	726.5
T15	LLESK	588.7	589.7	295.4	197.2
T16	CQ	249.1	250.1	125.6	84.0
T1-2	SEDRSR	748.8	749.8	375.4	250.6
T2-3	SRLLGAPVPVDENDEGLQR	2065.3	2066.3	1033.6	689.4
T3-4	LLGAPVPVDENDEGLQRALQFAMAEYNR	3117.5	3118.5	1559.8	1040.2
T4-5	ALQFAMAEYNRASNDK	1829.0	1830.0	915.5	610.7
T5-6	ASNDKYSSR	1027.1	1028.1	514.5	343.4
T6-7	YSSRVVR	866.0	867.0	434.0	289.7
T7-8	VVRVISAK	871.1	872.1	436.6	291.4
T8-9	VISAKR	672.8	673.8	337.4	225.3
T9-10	RQLVSGIK	900.1	901.1	451.1	301.0
T10-11	QLVSGIKYILQVEIGR	1816.2	1817.2	909.1	606.4
T11-12	YILQVEIGRTTCPK	1620.9	1621.9	811.5	541.3
T12-13	TTCPKSSGDLQSCEFHDEPE MAK	2540.8	2541.8	1271.4	847.9
T13-14	SSGDLQSCEFHDEPEMAKYTTCTFVVYSIP WLNQIK	4168.7	4169.7	2085.4	1390.6
T14-15	YTTCTFVVYSIPWLNQIKLL ESK	2747.3	2748.3	1374.6	916.8
T15-16	LLESKCQ	820.0	821.0	411.0	274.3

Kaiser and Metzka [45] too investigated the necessity of water in the reaction medium, with special focus on the methionine-serine and methionine-threonine sequences. They found, in accordance to the findings reported here, better cleavage yields under conditions where a higher water concentration is present. In addition, contrary to earlier reports [50], they concluded that the acidic strength of the reaction medium does not play a significant role in the CNBr cleavage efficiency. From Figure 7 it is also clear that the digestion yield increases with the use of FA instead of trifluoroacetic acid. Until now, there is no conclusive evidence why. These findings corroborate the report by Rodriguez *et al.* who also found that efficient CNBr cleavage is substantially compromized when 70% TFA is used in the reaction [50].

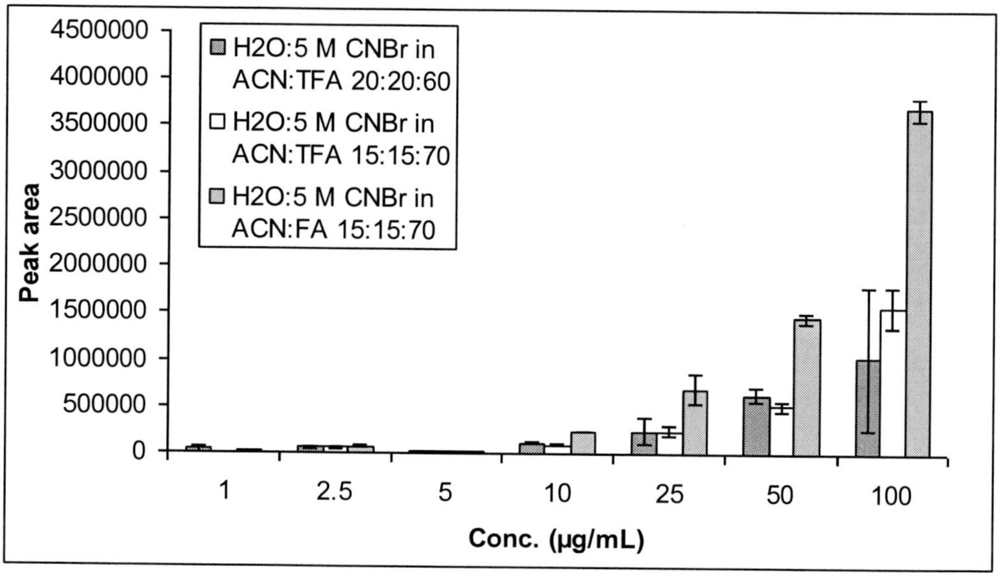

Figure 7. Mean (n=3) peak area (LC-MS/MS, TIC) of cystatin C marker-peptide M2 after proteolysis in the following reaction media: H2O:5 M CNBr in ACN:TFA 20:20:60, H2O:5 M CNBr in ACN:TFA 15:15:70, and H2O:5 M CNBr in ACN:FA 15:15:70. Error bars indicate repeatability.

These results are of particular interest, given the widespread use of 70% TFA as the medium of choice for CNBr cleavage of proteins [50-53]. One may speculate, based also on the findings by Rodriguez *et al.*, that different rates of cleavage may originate from a larger degree of exposure of methionine side chains in FA relative to TFA, as can be expected from the superior solubilizing properties of the former [50].

Figure 7 also contains repeatability (n=3) data for repeated CNBr proteolysis of cystatin C samples of different concentration. Repeatability of the raw peak areas indicates that chemical cleavage, as compared to in-solution trypsinization, produces peptides in a more reproducible way. CNBr proteolysis achieves CV%'s (peptide M2, n=3) of around 13.2%. To evaluate the absolute quantitative performance of CNBr proteolysis, 6 different calibration curves have been generated over 2 orders of magnitude (from 1.00 µg/mL to 100 µg/mL). Chicken egg white cystatin was introduced as internal standard and was proteolyzed simultaneously with the calibrators. Figure 8 shows the resulting concentration-response curve (n=6) as well as the measurement variation on the different calibrators. As can be seen, there is a clear linear correlation (R^2 of 0.9950) between the calibrator concentration and the cystatin C to IS peak area ratio. The trypsinization process, in contrast, proved to be inadequate, in terms of repeatability, to generate calibration curves over the same concentration range (see before in this chapter). If the calibration curves constructed using only absolute peak area values of the different calibrators (not compensated by the IS) are compared, it is clear that a similar linear trend is noticeable but the variability is larger. The overall coefficient of variation (CV%, n=6), expressed as the mean variation for the different calibrators increases from 15.4% ± 4.85 (mean ± SD) to 40.8% ± 10.2.

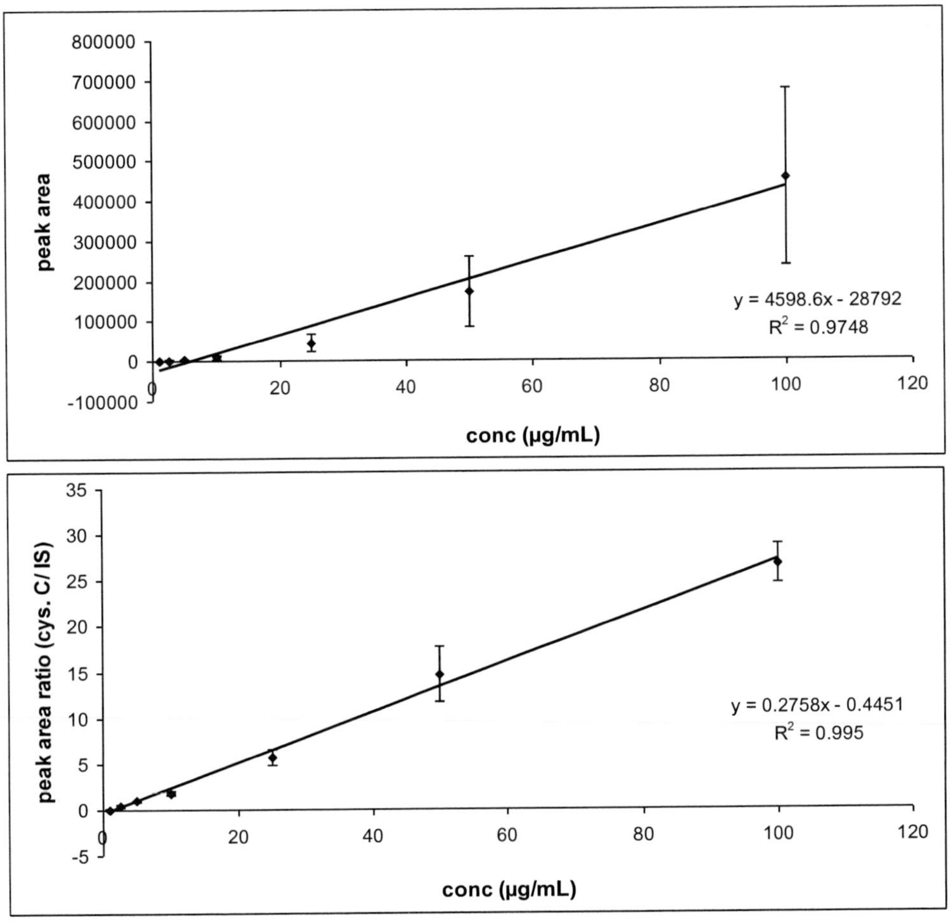

Figure 8. Concentration-response curve for cystatin C based on the CNBr (H2O: 5 M CNBr in ACN:FA 15:15:70) generated M2 peptide; without (upper pane) and with (lower pane) the use of the internal standard chicken egg white cystatin (CNBr generated M3 peptide).

One can conclude that the use of an IS which is able to compensate for differences in proteolysis efficiency, clearly has a positive effect on the precision of the method. A protein-related analogue internal standard perfectly serves this goal. Chemical proteolysis, in combination with the use of a protein internal standard, able to compensate for proteolysis efficiency variability, can be performed with the necessary reproducibility to generate calibrations, allowing the absolute quantitation of a given protein using marker-peptides. With tryptic marker-peptides, similar calibration curves are hard to obtain, possibly caused by insufficient trypsin performance at lower protein concentrations (<10 µg/mL).

Application of the Marker-Peptide Approach to Real Biological Samples: Issues to Consider

The ultimate goal of an absolute quantitative assay for proteins is to assay them in a biological system, i.e. within a complex mixture, next to an often overwhelming amount of other compounds, many of them proteins themselves. In essence this means that for a LC-MS(/MS) based quantitation method for proteins by means of marker-peptides, the applicability of the e.g. chemical proteolysis based methodology, should be tested in for example plasma samples. Plasma samples are a good test because of the complexity of this matrix. Continuing from cystatin C as model protein, the quantitation of endogenous cystatin C in plasma can be considered a final proof of the marker-peptide approach. Clearly, some form of sample clean-up is mandatory dealing with this level of sample complexity. Moreover, a sample clean-up step often coincides with a re-concentration step, providing enhanced sensitivity to the overall method. In a sample clean-up approach, the separation of cystatin C from other plasma proteins is obviously the prime objective. To fulfil this goal, the application of specific anti-human cystatin C antibodies could, theoretically, be considered the best option in terms of effectiveness and reproducibility. Inherently, this approach constitutes a major, sometimes prohibitive cost, especially when working with larger amounts of plasma. Moreover, specific antibodies are needed and one can start to question the added value of a LC-MS method part when these antibodies would quite easily be incorporated in a dedicated immunoassay. The opposite way of thinking, namely to remove the most abundant plasma proteins could be a promising alternative, especially taking into account that the 22 most abundant proteins are responsible for approximately 99% of the bulk mass of the total plasma proteome (Figure 9) [54, 55]. Such extraction procedures could be used for a broad range of proteins to be measured, and the effort of optimization can thus be spread over many more (eventually clinically related) applications. Indeed, many studies suggest that low and medium molecular mass proteins/peptides (respectively, LAP and MAP) in plasma, such as plasma hormones or small, secreted proteins, are often correlated with pathological conditions and present opportunities for potential clinical utility as therapeutic intervention or as diagnostic or prognostic biomarkers [56-61].

The technical challenge in the analysis of these LAP and MAP is that the plasma proteome covers a very broad concentration range, of which some proteins are so predominantly present, like albumin and the immunoglobulins, that they mask the detection of the other proteins [55, 62]. During the last decade(s), removal of these high abundance proteins out of plasma samples has become, albeit mostly for qualitative or semi-quantitative purposes, the method of choice in proteomics, to provide enhanced sensitivity and achieving a broader proteome coverage. Different special methodologies are nowadays available to serve the goal of high abundance protein depletion [54]. For instance, Pieper *et al.* in 2003 reported an approach that is capable of removing 10 high abundance proteins in a single step, based on immuno-affinity chromatography [63]. Most recently, commercial efforts too have intensified the search for adequate depletion procedures [54, 63-66]. For instance, the Genway supermix® system removes the 14 most abundant proteins and, in a next step, 77 of the medium abundant proteins out of human plasma based on immuno-affinity. Likewise, Agilent's' Multiple Affinity Removal Columns and Spin cartridges (respectively known as MARC and MARS) are capable of the simultaneous removal of the 6 most abundant proteins. These antibody based depletion systems have been demonstrated to be highly efficient in removing the specifically targeted proteins. They are, unfortunately, typically developed for proteomic applications using much smaller plasma volumes and questions still arise with regard to their reproducibility and selectivity in the framework of absolute quantitative work [64-66]. In particular, there are two primary questions: whether these systems are capable of removing their target proteins in a reproducible way, and whether there is any loss of non-targeted proteins (e.g. our analyte protein) along with the high abundance proteins through non-selective binding and/or physiological relevant association reactions [54]. Moreover, if these systems are applied to applications demanding higher plasma volumes, several depletion (spin-) columns will be required for one single sample and hence, not only their ease of handling will be compromized but also the inherent costs will become prohibitively high for routine work. Other depletion formats based on either ion-exchange, metal chelating or dye-ligands, also exist and have been commercially developed but are not protein specific and therefore of lower value [56]. Organic solvent extraction to remove HAP is another option. In doing so, it has been shown that two volumes of ACN added to plasma samples, eventually in the presence of low concentrations of ion-pairing agents like FA or TFA to produce a denser precipitate, efficiently precipitate HAP, while smaller proteins and peptides stay in solution [56]. Unfortunately, using this procedure a distinct separation boundary between the precipitate, composed out of the HAP, and the L/MAP filtrate is often hard to obtain.

This makes the procedure difficult to perform and prone to error or irreproducibility. Moreover, a substantial loss of the analyte protein, as in the case of cystatin C, is often encountered. It is likely that during solvent precipitation of the HAP, cystatin C is for a major part co-precipitated with the bulk of albumin and other HAP, a phenomenon which is known as the "albumin sponge effect". This is correlated to the capability of albumin, and other HAP, to bind peptides and proteins and hence, when these HAP are precipitated or removed, these bound peptides/proteins will equally be removed [64].

Nevertheless, from the point of view of generic application potential to many different protein quantitation tasks, an alternative approach to separate the HAP from the LAP based on ultrafiltration devices with molecular weight cut-off membranes could be considered. In the case of cystatin C (calculated average molecular mass of 13.347 kDa) for example, adequate choice of such membranes should allow it to be separated from at least the 6 most abundant proteins, of which the molecular mass ranges from minimally 46.737 (transferrin) to over 600.000 kDa for immunoglobulin complexes. For example (and taking cystatin C and the IS chicken egg white cystatin again as model proteins), a combination of two successive ultrafiltration steps could be envisaged. In the first step, the separation of cystatin C from other larger, and frequently more abundant proteins, is pursued.

This step should then be followed by a second ultrafiltration of the obtained filtrate, albeit this time over a smaller than the cystatin C mass range cut-off filter. As such, the first mass filter aims for the removal of most of the HAP, all characterized by a molecular mass over 45 kDa, while the second mass filter functions as a pre-concentration device hereby obstructing cystatin C from passage through the filter.

In a last step, the retained cystatin C, present on the second filter membrane, is e.g. chemically proteolyzed (overnight, 4°C) and the obtained marker-peptides can, after been reduced to dryness under a nitrogen stream and redissolved in mobile phase, be analyzed using LC-MS(/MS). The first filtration step is expected to play the most vital role in this proposed methodology.

According to the manufacturers of such ultrafiltration devices, a mass cut-off filter with a cut-off level at least three times higher than the mass range intended to allow passage through the membrane should be applied. Ideally, in the case of cystatin C, a mass cut-off filter of approximately 45 kDa should be used. Of course, membrane material is also of importance as different materials (cellulose triacetate, polyethersulfone, regenerated cellulose, Hydrosart …)

have different non-specific binding/adsorption characteristics. The Hydrosart (cf. Vivaspin® HY, Sartorius Stedim Biotech) membrane, for example, is a stable polymer that features a broad pH range. Hydrosart is also extremely hydrophilic, making it non-protein binding, and has an extremely high flux.

The ultrafiltration approach was investigated in a preliminary experiment. Plasma samples, spiked with cystatin C, were analyzed using such two successive ultrafiltration steps. The samples were first diluted with AcN to a final proportion of 20% (v/v, 500µL plasma + 125µL AcN, followed by 10 min of gentle shaking using a rotatory mixer).

Under these partly denaturing conditions, it is known that protein-protein interactions between the lower molecular mass proteins (e.g. cystatin C) and larger molecular mass carrier proteins like albumin and IgG are effectively disrupted. If not destroyed prior to the analysis, these protein complexes would be withheld during the ultrafiltration process and hence, the actual protein concentration would be underestimated. In a first step, the samples are ultrafiltrated (Vivaspin 2 HY 30k) for 60 min at 7500 *x g* (25°C) and the obtained filtrate is transferred to the second mass filter (Vivaspin 2 HY 5k), and again ultrafiltrated for 45 min at 7500 *x g* (25°C). The newly obtained filtrate is discarded and 500 µL of CNBr solution is added to the mass cut-off filter. Then, after overnight digestion (*vide infra*), the mass filter is backwise centrifuged at 2000 *x g* for 5 min., the recovered peptide solution is dried under a stream of nitrogen gas, redissolved in mobile phase and analyzed using LC-MS (see before in this chapter).

This procedure has been applied in the generation of cystatin C calibration curves, using chicken egg white cystatin as internal standard (10.0 µg/mL, equivalent to 760.6 pmol/mL), covering a concentration range from 0.50 (37.46 pmol/mL) to 20.0 µg/mL (14.98 x 10^2 pmol/mL). The analyte to IS peak area ratio was plotted against analyte concentration. No weighting has been applied to calculate the calibration curves. Figure 10 shows the corresponding calibration curves, measured using 4 different plasma lots.

As can be seen, although it is possible to create a calibration, there was a rather large variation in the slope of the different calibration lines (0.7905 ± 0.2748; mean ± sd, n=4). This already indicates that the fractionation/extraction procedure suffers from substantial relative matrix effects (different plasma lots have been used). Indeed, the difference in slope of calibration curves made up in different plasma lots can be used as a measure of the relative matrix effect often encountered in electrospray mass spectrometry [67]. The differences in intercept (4.011 ± 3.860; mean ± sd, n=4) could (partly) be explained by different endogenous cystatin C concentrations in the different plasma lots.

However, absolute recovery has additionally been assessed by spiking a quantity of cystatin C (2 concentration levels: 1.00 and 5.00 µg/mL) into a "blank" plasma (containing endogenous cystatin C) and comparing the peak areas to the peak areas obtained for blank plasma extracts spiked (post-extraction) to the same concentration. The endogenous cystatin C present in the plasma extracts (average cystatin C peak area present in 20 "blank" plasma samples not spiked with cystatin C) has been subtracted from the cystatin C areas measured in these spiked plasma extracts. Absolute recovery turned out to be extremely low (7.04 ± 0.4065 at 1.00 µg/mL and 3.20 ± 0.1582 at 5.00 µg/ml; mean% ± sd; n=3) and did absolutely not meet the requirements as generally postulated by bio-analytical method validation guidance protocols.

Based on these preliminary data, it seems that calibration curves for cystatin C can be generated using the general fractionation/extraction method, However, other preliminary validation data in terms of accuracy, precision and selectivity (data not shown) are borderline acceptable to unacceptable (e.g. recovery).

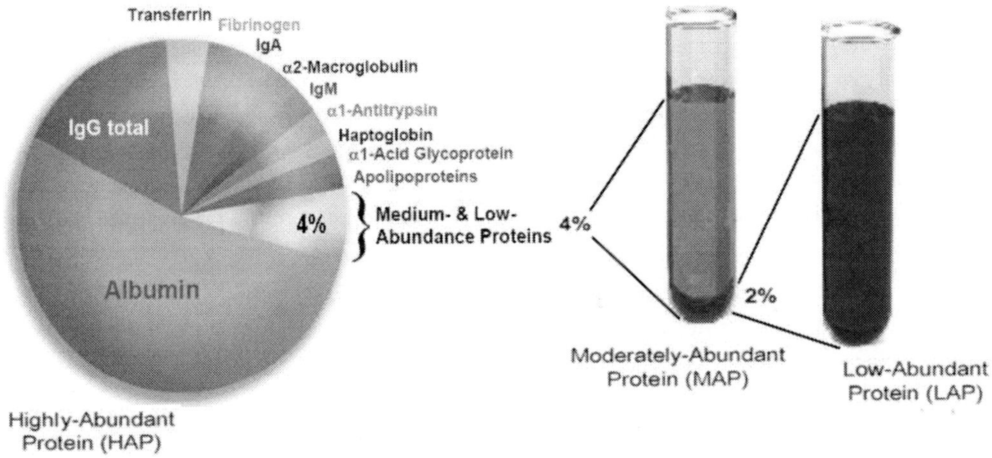

Figure 9. Composition of the human plasma proteome. The 14 most abundant proteins make up for 96% of the proteome (adapted from www.genwaybio.com).

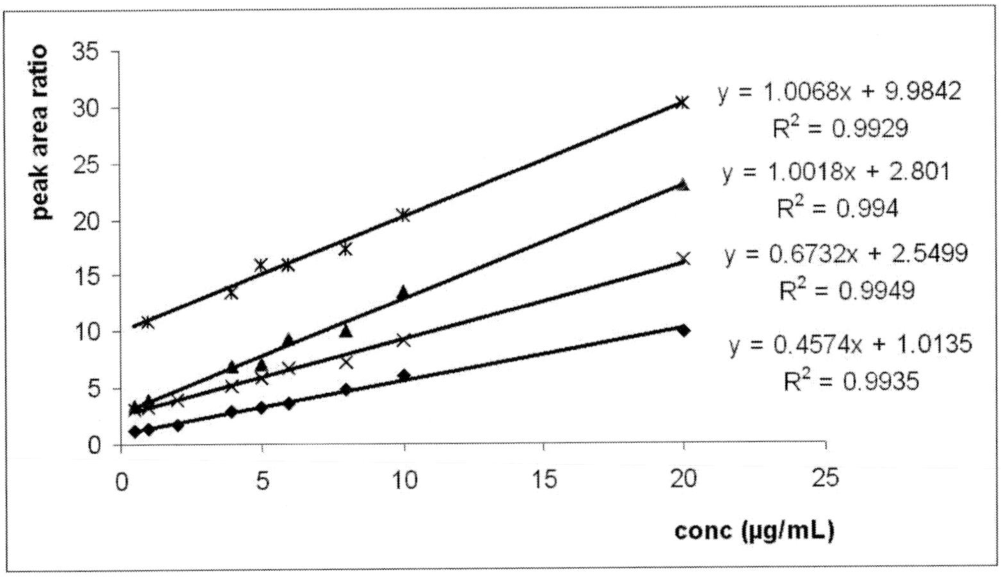

Figure 10. Calibration graphs and functions for cystatin C from 0.50 up to 20.0 µg/mL using a double ultrafiltration approach (30k + 5k) as fractionation procedure.

Substantially more optimization work is needed in order to either confirm or reject the applicability of ultrafiltration in biological (plasma) sample clean-up for quantitative protein analysis using marker proteins. It definitely remains to be seen whether the complexity of biological samples is not that high that even the formidable selectivity of LC-MS/MS still precludes the use of generic, unspecific sample preparation methods such as described here.

Conclusion

Proteins, either therapeutic or diagnostic, will become increasingly important in the bio-medical and pharmaceutical field. Consequently, their absolute quantitative measurement will become more and more of an issue. The present workhorse for these measurements are immunoassays. Nevertheless, more and more analysts are attracted to the quantitative potential of LC-MS in this field, not to the least driven by the success LC-MS techniques have had in the field of proteomics. LC-MS based approaches for whole protein quantitation are unfortunately hampered by many methodological difficulties. Due to these inconveniences, quantitative LC-MS of whole proteins, especially the bigger ones, is still rather a goal than a practice. In this perspective, the use of marker-peptides as a measure of the protein of interest as a whole is a potential alternative. In this chapter, we discussed different investigations into the potential of this approach, the optimisation of the methodology and its applicability in real quantitative measurements of a proof-of-concept protein cystatin C. It is clear that in such an approach reproducibility of the marker-peptide generation step is vital and special attention on internal standardization to compensate for differential proteolysis' efficiencies is mandatory. On using tryptic proteolysis in this respect, it was found that reproducibility was relatively poor and internal standardization, able to compensate for variation in the proteolysis step is inevitable. A major drawback is the substantial dilution which results from an enzymatic proteolysis protocol. The alternative cyanogen bromide mediated proteolysis requires, somewhat depending on the protein studied, less procedural steps, thus results in less dilution, and more importantly, provides enhanced reproducibility for the proteolysis step. Nevertheless, internal standardization remains indispensable when quantitative validation criteria are to be met. Both approaches succeeded in producing calibration curves which is the first (but certainly not the only) step in establishing the quantitative nature of a method. On comparing both approaches, the CNBr based method slightly outperforms tryptic proteolysis.

The ultimate goal of performing quantitative measurements of a protein in a biological matrix of course introduces many extra analytical aspects to tackle. We reported on some preliminary results of using a generic approach based on ultrafiltration and judicious selection of molecular mass cut-of membranes. Although some of the potential was illustrated, the results were still far from acceptable for absolute quantitative work e.g. in terms of recovery thus precision and accuracy. It remains to be established whether the use of generic, unspecific sample preparation methods will be sufficient to manage the challenges posed by such complex matrices as plasma.

Nevertheless, it is clear that the method of using marker-peptides for the absolute quantitative analysis of proteins has a definite potential. Further research is obviously needed, e.g. comparative investigations where the proteolysis step and ancillary procedural aspects is weighed against the drawbacks of whole protein separation and envelope formation.

References

[1] Fenselau, C. A review of quantitative methods for proteomic studies. *J. Chromatogr. B, Analyt. Technol. Biomed. Life Sci.*, 2007, 855/1, 14-20.

[2] Zhang, FG; Bartels, MJ; Stott, WT. Quantitation of human glutathione S-transferases in complex matrices by liquid chromatography/tandem mass spectrometry with signature peptides. *Rapid Commun. Mass Spectrom.*, 2004, 18/4, 491-498.
[3] Barber, M; Bordoli, RS; Sedgwick, RD; Tyler, AN. Fast Atom Bombardment of Solids (Fab) - A New Ion-Source for Mass-Spectrometry. *J. Chem. Soc. Chem. Commun.*, 1981, 7, 325-327.
[4] Fenn, JB; Mann, M; Meng, CK; Wong, SF. Whitehouse, CM. Electrospray Ionization for Mass-Spectrometry of Large Biomolecules. *Science*, 1989, 246/4926, 64-71.
[5] Rostom, AA; Robinson, CV. Detection of the intact GroEL chaperonin assembly by mass spectrometry. *J. Am. Chem. Soc.*, 1999, 121/19, 4718-4719.
[6] Paul, W; Steinwedel, H; Ein neues Massenspektrometer ohne Magnetfeld. *Z. Naturforschg.*, 1953, (8a), 448-450.
[7] Guilhaus, M; Mlynski, V; Selby,D. Perfect timing: Time-of-flight mass spectrometry. *Rapid Commun. Mass Spectrom*, 1997, 11/9, 951-962.
[8] March, RE. An introduction to quadrupole ion trap mass spectrometry. *J. Mass Spectrom*, 1997, 32/4, 351-369.
[9] Comisaro, MB; Marshall, AG. Fourier-Transform Ion-Cyclotron Resonance Spectroscopy. *Chem. Phys. Lett.*, 1974, 25/2, 282-283.
[10] Yost, RA; Enke, CG. Selected Ion Fragmentation with A Tandem Quadrupole Mass-Spectrometer. *J. Am. Chem. Soc.*, 1978, 100/7, 2274-2275.
[11] Morris, HR; Paxton, T; Dell, A; Langhorne, J; Berg, M; Bordoli, RS; Hoyes, J; Bateman, RH. High sensitivity collisionally-activated decomposition tandem mass spectrometry on a novel quadrupole/orthogonal-acceleration time-of-flight mass spectrometer. *Rapid Commun. Mass Spectrom.*, 1996, 10/8, 889-896.
[12] Hoffmann, E. Tandem mass spectrometry: A primer. *J. Mass Spectrom.*, 1996, 31/2, 129-137.
[13] McLafferty, FW. Tandem Mass Spectrometry. NY, Wiley-Interscience, 1983.
[14] Jonsson, AP. Mass spectrometry for protein and peptide characterisation. *CMLS, Cell. Mol. Life Sci.*, 2001, 58/7, 868-884.
[15] Fenn, JB; Mann, M; Meng, CK; Wong, SF; Whitehouse, CM. Electrospray Ionization-Principles and Practice. *Mass Spectrom. Rev.*, 1990, 9/1, 37-70.
[16] Mann, M. Electrospray - Its Potential and Limitations As An Ionization Method for Biomolecules. *Org. Mass Spectrom.*, 1990, 25/11, 575-587.
[17] Manisali, I; Chen, DDY; Schneider, BB. Electrospray ionization source geometry for mass spectrometry: past, present, and future. *Trends Analyt. Chem.*, 2006, 25/3, 243-256.
[18] Cole, RB. Some tenets pertaining to electrospray ionization mass spectrometry. *J. Mass Spectrom.*, 2000, 35/7, 763-772.
[19] Taylor, G. Disintegration of Water Drops in Electric Fields. *Proc. R. Soc. London*, 1964, 280/138, 383.
[20] Thomson, BA; Iribarne, JV. Field-Induced Ion Evaporation from Liquid Surfaces at Atmospheric-Pressure. *J. Chem. Phys.*, 1979, 71/11, 4451-4463.
[21] Dole, M; Mack, LL; Hines, RL. Molecular Beams of Macro-ions. *J. Chem. Phys.*, 1968, 49/5, 2240.

[22] Johnson, RS; Martin, SA; Biemann, K. Collision-induced fragmentation of $(M + H)^{\pm}$ ions of peptides. Side chain specific sequence ions. *Int. J. Mass Spectrom. Ion Proces.*, 1988, 86, 137-154.

[23] Kreunin, P; Urquidi, V; Lubman, DM; Goodison, S. Identification of metastasis-associated proteins in a human tumor metastasis model using the mass-mapping technique. *Proteomics*, 2004, 4/9, 2754-2765.

[24] Barr, JR; Maggio, VL; Patterson, DG; Cooper, GR; Henderson, LO; Turner, WE; Smith, SJ; Hannon, WH; Needham, LL; Sampson, EJ. Isotope dilution mass spectrometric quantification of specific proteins: Model application with apolipoprotein A-I. *Clin. Chem.*, 1996, 42/10, 1676-1682.

[25] Barnidge, DR; Goodmanson, MK; Klee, GG; Muddiman, DC. Absolute quantification of the model biomarker prostate-specific antigen in serum by LC-MS/MS using protein cleavage and isotope dilution mass spectrometry. *J. Proteome Res.,* 2004, 3/3, 644-652.

[26] Gerbes, AL; Gülberg, V; Bilzer, M; Vogeser, M. Evaluation of serum cystatin Cconcentration as a marker of renal function in patients with cirrhosis of the liver. *Gut*, 2002, 50, 106-110.

[27] Mussap, M; Plebani, M. Biochemistry and clinical role of human cystatin C. *Crit. Rev. Clin. Lab. Sci.* , 2004, 41/5-6, 467-550.

[28] Thielemans, N; Lauwerys, R; Bernard, A. Competition Between Albumin and Low-Molecular-Weight Proteins for Renal Tubular Uptake in Experimental Nephropathies. *Nephron*, 1994, 66/4, 453-458.

[29] Thakkar, H; Lowe, PA; Price, CP; Newman, DJ. Measurement of the kinetics of protein uptake by proximal tubular cells using an optical biosensor. *Kidney Int.,* 1998, 54/4, 1197-1205.

[30] Mannes, AJ; Martin, BM; Yang, HYT; Keller, JM; Lewin, S; Gaiser, RR; Ladarola, MJ. Cystatin C as a cerebrospinal fluid biomarker for pain in humans. *Pain*, 2003, 102/3, 251-256.

[31] Dubas, F. Cerebral Amyloid Angiopathy. *Presse Med.*, 1994, 23/20, 948-950.

[32] Barrett, AJ. Cystatin, the egg white inhibitor of cysteine proteinases. *Methods Enzymol.*, 1981, 80, 771-778.

[33] Barrett, AJ. The cystatins: a diverse superfamily of cysteine peptidase inhibitors. *Biomed. Biochim. Acta*, 1986, 45/11-12, 1363-1374.

[34] Rawlings, ND; Barrett, AJ. Evolution of Proteins of the Cystatin Superfamily. *J. Mol. Evol.*, 1990, 30/1, 60-71.

[35] Grubb, A; Lofberg, H. Human Gamma-Trace, A Basic Microprotein - Amino-Acid-Sequence and Presence in the Adenohypophysis. *Proc. Natl. Acad. Sci. USA*, 1982, 79/9, 3024-3027.

[36] Merz, GS; Benedikz, E; Schwenk, V; Johansen, TE; Vogel, LK; Rushbrook, JI; Wisniewski, HM. Human cystatin C forms an inactive dimer during intracellular trafficking in transfected CHO cells. *J. Cell Physiol.*, 1997, 173/3, 423-432.

[37] Bronstrup, M. Absolute quantification strategies in proteomics based on mass spectrometry. *Expert Rev. Proteomics*, 2004, 4, 503-512.

[38] Storme, ML; Sinnaeve, BA; Van Bocxlaer, JF. The use of tryptic marker-peptides for the quantitative analysis of cystatin C. *J. Sep. Sci.*, 2005, *28/14*, 1759-1763.

[39] Strader, MB; Tabb, DL; Hervey, WJ; Pan, CL; Hurst, GB. Efficient and specific trypsin digestion of microgram to nanogram quantities of proteins in organic-aqueous solvent systems. *Anal. Chem.*, 2006, 78/1, 125-134.

[40] Samyn, B, Sergeant, K, Van Beeumen, J. A method for C-terminal sequence analysis in the proteomic era (proteins cleaved with cyanogen bromide). *Nat. Protoc.*, 2006, 1/1, 318-323.

[41] Quadroni, M; James, P. Proteomics and automation. *Electrophoresis*, 1999, 20/4-5, 664-677.

[42] Russell, WK; Park, ZY; Russell, DH. Proteolysis in mixed organic-aqueous solvent systems: applications for peptide mass mapping using mass spectrometry. *Anal. Chem.*, 2001, 73/11, 2682-2685.

[43] Ekstrom, S; Onnerfjord, P; Nilsson, J; Bengtsson, M; Laurell, T; Marko-Varga, G. Integrated microanalytical technology enabling rapid and automated protein identification. *Anal. Chem.*, 2000, 72/2, 286-293.

[44] Medzihradszky, KF. In-solution digestion of proteins for mass spectrometry. *Meth. Enzymol.*, 2005, 405, 50-65.

[45] Kaiser, R; Metzka, L. Enhancement of cyanogen bromide cleavage yields for methionyl-serine and methionyl-threonine peptide bonds. *Anal. Biochem.*, 1999, 266/1, 1-8.

[46] Samyn, B; Sergeant, K; Castanheira, P; Faro, C; Van Beeumen, J. A new method for C-terminal sequence analysis in the proteomic era. *Nat. Methods*, 2005, 2/3, 193-200.

[47] Hardeman, K; Samyn, B; Van der Eycken, J; Van Beeumen, J. An improved chemical approach toward the C-terminal sequence analysis of proteins containing all natural amino acids. *Protein Sci.*, 1998, 7/7, 1593-1602.

[48] Aebersold, R; Mann, M. Mass spectrometry-based proteomics. *Nature*, 2003, 422/6928, 198-207.

[49] Itakura, K; Hirose, T; Crea, R; Riggs, AD; Heyneker, HL; Bolivar, F; Boyer,H.W. Expression in Escherichia-Coli of A Chemically Synthesized Gene for Hormone Somatostatin. *Science*, 1977, 198/4321, 1056-1063.

[50] Rodriguez, JC; Wong, L; Jennings, PA. The solvent in CNBr cleavage reactions determines the fragmentation efficiency of ketosteroid isomerase fusion proteins used in the production of recombinant peptides. *Protein Expr. Purif.*, 2003, 28/2, 224-231.

[51] Morrison, JR; Fidge, NH; Grego, B. Studies on the Formation, Separation, and Characterization of Cyanogen-Bromide Fragments of Human AI Apolipoprotein. *Anal. Biochem.*, 1990, 186/1, 145-152.

[52] Goodlett, DR; Armstrong, FB; Creech, RJ; Vanbreemen, RB. Formylated Peptides from Cyanogen-Bromide Digests Identified by Fast Atom Bombardment Mass-Spectrometry. *Anal. Biochem.*, 1990, 186/1, 116-120.

[53] Zhang, XY; Dillen, L; Vanhoutte, K; Vandongen, W; Esmans, E; Claeys, M. Characterization of unstable intermediates and oxidized products formed during cyanogen bromide cleavage of peptides and proteins by electrospray mass spectrometry. *Anal. Biochem.*, 1996, 68/19, 3422-3430.

[54] Liu, T; Qian, WJ; Mottaz, HM; Gritsenko, MA; Norbeck, AD; Moore, RJ; Purvine, SO; Camp, DG; Smith, RD. Evaluation of multiprotein immunoaffinity subtraction for plasma proteomics and candidate biomarker discovery using mass spectrometry. *Mol. Cell. Proteomics*, 2006, 5/11, 2167-2174.

[55] Anderson, NL; Anderson, NG. The Human Plasma Proteome. History, Character, and Diagnostic Prospects. *Mol. Cell. Proteomics*, 2002, 1, 845-867.

[56] Luque-Garcia, JL; Neubert, TA. Sample preparation for serum/plasma profiling and biomarker identification by mass spectrometry. *J. Chromatogr. A*, 2007, 1153/1-2, 259-276.

[57] Petricoin, EF; Ardekani, AM; Hitt, BA; Levine, PJ; Fusaro, VA; Steinberg, SM; Mills, GB; Simone, C; Fishman, DA; Kohn, EC; Liotta, LA. Use of proteomic patterns in serum to identify ovarian cancer. *Lancet*, 2002, 359/9306, 572-577.

[58] Tirumalai, RS; Chan, KC; Prieto, DA; Issaq, HJ; Conrads, TP; Veenstra, TD. Characterization of the low molecular weight human serum proteome. *Mol. Cell. Proteomics*, 2003, 2/10, 1096-1103.

[59] Zhang, Z; Bast, RC; Yu, YH; Li, JN; Sokoll, LJ; Rai, AJ; Rosenzweig, JM; Cameron, B; Wang, YY; Meng, XY; Berchuck, A; van Haaften-Day, C; Hacker, NF; de Bruijn, HWA; van der Zee, AGJ; Jacobs, IJ; Fung, ET; Chan, DW. Three biomarkers identified from serum proteomic analysis for the detection of early stage ovarian cancer. *Cancer Res.*, 2004, 64/16, 5882-5890.

[60] Mian, S; Ugurel, S; Parkinson, E; Schlenzka, I; Dryden, I; Lancashire, L; Ball, G; Creaser, C; Rees, R; Schadendorf, D. Serum proteomic fingerprinting discriminates between clinical stages and predicts disease progression in melanoma patients. *J. Clin. Oncol.*, 2005, 23/22, 5088-5093.

[61] Terracciano, R; Gaspari, M; Testa, F; Pasqua, L; Tagliaferri, P; Cheng, MMC; Nijdam, AJ; Petricoin, EF; Liotta, LA; Cuda, G; Ferrari, M; Venuta, S. Selective binding and enrichment for low-molecular weight biomarker molecules in human plasma after exposure to nanoporous silica particles. *Proteomics*, 2006, 6/11, 3243-3250.

[62] Qin, SZ; Ferdinand, AS; Richie, JP; O'Leary, MP; Mok, SC; Liu, BCS. Chromatofocusing fractionation and two-dimensional difference gel electrophoresis for low abundance serum proteins. *Proteomics*, 2005, 5/12, 3183-3192.

[63] Pieper, R; Su, Q; Gatlin, CL; Huang, ST; Anderson, NL; Steiner, S. Multi-component immunoaffinity subtraction chromatography: An innovative step towards a comprehensive survey of the human plasma proteome. *Proteomics*, 2003, 3/4, 422-432.

[64] Zalotarjova, N; Martosella, J; Nicol, G; Bailey, J; Boyes, BE; Barrett, WC. Differences among techniques for high-abundant protein depletion. *Proteomics*, 2005, 5/13, 3304-3313.

[65] Huang, L; Harvie, G; Feitelson, JS; Gramatikoff, K; Herold, DA; Allen, DL; Amunngama,R; Hagler, RA; Pisano, MR; Zhang, WW; Fang, XM. Immunoaffinity separation of plasma proteins by Ig Y microbeads: Meeting the needs of proteomic sample preparation and analysis. *Proteomics*, 2005, 5/13, 3314-3328.

[66] Brand, J; Haslberger, T; Zolg, W; Pestlin, G; Palme, S. Depletion efficiency and recovery of trace markers from a multiparameter immunodepletion column. *Proteomics*, 2006, 6/11, 3236-3242.

[67] Matuszewski, BK; Constanzer, ML; Chavez-Eng, CM. Matrix effect in quantitative LC/MS/MS analyses of biological fluids: A method for determination of finasteride in human plasma at picogram per milliliter concentrations. *Anal. Chem.*, 1998, 70/5, 882-889.

Index

A

B

C

D

E

F

G

H

I

J

K

L

M

W

Y

Z